Pharmacodynamics and Pharmacokinetics

Pharmacodynamics and Pharmacokinetics

Edited by Tyler Morrow

hayle medical
New York

Hayle Medical,
750 Third Avenue, 9th Floor,
New York, NY 10017, USA

Visit us on the World Wide Web at:
www.haylemedical.com

ISBN: 978-1-63241-782-4

The publisher's policy is to use permanent paper from mills that operate a sustainable forestry policy. Furthermore, the publisher ensures that the text paper and cover boards used have met acceptable environmental accreditation standards.

Printed in China.

Cataloging-in-Publication Data

Pharmacodynamics and pharmacokinetics / edited by Tyler Morrow.
p. cm.
Includes bibliographical references and index.
ISBN 978-1-63241-782-4
1. Drugs--Physiological effect. 2. Pharmacokinetics. 3. Pharmacology.
4. Drugs--Metabolism. I. Morrow, Tyler.
RM300 .P43 2019
615--dc23

Table of Contents

Preface IX

Chapter 1 **The Effect of Various Vehicles on the Naproxen Permeability through Rat Skin: A Mechanistic Study by DSC and FT-IR Techniques** 1
Anayatollah Salimi, Najme Hedayatipour and Eskandar Moghimipour

Chapter 2 **Anticonvulsant and Antioxidant Effects of Pitavastatin against Pentylenetetrazol-Induced Kindling in Mice** 9
Nastaran Faghihi and Mohammad Taghi Mohammadi

Chapter 3 **The Effects of Cetirizine on P-glycoprotein Expression and Function *In vitro and In situ*** 17
Mehran Mesgari Abbasi, Hadi Valizadeh, Hamed Hamishekar, Leila Mohammadnejad and Parvin Zakeri-Milani

Chapter4 **In vitro Cytotoxicity Effects of ^{197}Au/PAMAMG4 and ^{198}Au/PAMAMG4 Nanocomposites against MCF7 and 4T1 Breast Cancer Cell Lines** 25
Simin Janitabar-Darzi, Reza Rezaei and Kamal Yavari

Chapter 5 **Optimization of Chitosan and Cellulose Acetate Phthalate Controlled Delivery of Methylprednisolone for Treatment of Inflammatory Bowel Disease** 34
Swati Jagdale and Apoorva Chandekar

Chapter 6 **The Effect of Particle Size on the Deposition of Solid Lipid Nanoparticles in Different Skin Layers** 45
Zahra Mardhiah Adib, Saeed Ghanbarzadeh, Maryam Kouhsoltani, Ahmad Yari Khosroshahi and Hamed Hamishehkar

Chapter 7 **Evaluating Adherence of Health-Care Team to Standard Guideline of Colistin use at Intensive Care Units of a Referral Hospital** 51
Afsaneh Vazin, Iman Karimzadeh, Atiyeh Zand, Nazafarin Hatami-Mazinani and Dena Firouzabadi

Chapter 8 **Pharmacokinetic Parameters and Over-Responsiveness of Iranian Population to Propranolol** 58
Ebrahim Salehifar, Shima Ebrahim, Mohammad-Reza Shiran, Fatemeh Faramarzi, Hossein Askari Rad, Razieh Avan, Asadollah Mohseni Kiasari and Pouneh Ebrahimi

Chapter 9 **Hybrid Scaffolds of Hyaluronic Acid and Collagen Loaded with Prednisolone: an Interesting System for Osteoarthritis** 66
Farhad Mohammadi, Soliman Mohammadi Samani, Nader Tanideh and Fatemeh Ahmadi

Chapter 10 **Comparative Study of Different Combinational Mucoadhesive Formulations of Sumatriptan-Metoclopramide** 75
Mitra Jelvehgari, Hadi Valizadeh, Sanam Ziapour, Mahdieh Rahmani, Seyed Hassan Montazam and Saieede Soltani

Chapter 11 **Sustained release Curcumin loaded Solid Lipid Nanoparticles** 87
Parisa Jourghanian, Solmaz Ghaffari, Mehdi Ardjmand, Setareh Haghighat and Mahdieh Mohammadnejad

Chapter 12 **Investigating Effect of Rapamycin and Metformin on Angiogenesis in Hepatocellular Carcinoma Cell Line** 92
Mandana Rastegar, Haji-Amin Marjani, Yaghoub Yazdani, Majid Shahbazi, Masoud Golalipour and Touraj Farazmandfar

Chapter 13 **Interactions Between Sirolimus and Anti-Inflammatory Drugs: Competitive Binding for Human Serum Albumin** 98
Arash Khodaei, Soheila Bolandnazar, Hadi Valizadeh, Leila Hasani and Parvin Zakeri-Milani

Chapter 14 **Aggregated Nanotransfersomal Dry Powder Inhalation of Itraconazole for Pulmonary Drug Delivery** 105
Mehdi Hassanpour Aghdam, Saeed Ghanbarzadeh, Yousef Javadzadeh and Hamed Hamishehkar

Chapter 15 **Studying the Effect of Sertraline in Reducing Aggressive Behavior in Patients with Major Depression** 113
Alireza Farnam, Arezoo MehrAra, Hossein Dadashzadeh, Golamreza Chalabianlou and Salman Safikhanlou

Chapter 16 **Comparative Evaluation of Dexmedetomidine and Magnesium Sulphate on Propofol Consumption, Haemodynamics and Postoperative Recovery in Spine Surgery** 118
Vinit K. Srivastava, Abhishek Mishra, Sanjay Agrawal, Sanjay Kumar, Sunil Sharma and Raj Kumar

Chapter 17 **Bacteriophage Isolated from Sewage Eliminates and Prevents the Establishment of *Escherichia Coli* Biofilm** 125
Karla Veloso Gonçalves Ribeiro, Cleberson Ribeiro, Roberto Sousa Dias, Silvia Almeida Cardoso, Sérgio Oliveira de Paula, Jose Cola Zanuncio and Leandro Licursi de Oliveira

Chapter 18 **Protective Effect of Gemfibrozil on Hepatotoxicity Induced by Acetaminophen in Mice: the Importance of Oxidative Stress Suppression** 136
Hojatolla Nikravesh, Mohammad Javad Khodayar, Masoud Mahdavinia, Esrafil Mansouri, Leila Zeidooni and Fereshteh Dehbashi

Chapter 19 ***Teucrium polium* Extract Enhances the Anti-Angiogenesis Effect of Tranilast on Human Umbilical Vein Endothelial Cells** 145
Fatemeh Sheikhbahaei, Mozafar Khazaei and Seyed Noureddin Nematollahi-Mahani

Chapter 20 **Preparation and Statistical Modeling of Solid Lipid Nanoparticles of Dimethyl Fumarate for Better Management of Multiple Sclerosis** 154
Smriti Ojha and Babita Kumar

Chapter 21 **Combination of Vildagliptin and Ischemic Postconditioning in Diabetic Hearts as a Working Strategy to Reduce Myocardial Reperfusion Injury by Restoring Mitochondrial Function and Autophagic Activity** 163
Goltaj Bayrami, Alireza Alihemmati, Pouran Karimi, Aniseh Javadi, Rana Keyhanmanesh, Mustafa Mohammadi, Milad Zadi-Heydarabad and Reza Badalzadeh

Chapter 22 **The Eeffect of Metformin Combined with Calcium-Vitamin D_3 against Diet-Induced Nonalcoholic Fatty Liver Disease** 174
Sara Shojaei Zarghani, Samin Abbaszadeh, Mohammad Alizadeh, Maryam Rameshrad, Alireza Garjani and Hamid Soraya

Chapter 23 **Nanotechnology in Wound Healing; Semisolid Dosage Forms Containing Curcumin-Ampicillin Solid Lipid Nanoparticles, *in-Vitro, Ex-Vivo* and *in-Vivo* Characteristics** 183
Solmaz Ghaffari, Faezeh Alihosseini, Seyed Mahdi Rezayat Sorkhabadi, Sepideh Arbabi Bidgoli, Seyyedeh Elaheh Mousavi, Setareh Haghighat, Ahoo Afshar Nasab and Nooshin Kianvash

Chapter 24 **Effects of Pharmacologic Dose of Resveratrol Supplementation on Oxidative/Antioxidative Status Biomarkers in Nonalcoholic Fatty Liver Disease Patients** 189
Somayyeh Asghari, Maryam Rafraf, Laleh Farzin, Mohammad Asghari-Jafarabadi, Seyed-Mostafa Ghavami and Mohammad-Hossein Somi

Chapter 25 **Enhanced Intestinal Permeation of Doxorubicin using Chitosan Nanoparticles** 200
Marziyeh Zare, Soliman Mohammadi Samani and Zahra Sobhani

Permissions

List of Contributors

Index

Preface

The study associated with the biochemical and physiological effects of pharmaceutical drugs is known as pharmacodynamics. The field of pharmacology which studies the way a living organism affects the drug administered to it, is called pharmacokinetics. It is concerned with the analysis of the chemical metabolism, and the discovery of the fate of the drug administered to the body from the time of its administration up to the point of its complete elimination from the body. The technique combining both pharmacokinetics and pharmacodynamics is called pharmacokinetic/pharmacodynamic modelling or PK/PD modelling. This book is a compilation of chapters that discuss the most vital concepts and emerging trends in the areas of pharmacodynamics and pharmacokinetics. The various advancements in these fields are glanced at herein and their applications as well as ramifications are looked at in detail. The extensive content of this book provides the readers with a thorough understanding of these disiplines.

This book is the end result of constructive efforts and intensive research done by experts in this field. The aim of this book is to enlighten the readers with recent information in this area of research. The information provided in this profound book would serve as a valuable reference to students and researchers in this field.

At the end, I would like to thank all the authors for devoting their precious time and providing their valuable contribution to this book. I would also like to express my gratitude to my fellow colleagues who encouraged me throughout the process.

Editor

The Effect of Various Vehicles on the Naproxen Permeability through Rat Skin: A Mechanistic Study by DSC and FT-IR Techniques

Anayatollah Salimi*, Najme Hedayatipour, Eskandar Moghimipour

Nanotechnology Research Center, Department of Pharmaceutics, Ahvaz Jundishapur University of Medical Sciences, Ahvaz, Iran.

Keywords:
- Naproxen
- Permeability
- Mean transition temperature
- Thermotropic behavior
- Diffusion coefficient
- Flux

Abstract

Purpose: The purpose of the present investigation was to evaluate the effectiveness of different vehicles on drug permeability and microstructure of intercellular or lipids in SC layer of skin.

Methods: Pre-treated skin of rat using some vehicles including Labarac PG ,Transcutol P, tween 80, span 80 and propylene glycol (PG), were mounted on specialized design franz-diffusion cell was used to assess naproxen permeation and parameters such as permeability coefficients and state flux (J_{ss}) were evaluated. Any differences in peak position and also change in symmetric and asymmetric stretching of C-H bond, lipid ester carbonyl stretching in SC, C=O stretching (Amide I) and C-N stretching of keratin (Amide II) absorbance using Fourier transform infrared spectroscopy (FTIR) were considered to investigate the enhancing mechanism. DSC method was utilized to compare their mean transition temperature (Tm) and enthalpies (ΔH).

Results: Steady-state flux (Jss), permeability coefficient (Kp) and diffusion coefficient (D) were significantly ($p<0.05$) increased by using their span80 showed the biggest enhancement ratio (ER_{flux}) and Transcutol P, Labrafac PG, Tween 80 and Propylene glycol were at the next levels. In comprised to hydrated rat skin the maximum increase in diffusion coefficient was for Tween 80($p<0.05$), Lipid fluidization, lipid disruption structure and the irreversible denaturation of proteins in the SC layer of skin by span 80, Tween 80, Labrafac PG, Transcutol P and propylene glycol, were indicated by FT-IR and DSC techniques.

Conclusion: It is concluded that naproxen permeation through rat skin may be facilitated by utilizing the vehicle systems. Lipid fluidization and lipid extraction are among suggested mechanisms.

Introduction

Nowadays, dermal delivery of drugs is considered as an important way for administration of drugs. There are many advantages with transdermal drug delivery(TDD), although only a few drugs with acceptable release profiles have used in therapy. Utilization of vehicles that affect the skin barrier function is one of the classic strategies of permeation enhancement. Some of these vehicles have well characterized actions on the stratum corneum, but the majority is still selected using empirical criteria. The skin, our body's largest organ, is generally considered as an impermeable protective barrier against mechanical, chemical, microbial, and physical hazards. The success of a topical drug to be used for systemic drug delivery depends on the ability of the drug to penetrate via skin in sufficient quantities to achieve the desired effect.[1]

Avoiding first pass metabolism , sustained and controlled delivery of drugs, decrease of dose frequency, proper patient compliance and localization of drugs in target site, avoidance of the risks of injections, and reduction in toxic level of drugs are among TDD advantages.[2-6]

Skin permeation of drugs is an essential stage percutaneous absorption. Permeation is the penetration from one layer into another layer of skin. The lipid matrix of stratum corneum layer acts a meaningful role in determining the permeability of substances through the skin. The physicochemical properties of both drug and vehicle play an important role in determining percutaneous absorption.[7]

Skin permeation can be improved by the several strategies: increasing the diffusivity in the skin by disturbance of SC lipid matrix, strengthening drug solubility in the skin, enhancing the degree of saturation of the drug in formulation.[8]

The main principle of transdermal drug delivery is passive permeation of drug through skin ,that often depends the solubility and partition coefficient of the drug molecule. Two main strategies for improvement permeation of drugs are reversible enhancing effect of vehicle and modifications of drug thermodynamic property.[7] So, selection of a suitable vehicle for the preparation of topical formulations greatly affects on the drug delivery.

Several vehicles including oleic acid, propylene glycol and water are considered as permeation enhancers working by some mechanisms including disruption of the

***Corresponding author:** Anayatollah Salimi, Email: salimi_a@ajums.ac.ir organized intercellular lipid structure of the stratum corneum, fluidization of the stratum corneum lipids, cellular proteins alteration, and extraction of intercellular lipids by non-polar solvents.[6-8]

To develop transdermal drug delivery systems, investigation of microstructure of intercellular or lipids in SC layer of skin is required. In the recent studies, organization of lipids and skin microstructure have been examined using various techniques including differential scanning calorimetry(DSC) and Fourier transform infrared spectroscopy (FT-IR).[9] The FTIR analysis of skin can be practical tool for studying the interaction between chemical enhancers materials with SC that provides bands at different wave numbers.[10,11]

Several infrared spectral bands of the skin are attributed to vibration of protein and lipid molecules in the SC.[12] The lipid vibration are a good index from which to evaluate the microstructure of the lamellar lipids form in the intercellular area in the SC layer of skin .Some different spectral regions of the SC was expected to have various bands, -CH2 symmetric vibration (near 2850 cm^{-1}) and –CH2 asymmetric vibration (near 2920cm^{-1}) and amide I (about 1650cm^{-1}) and amide II (near 1550cm^{-1}) stretching vibrations of SC protein have been reported. An increase in wave number and width of –CH2 stretching peaks is due fluidization of the stratum corneum lipids.[13-15] The frequencies of amide I and amide II bands, especially amide I band, are sensitive and shift to lower or higher frequencies according to the change in protein conformation. Alteration of the amide I (C=O stretching) bands shows secondary structure of keratin, which may interference with H-O-H bending vibrationof water at 1645cm^{-1}. The amide bonds along with 1645cm^{-1} band are sensitive to H-bond change in the SC.[13]

To recognize the mechanism by which the properties of enhancers/retardants change in a given vehicle, molecular studies of whole rat skin was carried out using DSC and FTIR.

The rationale for use of FTIR technique to understand mechanism of penetration modifier was that the treatment with enhancers/retardants, sometimes yield a shift in specific band position to higher or lower wavenumber or lead to change in the intensity of the signal observed at that band position.

If the shift is to higher wavenumber (blue shift), it indicates SC membrane (lipid bilayer) fluidization that in change contribute to disruption of the barrier properties that probably causes the substance permeation enhancement through the SC.[16] On the other hand, lipid groups are oriented again, a phenomenon that that causes a shift to lower wave number (e.g. red shift) and strengthening of subcutaneous barrier properties which finally slows down the entrance of permeant through the skin.[16] If the penetration modifier performs by affecting on lipid pathway, the phase transition of the lipids is showed by increase/decrease in the band position (wavenumber) of the signals at 2920, 2850, and near1738 cm^{-1}.

The quantity of proteins and lipids in SC layer is presented by area or height of the bands and any alteration in the intensity of the peaks may be due to strengthening or extraction of subcutaneous lipids. The mechanism is also suggested for the treatment with penetration enhancers. They may also increase the intensity at specific band indicating retardation when retardants are utilized.[16]

Thermal analysis methods such as differential scanning calorimetry (DSC) have been utilized to investigate thermal transitions in mammalian stratum corneum. The stratum corneum (SC) is the outermost layer of the epidermis and is primarily responsible for the skin's barrier function.[11]

The DSC technique is widely used for characterization the melting of lipids and the phase transition of lipid bilayers and protein denaturation in SC layer. To obtain more detailed information about lipid components and protein conformational stability of the whole skin rat treated with pure vehicle, a DSC study was programmed. By comparing mean transition temperature (T_m) and enthalpies (H), thermotropic behavior of treated skin was assessed. Any transition in T_m to lower degrees may be due to lipid disruption in bilayer and irreversible protein denaturation in SC. While, enthalpy decrease was related to lipid fluidization in lipid bilayers and protein – lipid complexes.[13-15,17-19] Naproxen is a propionic acid derivative drug widely used as analgesic, antipyretic and for relief of symptoms of dysmenorrheal pain.[12] Common adverse effect of NSAIDs including, GI ulcer, accompanied by anemia as a result of bleeding. To reduce the risk of gastric irritation and toxicity, and also to gain a more effective therapy, transdermal administration is a promising route. It also enables sustained and controlled release of drugs and increases patient compliance.[20]

The study was aimed to evaluate the effectiveness of some hydrophobic and hydrophilic vehicles on naproxen *in vitro* skin permeability of through Excised Whole Rat Skin and also the study of biophysical characteristics of Rats' stratum corneum by FT-IR and DSC techniques in order to design a new drug delivery system for skin delivery of naproxen.

Materials and Methods

Naproxen was obtained from Pars Darou (Iran), Propylene glycol dicaprylocapraye (Labrafac PG, Diethylene glycol monoethyl ether (Transcutol P) was donated as gift by GATTEFOSSE Company (France). Span 80, Propylene glycol(PG), and Tween 80 were purchased from Merck (Germany). All solvents and chemicals were of analytical grade. Also, Freshly double distilled water was used in the experiments

Solubility Tests

The solubility of naproxen was determined in Transcutol p, Labrafac PG, Tween 80, Span 80 and PG. A definite quantity of naproxen was added to 5 ml of the solvent. The mixture was immersed in a water bath and equilibrated at 37 °C for 24 hrs. Then, suspension was centrifuged for 10 min at 3000 rpm, filtered, diluted and the dissolved drug was quantified spectrophotometrically at 271 nm.[21]

Animal Studies

Male adult Wistar rats (weighing 175 - 225 g) and aged 8-10 weeks were prepared from Animals Laboratory, Jundishapur University of Medical Sciences, Ahvaz, Iran. Their abdominal skin was shaved using an electric clipper, taking care not to damage the skin. Prior to sacrificing, they were anaesthetized with ether. Abdominal full-thickness skin was removed and using cooled pure acetone solution with 4 °C any extraneous subcutaneous fats cleaned from the dorsal side. The thickness of whole skin was determined using a digital micrometer (AAOC, France). The animals were treated according to the principles for the care and use of laboratory animals and the procedures followed with standard international guidelines.[22]

Differential scanning calorimetry (DSC)

The solvents, which induced skin structural alteration, were determined using a DSC instrument (DSC[1] system, Mettler Toledo). About 5-10 mg of each skin sample was placed in a hermetically sealed aluminum pan. Simultaneously, an empty sealed pan was concurrently utilized as reference. Skin samples were exposed to heat ranging from 20 to 200°C (scan rate: 5 °C/min). Enthalpy (ΔH) values were determined from endothermic and exothermic transitions of the thermo grams.[2]

FT-IR spectroscopy

Skin samples were treated by Labrafac PG, Transcutol P, Span 80, Tween 80, PG for 24 hrs,then vacuum-dried (650 mm Hg, 25 ± 1 °C) for 1 h and finally stored in desiccators to remove traces of solvent . The skin samples were analyzed in 4000 to 500 cm^{-1} scan range using an FT-IR facility (Uker, Vertex70, Germany).[2]

Permeability Experiments

Specially designed vertical diffusion cells (with an effective diffusion area of approximately 4.9 cm^2) were utilized to evaluate in vitro naproxen permeation. The receptor compartment was filled with 25ml phosphate buffer solution (PBS, pH 7.4). Whole skin sample, hydrated prior to use, was mounted between the donor and receptor compartments of the cell with the stratum corneum facing the donor medium. 1 % (w/v) solution of naproxen in each solvent was placed in donor compartment. The diffusion cells were placed on a heater-stirrer (37 ± 0.5 °C) and the receptor phase was stirred continuously at 200 rpm using small magnetic bars . At each interval time (0.5, 1, 2, 3, ..., 56 h), a 2ml sample was withdrawn from the receptor phase, and replaced by an equivalent volume of PBS to maintain sink condition. A UV spectrophotometer was utilized to detect the permeated amount of naproxen in derived samples.[2,22]

Data analysis and statistics

Cumulative permeated naproxen per unit area was calculated by dividing the corrected naproxen concentration by the area of the exposed area of the skin to donor solution. Steady-state flux ($mg/cm^2/h$) was calculated from the linear portion of the slope of the permeation curve. Permeability coefficient(Kp, cm/h) through the skin for naproxen was calculated as in Eq1.[23,24]: naproxen concentration was corrected for sampling effects according to Eq1.[23,24]

$Kp = J_{ss}/C_v$. .... (1)

where is Jss and Cv were steady-state flux and naproxen concentration in donor phase,respectively.

All of the experiments were carried out in triplicateand the results were presented as mean±SE, using one-way analysis of variance (ANOVA), the data were statiscally analyzed and p values less than 0.05 were considered as significant differences.

Results and Discussion

Solubility Study

Table 1 shows the solubilities of naproxen in different vehicles. Its solubilities in Span 80, Propylene glycol, Transcutol P, Labrafac PG, Tween 80 and water was 15.033 mg/ml, 14.12mg/ml,13.87 mg/ml, 13.697mg/ml, 0.567mg/ml and 0.036 mg/ml, respectively .

Table1. Solubility of naproxen in various solvents at 37°C (mean±SD,n=3)

vehicle	Solubility(mg/ml)
Span 80	15.033±0.208
Propylene glycol	14.120±0.368
Transcutol p	13.87±0.023
Labrafac PG	13.697±0.536
Tween 80	0.567±0.012
Water	0.036±0.002

FT-IR Spectroscopy

Figure 1, Table 2, Table 3 and Table 4 show spectral analysis of samples, regarding any change in position of peaks and also their intensities from intensities from 4000cm^{-1}-500cm^{-1}.

Any O-H and N-H stretches from protein, water and lipid are observed between 3000-3600cm^{-1}, while symmetric and asymmetric stretching bonds of terminal methyl groups of dermal lipids are presented around 2948.02 and 2821.65 cm^{-1}. The lipid ester carbonyl stretching in SC showed at 1723.62 cm^{-1} position. Also, the stretching of lipid ester in stratum corneum and amide I (C=O stretching) and amide II (C-N stretching) linkage of the helical secondary structure found in epidermal keratin are presented at 1652.78 and 1572.27 cm^{-1}.[15-17]

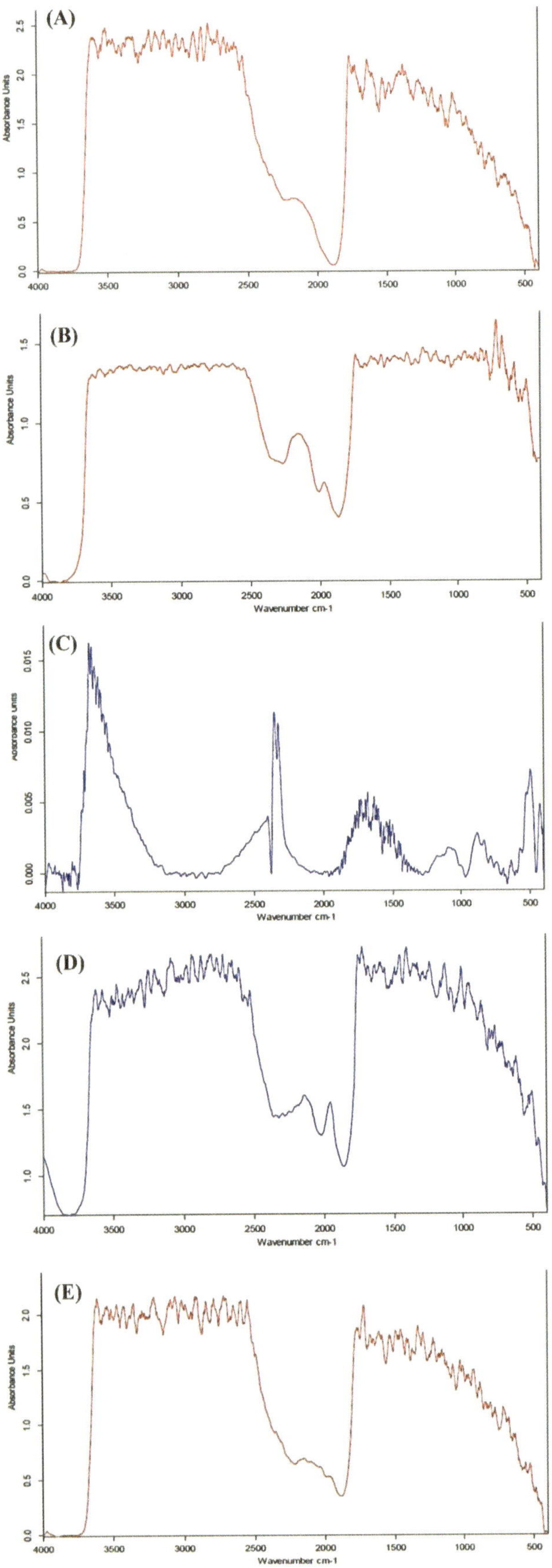

Figure 1. FT-IR spectra of whole skin abdominal rat after treatment with (A): Propylene glycol, (B): Labrafac PG, (C): Span 80, (D): Transcutol p, (E): Tween 80.

The spectra of PG treated rat skin show changes in peak height and wave numbers. The lack of significant correlation between drug solubility in PG and ER_{flux} probably indicates that the high hydrogen bonding capacity of PG decreased affinity of skin for bonding with naproxen during treatment with this vehicle. Hence, the effect of vehicles on drug solubility in stratum corneum and hydrogen bonding formation between skin and drug are important factors for drug partitioning. ER_D results after skin treatment with PG correlate with FT-IR and DSC observations so that propylene glycol interacts mainly with proteins in stratum corneum layer, Red shift was observed in PG-treated rat skin at wave number (2929.5cm$^{-1)}$, indicating reorientation within the lipid groups that causes strengthening of SC barrier properties, thus resulting in decrease in naproxen transport across the skin. Relatively red shift in 1722.7cm^{-1} band was observed in PG treated skin rat ,indicating formation of strong hydrogen bonds within the lipid structures. Skin treatment with permeation modifiers might have led to lipid extraction from SC layer, or might have increased the intensity at the particular band indicating retardation in the case of retardants.[13]

IR spectra of Tween 80 treated rat skin represented blue shifts and significant decreases in height of peaks height in the 3010.75, 2840.74, 1770.18, 1653, 1591.73 cm^{-1} wave numbers.

Red shifts was observed in labrafac PG-treated rat skin and height of peaks at wave numbers (2895.27, 2778, 1716.94 cm^{-1}) decreased significantly, and blue shift in which peak height of the wave numbers (1669.4 and 1591.82cm^{-1}) decreased significantly. Relatively red shift in band 1716.94 cm^{-1} was observed in labrafac PG treated skin rat, indicating formation strong hydro genic bonds within the lipid molecules that causes strengthening of SC barrier properties, thus resulting in decrease in diffusion coefficient than tween 80. Height of peaks of wave numbers (2860.64, 1764.86, 1694.84, 1599.9 cm^{-1}) were significantly decreased when the skin was treated with span 80 and blue shifts at 2860.64, 1764.86, 1694.84, 1599.9 cm^{-1}and disappeared at 29486.02cm^{-1}. The spectra for rat skin treated with transcutol P indicate red shifts with lowering of in peak height of the wave number (2836.97cm^{-1}) and blue shift in which height of peak numbers (2895.24, 1729.69 and 1579.46 cm^{-1}) decrease.

Lipid fluidization, lipid disruption and the irreversible denaturation of proteins in the SC layer of skin by tween 80, span 80 and labrafac PG as indicated by FT-IR and DSC, is the main factor for higher ER_{flux} and ER_D ratios in comparison with control.

Differential Scanning Calorimetery (DSC)

Mean transition temperature (T_m) and their enthalpies (ΔH) were used to evaluate thermotropic behavior of treated skin. Table 5 shows transition temperatures and enthalpies while Figure 2 shows thermograms. Tm_1 and Tm_2 resulted from hydrated rat skin were 67.5 and 112°C, respectively, indicated melting of lipids and intracellular keratin irreversible denaturation.[2] Vaddi et al were obtained three endothermic transition at 62, 79, and 95°C in the thermotropic behavior of rat skin[21] while Shakeel et al.[24] observed four endothermic transitions at 34, 82, 105, and 114°C. Kaushik et al reported in human dermal DSC graphs and observed three endothermic transition peaks at temperatures 59-63°C (Tm_1), 75-82°C (Tm_2) and 99.5-120°C (Tm_3).[16] They suggested that Tm_1 was due to transformation of lipid forms from a lamellar to disordered state, Tm_2 corresponds to protein-lipid complex melting point,[16] or the disruption of polar head groups of lipids[14-16] and Tm_3 is known to occur during the proteins irreversible denaturation,[14] respectively. It was observed that span 80, labrafac PG to lower melting points and ΔH_1 decreased in comparison with hydrated rat skin, shifted Tm1. In addition, Tm_1 and Tm_2 were disappeared by tween 80, while Tm_1 was shifted by PG and transcutol P to higher melting point and ΔH_1 increased in transcutol P when compared with control. Also, all the vehicles shifted Tm_2 indicating increase in melting point (with the exception of Tween 80 and Transcutol P) and decrease enthalpies that may be due to protein denaturation.

Table 2. Decrease in mean peak height (± SD), compared with control (untreated skin) of asymmetric (Asy) and symmetric (Sym) C-H stretching and C=O stretching absorbance of abdominal hydrated whole skin rat following treatment with different vehicles (mean ± SD, n = 3)

vehicles	Asymmetric C-H stretching		Symmetric C-H stretching		C=O stretching of lipid ester	
	Peak height	%D	Peak height	%D	Peak height	%D
Control	4.877±0.0015	-	5.026+0.0026	-	4.999±0.0065	-
PG	0.021±0.002	99.56±1.05	0.023+0.0041	99.54±1.547	0.013±0.002	99.73±1.41
Span 80	0	100	1.95+0.041	61.2±1.004	1.874±0. 018	62.5±1.015
Tween 80	2.129±0.066	56.34±1.84	2.115±0.055	57.91±1.804	1.872±0.025	62.55±1.215
Labrafac PG	2.092 ±0.008	57.1 ±1.93	1.999±0.078	59.01±2.11	1.944±0.045	61.1±1.312
Transcutol P	1.888±0.012	61.28±2.01	1.850±0.114	63.19±2.29	1.640±0.051	67.19±1.493

*%Decrease in peak height(%D) =(peak height from untreated whole skin - peak height from solvent treated whole skin)/ peak height from untreated whole skin x 100

Table 3. Decrease in mean peak height (± SD), compared with control (untreated skin) of C=O stretching (Amide I)and C-N stretching of keratin(Amide II)absorbance of abdominal hydrated whole skin rat following treatment with different vehicles (mean ± SD, n = 3)

vehicles	C=O stretching of keratin		C-N stretching of keratin	
	Peak height	%D	Peak height	%D
Control	4.952±0.021	-	4.840+0.045	-
PG	0.012±0.002	99.75±1.211	0.007±0.0003	99.85±2.18
Span 80	1.725±0.089	65.16±1.15	1.953±0.053	59.64±1.71
Tween 80	1.774±0.011	64.17±2.05	1.806±0.007	62.68±1.92
Labrafac PG	1.806±0.026	63.52±1.88	1.857±0.013	61.63±1.58
Transcutol P	1.555±0.064	68.598±2.014	1.719±0.037	64.48±1.71

Table 4. FT-IR Peak wave numbers(cm^{-1}) changes compared with control (untreated skin) and abdominal hydrated whole skin rat following treatment with different vehicles. (mean ± SD, n = 3)

vehicles	C-H stretching Asy	C-H stretching Sym	C=O stretching of lipid ester	Amide I	Amide II
Control	2948.02±0.115	2821.65±0.42	1723.65±0.55	1652.78±0.35	1572.27±0.22
PG	2952.9±0.6	2754.62±0.53	1724.34±0.45	1677.75±0.47	1539.97±0.45
Span 80	Deleted	2860.64±22	1764.86±0.42	1694.84±0.38	1599.9±0.62
Tween 80	3010.75±1.02	2840.74±0.27	1770.18±0.19	1653±0.9	1591.73±0.58
Labrafac PG	2895.27±0.62	2778±1.2	1716.94±0.62	1669.4±0.56	1591.82±0.72
Transcutol P	2936.97±0.35	2895.24±1.4	1729.69±0.48	1652.58±0.81	1579.46±0.63

Table 5. Effect of vehicles on the thermal properties of hydrated whole abdominal rat skin (mean ± SD, n = 3)

Treatment	Transition temperature (°C)		Enthalpy (mj/mg)	
	Tm_1	Tm_2	ΔH_1	ΔH_2
Hydrated control	67.5±2.1	112±6.6	7.01±0.4	552.1±19.5
PG	77.5±4.2	132±5.9	6.05±0.6	16.4± 2.2
Span 80	38±0.53	117±2.1	0.051±0.006	0.711±0.012
Tween 80	deleted	deleted	0	0
Labrafac PG	44.6±0.63	120±2.6	0.103±0.075	2.573±1.25
Transcutol P	68±2.12	deleted	8.925±2.658	-

Tm_1 = mean transison temperature of lipids; $SCTm_2$= mean transition temperature of irreversible denaturation of intracellularstratum corneum keratin; ΔH_1 = transition enthalpy of lipid phase $SC\Delta H_2$ = transition enthalpy of keratin phase SC

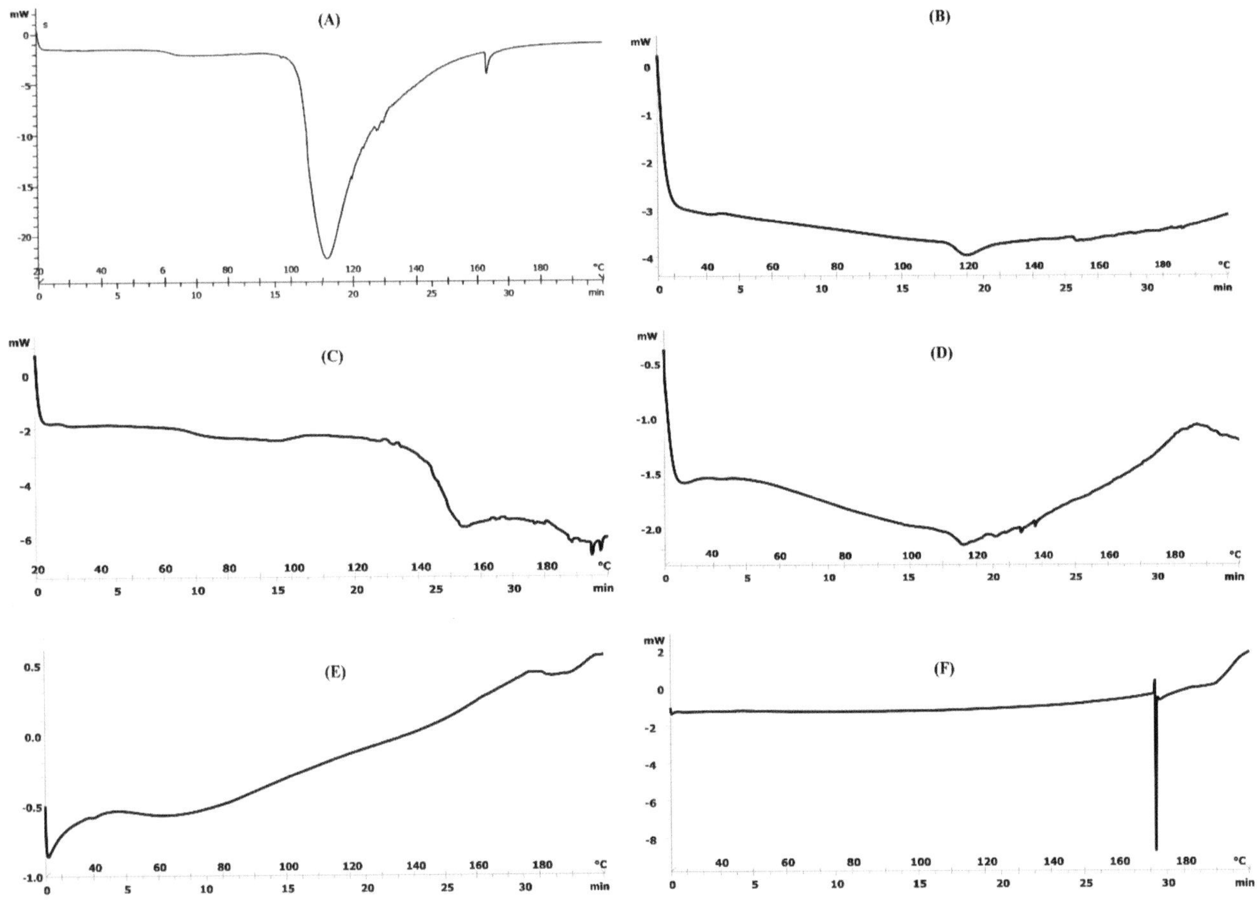

Figure 2. DSC Thermograms of whole skin abdominal rat after treatment with (A) Water (B) Labrafac PG (C) Propylene glycol (D) Span 80 (E) Transcutol P (F) Tween 80

In vitro permeability experiments

The effect of vehicles on naproxen permeability (hydrated skin as control) is expressed in Table 6 as ER_{flux}, was considered to express the impact of different vehicles on the drug permeability. Hydrated rat skin was used as blank, ER_D (drug diffusion coefficient after and before skin pretreatment with vehicle) and ER_p (ratio of drug permeability coefficient after and before skin pretreatment with vehicle). Figure 3 is shown the amount of naproxen permeated from various vehicles across the rat abdominal skin. The results indicated that in comparison to control, naproxen permeation through rat skin was increased in presence of all of vehicles. The drug diffusion coefficients are significantly increased by solvents, with the highest value of ER_D for Tween 80 and followed by Transcotul P, labrafac PG, PG, and Span 80, indicating that their flux was more significantly increased than diffusion coefficient values.

Table 6. Effect of vehicles on derived permeation parameters for naproxen (mean ± SD, n = 3)

Solvent	ER_{flux}	ER_D	ER_P
Span 80	5.364±0.014	1.150±0.004	5.408±0.117
Transcutol P	4.455±0.071	3.116±0.070	4.476±0.053
Labrafac PG	4.424±0.081	2.021±0.073	4.443±0.139
Tween 80	3.970±0.147	16.176±1.267	3.975±0.091
PG	2.909±0.180	1.228±0.138	2.913±0.011

ER_{flux} = ratio of flux after and before treatment with vehicle;
ER_D = ratio of diffusion coefficient after and before treatment with vehicle
ER_P= ratio of permeabilitycoefficient after and before treatment with vehicle

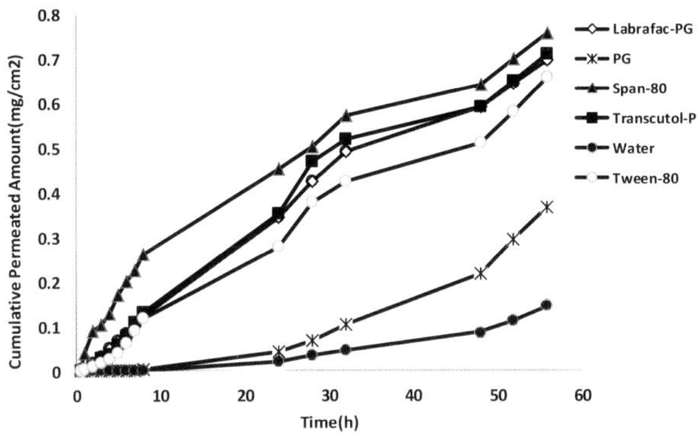

Figure 3. The amount of naproxen permeated from various vehicles across the rat abdominal skin

All of the vehicles significantly increased permeability coefficient compared with water solution of naproxen ($p<0.05$). It can be deduced that the applied vehicles with different lipophilic characteristics increased naproxen solubility in stratum corneum and increased partitioning, flux and permeability. The best enhancing effect was observed by Span 80, followed by Transcutol P, Labrafac PG, Tween 80, and propylene glycol. All of the vehicles significantly increased the diffusion coefficient ($p<0.05$). The best ER_D was observed by tween 80 followed by Transcutol P, Labrafac PG, propylene glycol and span 80. ER_P for all the vehicles was equal increasing ER_{flux}. Span 80provide the best effect on naproxen flux and permeability and tween 80 provide the best effect on diffusion coefficient.

Naproxen belongs to Biopharmaceutical Classification System (BCS) class II so that the low solubility of naproxen in water suggests that the rate-limiting phase is partitioning from stratum corneum to vital epidermis so, the vehicles having various lipophilicities increased partitioning and increased flux from stratum corneum to vital epidermis. It is indicated that there is the drug solubilities in different solvents and ER_D (9.7-1.07) are significantly correlated, so that any decrease in drug solubility is led to ER_D increase. The results of this study indicates significant correlation between drug solubility in various solvents and ER_D (ER_D = 16.8-1.5 drug solubility amount in solvents, p=0.001) so that with decrease of drug solubility in solvent, ER_D value is increased. The low solubility of drug in solvents might have led to higher thermodynamic activity and hence less resistance of skin, thus resulting increase in diffusion coefficient.

Conclusion

The results obtained indicate that the used vehicles increased the drug transport through rat skin. Different mechanisms including Lipid fluidization , disruption lipid structure, lipid extraction and also irreversible protein denaturation in stratum corneum by span 80, Tween 80, Labrafac PG, Transcutol P and propylene glycol are the main probable mechanisms for higher ER_{flux} and ER_D ratios compared to control.

Acknowledgments

This paper is derived from the pharm D thesis of one of the authors (najme hedayati pour). Ahvaz Jundishapur University of Medical Sciences is acknowledged for providing financial support.

Ethical Issues

Not applicable.

Conflict of Interest

The authors report no conflicts of interest.

References

1. Benson HA. Transdermal drug delivery: Penetration enhancement techniques. *Curr Drug Deliv* 2005;2(1):23-33.
2. Moghimipour E, Salimi A, Sharif Makhmal Zadeh B. Effect of the various solvents on the *in vitro* permeability of vitamin B_{12} through excised rat skin. *Trop J Pharm Res* 2013;12(5):671-77.doi: 10.4314/tjpr.v12i5.2.
3. Subedi RK, Oh SY, Chun MK, Choi HK. Recent advances in transdermal drug delivery. *Arch Pharm Res* 2010;33(3):339-51. doi: 10.1007/s12272-010-0301-7
4. Rosado C, Rodrigues LM. Solvent effects in permeation assessed in vivo by skin surface biopsy. *BMC Dermatol* 2003;3:5. doi: 10.1186/1471-5945-3-5
5. Trommer H, Neubert RH. Overcoming the stratum corneum: The modulation of skin penetration. A review. *Skin Pharmacol Physiol* 2006;19(2):106-21. doi: 10.1159/000091978
6. Kumar R, Philip A. Modified transdermal technologies: Breaking the barriers of drug permeation via the skin. *Trop J Pharm Res* 2007;6(1):663-44.doi:10.4314/tjpr.v6i1.14641.
7. Salimi A, Sharif Makhmal Zadeh B, Safavi G. Effect of formulation components on the *in vitro* skin permeation of micro emulsion drug delivery system of piroxicam. *Int Res J Pharm Appl Sci* 2013;3(4):152-60.
8. Moser K, Kriwet K, Naik A, Kalia YN, Guy RH. Passive skin penetration enhancement and its

quantification in vitro. *Eur J Pharm Biopharm* 2001;52(2):103-12.

9. Schulman JH, Hoar TP. Transparent water-in-oil dispersions: The oleopathic Hydro micelle. *Nature* 1943;152(3847):102-3. doi: 10.1038/152102a0.
10. Obata Y, Utsumi S, Watanabe H, Suda M, Tokudome Y, Otsuka M, et al. Infrared spectroscopic study of lipid interaction in stratum corneum treated with transdermal absorption enhancers. *Int J Pharm* 2010;389(1-2):18-23. doi: 10.1016/j.ijpharm.2010.01.007
11. Boncheva M, Damien F, Normand V. Molecular organization of the lipid matrix in intact stratum corneum using atr-ftir spectroscopy. *Biochimica et biophysica acta* 2008;1778(5):1344-55. doi: 10.1016/j.bbamem.2008.01.022
12. Songkro S. An overview of skin penetration enhancers: penetration enhancing activity, skin irritation potential and mechanism of action. *Songklanakarin J Sci Technol* 2009;31(3):299-321.
13. Vaddi HK, Ho PC, Chan SY. Terpenes in propylene glycol as skin-penetration enhancers: Permeation and partition of haloperidol, fourier transform infrared spectroscopy, and differential scanning calorimetry. *J Pharm Sci* 2002;91(7):1639-51. doi: 10.1002/jps.10160
14. Golden GM, Guzek DB, Harris RR, Mckie JE, Potts RO. Lipid thermotropic transition in human stratum corneum. *J Invest Dermatol* 1986;86(3):255-9. doi: 10.1111/1523-1747.ep12285373
15. Marjukka Suhonen T, Bouwstra JA, Urtti A. Chemical enhancement of percutaneous absorption in relation to stratum corneum structural alterations. *J Control Release* 1999;59(2):149-61.
16. Kaushik D, Michniak-Kohn B. Percutaneous penetration modifiers and formulation effects: Thermal and spectral analyses. *AAPS Pharm Sci Tech* 2010;11(3):1068-83. doi: 10.1208/s12249-010-9469-x
17. Al-Saidan SM, Barry BW, Williams AC. Differential scanning calorimetry of human and animal stratum corneum membranes. *Int J Pharm* 1998;168(1):17-22. doi: 10.1016/S0378-5173(98)00078-7
18. Van Duzee BF. Thermal analysis of human stratum corneum. *J Invest Dermatol* 1975;65(4):404-8. doi: 10.1111/1523-1747.ep12607656
19. Barry BW. Mode of action of penetration enhancers in human skin. *J Control Release* 1987;6(1):85-97. doi: 10.1016/0168-3659(87)90066-6
20. Moghimipour E, Salimi A, Eftekhari S. Design and characterization of microemulsion systems for naproxen. *Adv Pharm Bull* 2013;3(1):63-71. doi: 10.5681/apb.2013.011
21. Salimi A, Sharif Makhmal Zadeh B, Moghimipour E. Preparation and characterization of cyanocobalamin (vit b12) microemulsion properties and structure for topical and transdermal application. *Iran J Basic Med Sci* 2013;16(7):865-72.
22. Sharif Makhmal Zadeh B, Hasani MH. The effect of chemical and physical enhancers on trolamine salicylate permeation through rat skin. *Trop J Pharm Res* 2011;9(6):541-8. doi: 10.4314/tjpr.v9i6.63552
23. Salimi A, Moghimipour E, Tavakolbekhoda N. Transdermal delivery of celecoxib through rat skin from various microemulsions. *Int Res J Pharm Appl* 2013;3(4):173-81.
24. Shakeel F, Baboota S, Ahuja A, Ali J, Shafiq S. Skin permeation mechanism and bioavailability enhancement of celecoxib from transdermally applied nanoemulsion. *J Nanobiotechnology* 2008;6:8. doi: 10.1186/1477-3155-6-8

2

Anticonvulsant and Antioxidant Effects of Pitavastatin Against Pentylenetetrazol-Induced Kindling in Mice

Nastaran Faghihi, Mohammad Taghi Mohammadi*

Department of Physiology and Biophysics, Faculty of Medicine, Baqiyatallah University of Medical Sciences, Tehran, Iran.

Keywords:
- Seizure
- Oxidative damage
- Nitrosative damage
- Pentylenetetrazole
- Pitavastatin

Abstract

Purpose: The pleiotropic effects of statins (antioxidant and anti-inflammation) have been reported by previous studies. Therefore, we aimed to determine whether pitavastatin has protective effects against pentylenetetrazol (PTZ)-induced kindling in mice and also whether pitavastatin improves the brain antioxidant capacity and attenuates the oxidative injuries in kindled mice.

Methods: Twenty-four mice were randomly divided into four groups (each group n=6); control, PTZ-kindling and PTZ-kindled rats treated with pitavastatin (1&4 mg/kg). PTZ kindling seizures were induced by repetitive intraperitoneal injections of PTZ (65 mg/kg) every 48 hours till day twenty-one. Animals received daily oral pitavastatin for twenty-one days. Latency, score and duration of the seizures were recorded. The activities of catalase (CAT) ad superoxide dismutase (SOD), and likewise the contents of malondialdehyde (MDA) and nitrate were assessed in the brains of all rats.

Results: There was a progressive reduction in latency of the kindled rats in the next injections of PTZ. Pitavastatin reduced this value (latency) particularly at higher dose. Seizures duration and score also decreased in treatment groups. SOD and CAT activities significantly decreased in PTZ-kindling group by 62% and 64%, respectively, but pitavastatin did not significantly change the SOD and CAT activities. Brain MDA and nitrate significantly increased in PTZ-kindling group by 53% and 30%, respectively. Pitavastatin at higher dose significantly decreased the MDA and nitrate contents of PTZ-kindling rats by 45% and 32%, respectively.

Conclusion: Our findings revealed that pitavastatin can improve the behavioral expression of the PTZ-kindling rats and attenuate the seizure-induced oxidative/nitrosative damage.

Introduction

Epilepsy, the condition of recurrent unprovoked seizures, is one of the most common and serious brain disorders, which involves about 1% of individuals in worldwide.[1] It's characterized by abnormal hypersynchronous paroxysmal cerebral discharges from a circumscribed region or large portions of the brain.[2] Seizures frequently result from an imbalance of excitation and inhibition due to a failure of inhibitory neurotransmission.[3,4] The evidence linking epilepsy with dysfunction of GABAergic inhibition is substantial and $GABA_A$ receptor is a major target of antiepileptic drugs (AED).[5] Using the drugs that impacts the ion channels of cell membranes such as GABA receptors is useful to control the seizures in approximately 70 percent of epileptic patients.[1,5] However, for remaining patients that have intractable seizures (30 percent) new antiepileptic drugs have slight effects.[6] Therefore, new attitudes are needed to treat these patients.

Several animal models and genetic studies have confirmed the connection between oxidative stress and seizure.[7,8] Previously, studies have proven that status epilepticus alter the redox potential and reduce the level of ATP, which can result in failure of brain energy production and supply.[9,10] Recently, Waldbaum *et al.* reported acute injuries induced by reactive oxygen species (ROS) contribute to formation of chronic epilepsy.[11] Likewise, ROS accumulation, mitochondrial dysfunction, lipid peroxidation and brain edema have been observed following prolonged epileptic seizures.[8,9] Lipid peroxidation in patients with seizure is significantly higher compared to normal people.[7,12] Liang and Patel have also verified oxidative damage to susceptible targets (protein, lipids, and DNA) caused by seizure.[13,14] Therefore, reducing oxidative damage may ameliorate tissue damage and occurrence of seizure.

Statins are competitive inhibitors of HMG-CoA (3-hydroxyl-3-methyl-glutaryl coenzyme A) reductase, which inhibit the rate-limiting enzyme of the mevalonate pathway for cholesterol biosynthesis. Pleiotropic effects of statins are other important advantages of using these drugs that are including the improving endothelial function, anti-oxidative stress, neuroprotection, anti-

***Corresponding author:** Mohammad Taghi Mohammadi, Emails: Mohammadi.mohammadt@yahoo.com, Mohammadimohammadt@bmsu.ac.ir inflammation, and anti-neurotoxicity.[15,16] Recently, studies have suggested the anticonvulsive effects of statins. It has been shown that atorvastatin efficiently reduces the kainic acid-induced seizure activities, hippocampal neuronal death and pro-inflammatory genes expression.[17] Also, oral atorvastatin treatment has increased the latency to pentylenetetrazol (PTZ)-induced generalized seizures.[18] The findings of Rangel *et al.* indicated that lovastatin exerted a neuroprotective role in attenuation of brain damage after pilocarpine-induced status epilepticus.[19] Moreover, Xie *et al.* reported simvastatin suppressed cytokines expression and reactive astrocytosis and also decreased the frequency of discharges of epileptic brain.[20] These observations suggest a potential for use of statins in modulation of seizure behaviors. However, there is no study to show the effects of pitavastatin on seizure or epilepsy.

In the present study, we aimed to examine the protective effects of pitavastatin in PTZ kindling model of seizure in mice. Furthermore, the purpose of our study was to determine whether pitavastatin improve the antioxidant capacity of cerebral tissues and reduce oxidative/nitrosative damages during seizure.

Materials and Methods

Animals

The protocols of all experiments were approved by institutional Animal Ethics Committee of Baqiyatallah University of Medical Sciences (Tehran, Iran). Adult male NMRI mice (7-8 weeks old, 23±7 gr) were obtained from Animal House Facility of the University of Baqiyatallah Medical Sciences. The mice were kept in standard cages in a room with controlled light period (07.00 a.m. to 19.00 p.m.), humidity (40-60%), temperature (22-24°C), and also rats were given *ad libitum* access to rat chow and water.

Chemicals

Pitavastatin was purchased from Kowa Pharmaceutical Co Ltd, Tokyo, Japan. Pentylenetetrazole (PTZ) was obtained from Sigma, Germany. PTZ was dissolved in physiological saline solution for intraperitoneal (*i.p.*) injection. Pitavastatin was dissolved in sterile distilled water and administrated orally (by gavage) in treatment groups, while untreated mice received sterile distil water in same volume.

Experimental design

Four groups of mice (N=24) were used in the present study (for each group; n= 6). The mice were randomly divided into Control, PTZ (PTZ kindling model of seizure) and two PTZ groups treated with pitavastatin (1 and 4 mg/kg). Seizures were induced in mice by the repeated intraperitoneal injections of PTZ (65 mg/kg) every 48 hours.[21,22] PTZ injection was continued till day 21. Treated mice received orally pitavastatin 5 days before induction of seizures till day 21 at doses of 1 and 4 mg/kg/day. Moreover, untreated mice received saline solution (*i.p.*) like treated mice in same volume.

Determination of score, latency and duration of seizures

Immediately after PTZ injection in PTZ kindling model of seizure, the animals were transferred to a round open filed and seizure score was monitored. Latency or the time elapsed between injection of a convulsive dose of PTZ (65 mg/kg) and beginning of seizure was recorded. The seizures scores were classified as followed stage 0: no response, stage 1: eat and facial twitching, stage 2: myoclonic body jerks, stage 3: forelimb clonus, rearing, stage 4: clonic convulsions, turn onto the side and stage 5: generalized clonic convulsions, turn onto the back. Finally, the length of seizures was recorded as the seizure duration.[23]

Preparation of brain tissues

The brain tissues of mice were rapidly removed under deep anesthesia to determine the brain contents of nitrate and malondialdehyde (MDA) as well as to assay the activities of catalase (CAT) and superoxide dismutase (SOD) enzymes. The brains were quickly washed in ice-cold phosphate buffer saline (PBS) and immediately frozen by liquid nitrogen. The frozen tissues were rapidly weighed and homogenized in ice-cold PBS (1:10). After centrifuging (14000×g for 15 min at 4°C), the supernatants were used to determine the brain contents of nitrate, MDA and protein as well as the enzymes activities of SOD and CAT.

Determination of superoxide dismutase (SOD) activity

According to the ability of SOD to inhibit the reduction of nitroblue tetrazolium (NBT; Sigma, Germany) by superoxide, the activity of SOD was determined. "For assay, 0.067 M potassium phosphate buffer, pH 7.8 was added to 0.1 M EDTA containing 0.3 mM sodium cyanide, 1.5 mM NBT and 0.1 mL of sample. Then, 0.12 mM riboflavin (Sigma, Germany) was added to each sample to initiate the reaction and was incubated for 12 min. The absorbance of samples was read on a Genesys 10 UV spectrophotometer (CECIL-2501, England) at 560 nm for 5 min. The amount of enzyme required to produce 50% inhibition was taken as 1 U and results were expressed as U/mg protein".[24]

Determination of catalase (CAT) activity

To determine the brain activity of catalase (CAT), "reaction mixture, containing 0.85 mL potassium phosphate buffer 50 mM (pH; 7.0) and 0.1 mL tissue homogenate, was incubated at room temperature for 10 min. Reaction was initiated by addition of 0.05 mL H_2O_2 (30 mM prepared in potassium phosphate buffer 50 mM, pH 7.0) and the decrease in absorbance was recorded for 3 min at 240 nm. Specific activity is expressed as 1μmol H_2O_2 decomposed U/mg protein".[25]

Assessment of malondialdehyde (MDA)

The brain content of MDA (end product of lipid peroxidation) was measured as the index of oxidative stress. First, "0.5 mL of tissue homogenate was added to 1.5 mL of 10% TCA (trichloroacetic acid; Sigma,

Germany), vortexed and incubated for 10 min at room temperature. 1.5 mL of supernatant and 2 mL of thiobarbituric acid (0.67%; Sigma, Germany) were added and placed in a boiling water bath in sealed tubes for 30 min. The samples were allowed to cool at room temperature. 1.25 mL of n-butanol (Sigma, Germany) was added, vortexed and centrifuged at 2000 g for 5 min. The resulting supernatant was removed and measured at 532 nm on a spectrophotometer. MDA concentrations were determined by using 1,1,3,3-tetraethoxypropane as the standard. Finally, the MDA concentration was expressed as µg/mg protein".[26]

Assessment of nitrate content

The nitrate content (the main metabolite of nitric oxide, NO) of brain, as the index of NO, was determined by the colorimetric reaction of Griess reagent. "0.1 mL of homogenate solution was deproteinized by adding 0.2 mL of zinc sulfate solution and centrifuged for 20 min at 4000 g and 4 °C to separate supernatant for nitrate assay. 0.1 mL of supernatant (as sample) or pure water (as blank) or sodium nitrite (as standard; Sigma, Germany) was mixed with 0.1 mL vanadium III chloride (Sigma, Germany). 0.05 mL sulfanilamide (0.01 %; Sigma, Germany) and 0.05 mL N-[1-naphthyl] ethylene-diamin-dihydrochloride (NED, 0.01 %; Sigma, Germany) were incubated for 30 min in dark place at 37 °C. Thereafter, the absorbance of solution was determined at wave length of 540 nm. Nitrate concentration was estimated from a standard curve generated from absorbance of each sodium nitrite solution. Finally, the nitrate content was expressed as µg/mg protein".[27]

Assessment of protein concentration

Based on Bradford method, protein levels of the brain tissues were determined.[28] To calculate the protein concentration, bovine serum albumin (BSA; Sigma, Germany) was used as a standard.

Statistical analysis

SPSS (V.21) was used for statistical analysis. All data were presented as mean±SEM. One-way variance (ANOVA) and Tukey's Post-Hoc test was used to compare the data between control and PTZ (treated and untreated kindled mice) groups. Also, repeated measure was used to analyze the data of different times for latency, duration and score of seizures in each group. All states, $p<0.05$ was considered as significant difference.

Results

Effect of pitavastatin on latency time

Latency or the time elapsed between injection of a convulsive dose of PTZ (65 mg/kg) and beginning of seizure is presented in Figure 1. The latency of PTZ group (untreated kindled mice) was 229±13 Sec at day one that decreased progressively in the next injections of PTZ. So the reduction of latency at days of 14 (90±10 Sec) and 21 (52±10 Sec) statistically differed compared with day one. Likewise, the progressive reduction of latency was observed in kindled mice treated with 1 mg/kg pitavastatin but this reduction was mild. The value of latency for this group was 142±6 and 138±6 Sec at days 14 and 21, respectively, that statistically differed compared to PTZ group. However, pitavastatin at dose of 4 mg/kg prevented the progressive reduction of latency in kindled mice. This value was 229±16, 244±9 and 231±9 Sec at days 7, 14 and 21, respectively, which were near to the latency of day one (197±6 Sec).

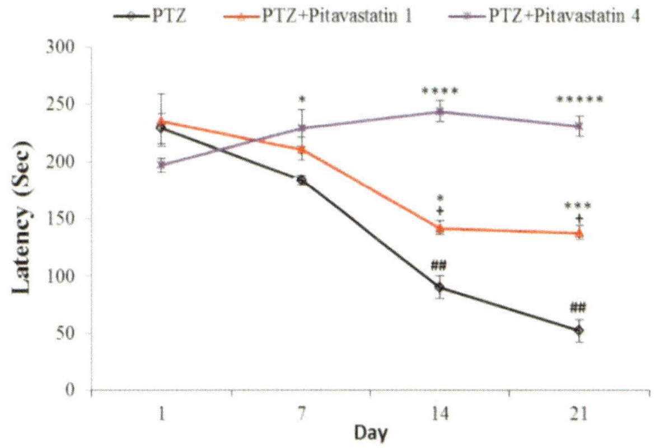

Figure 1. The latency of untreatment kindled group (PTZ) and kindled mice treated with 1 mg/kg (PTZ+Pitavastatin 1) and 4 mg/kg (PTZ+Pitavastatin 4) pitavastatin. All values are presented as Mean±SEM.

*P<0.05, ***P<0.001, ****P<0.0001 and *****P<0.00001 as significant difference compared to PTZ group for own day

##P<0.01 and ###P<0.001 as significant difference compared to PTZ group at day one

+P<0.05 as significant difference compared to kindled mice treated with 1 mg/kg day one

Effect of pitavastatin on seizure length

Figure 2 is showing the seizure length of kindled mice during the test. The seizure length of PTZ group (untreated kindled mice) was 40±1 at day one. This value did not significantly alter in the next injections of PTZ. Administration of pitavastatin considerably decreased the values of seizure length in both treatment kindled groups during the test. This reduction was same in both kindled groups treated with pitavastatin and there was no significant difference between them.

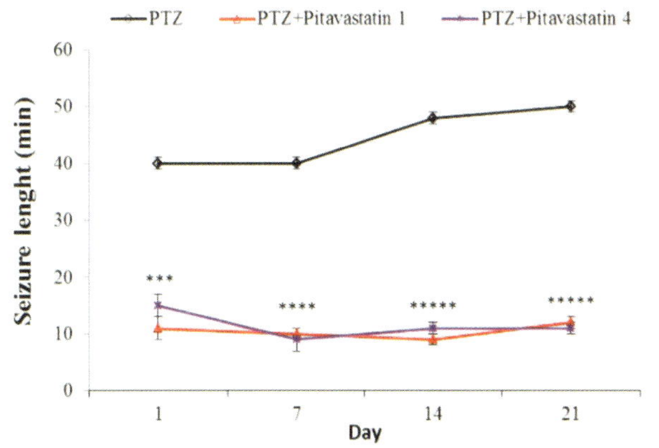

Figure 2. Seizure length of untreatment kindled group (PTZ) and kindled mice treated with 1 mg/kg (PTZ+Pitavastatin 1) and 4 mg/kg (PTZ+Pitavastatin 4) pitavastatin. All values are presented as Mean±SEM.

***P<0.001, ****P<0.0001 and *****P<0.00001 as significant difference compared to PTZ group for own day

Effect of pitavastatin on seizure score

Seizure score, the severity of seizure in kindled mice, is shown in Figure 3. The control mice did not show any seizure signs during the test. Mean value of seizure score in untreatment kindled mice (PTZ group) was 3.75±0.25 at day one. The value of seizure score did not change in the next injections of PTZ in PTZ group. Pitavastatin administration at dose of 1 mg/kg decreased the values of seizure score in the next injections. The values of days 7 and 14 significantly differed compared to PTZ group. Likewise, pitavastatin at dose of 4 mg/kg reduced the values of seizure score in the next injections of PTZ more than 1 mg/kg.

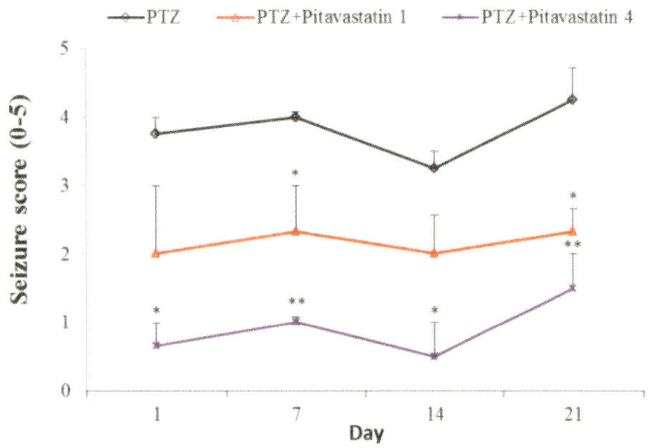

Figure 3. Score of seizure (0-5) in untreatment kindled group (PTZ) and kindled mice treated with 1 mg/kg (PTZ+Pitavastatin 1) and 4 mg/kg (PTZ+Pitavastatin 4) pitavastatin. All values are presented as Mean±SEM.
*P<0.05 and **P<0.01as significant difference compared to PTZ group for own day

Effect of pitavastatin on SOD activity

The activity of brain SOD is presented in Figure 4 at termination of the experiment. The value of SOD significantly reduced in untreatment kindled mice (1.37±0.39 U/mg protein) in comparison with control mice (3.60±1.03U/mg protein). Pitavastatin at doses of 1 and 4 mg/kg did not significantly decrease the SOD activity of brain in treatment kindled mice compared to untreatment kindled mice. The value of SOD was 2.13±0.32 and 2.10±0.28 U/mg protein for treatment kindled groups at doses of 1 and 4 mg/kg pitavastatin, respectively.

Effect of pitavastatin on CAT activity

Figure 5 shows the activity of brain CAT at termination of the experiment. This value significantly decreased in untreatment kindled mice (0.30±0.12 U/mg protein) in comparison with control mice (0.85±0.08 U/mg protein). Pitavastatin at doses of 1 and 4 mg/kg did not significantly decrease the CAT activity of brain in treatment kindled mice compared to untreatment kindled mice. This value was 0.38±0.10 and 0.60±0.14 U/mg protein for kindled groups treated with 1 and 4 mg/kg pitavastatin, respectively.

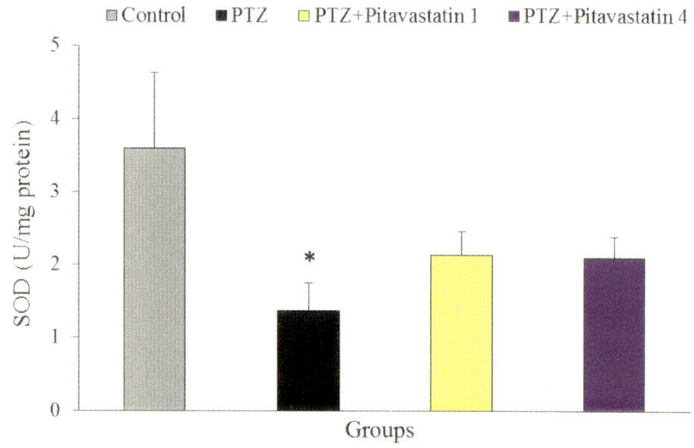

Figure 4. Brain activity of superoxide dismutase, SOD, (U/mg protein) at the end of experiment in groups of control, untreatment kindled group (PTZ) and kindled mice treated with 1 mg/kg (PTZ+Pitavastatin 1) and 4 mg/kg (PTZ+Pitavastatin 4) pitavastatin. All values are presented as Mean±SEM.
* As significant difference compared to control (P<0.05)

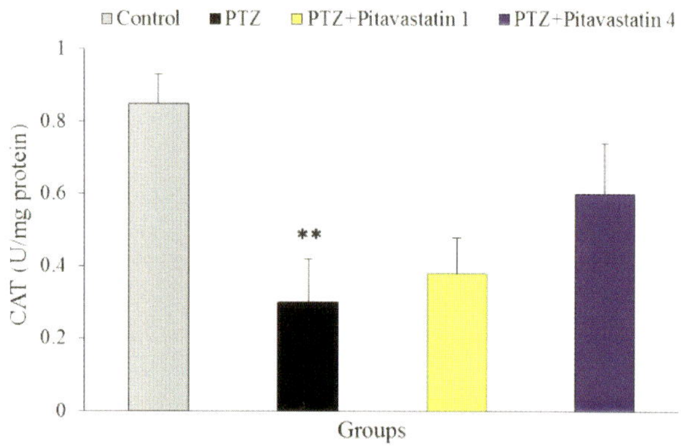

Figure 5. Brain activity of catalase (CAT, U/mg protein) at the end of experiment in groups of control, untreatment kindled group (PTZ) and kindled mice treated with 1 mg/kg (PTZ+Pitavastatin 1) and 4 mg/kg (PTZ+Pitavastatin 4) pitavastatin. All values are presented as Mean±SEM.
** as significant difference compared to control (P<0.05)

Effect of pitavastatin on MDA content

The relative concentration of brain MDA (Control %), as an index of lipid peroxidation, was shown in Figure 6 at termination of the experiment. The value of MDA significantly increased in untreatment kindled mice (PTZ group) by 53% compared to the control mice. Pitavastatin at dose of 1 mg/kg did not noticeably decrease the value of brain MDA of treatment kindled mice. However, pitavastatin at dose of 4 mg/kg significantly decreased the value of MDA in treatment kindled mice by 45% compared to untreated PTZ group.

Effect of pitavastatin on nitrate content

Figure 7 is showing the relative content of brain nitrate (Control %) at the end of experiment. The value of nitrate, as the index of NO production, significantly increased in untreatment kindled mice (PTZ group) by 30% compared to the control mice. Pitavastatin significantly decreased the value of brain nitrate in both treatment kindled groups (1 and 4 mg/kg) compared to PTZ group by 31% and 32%, respectively.

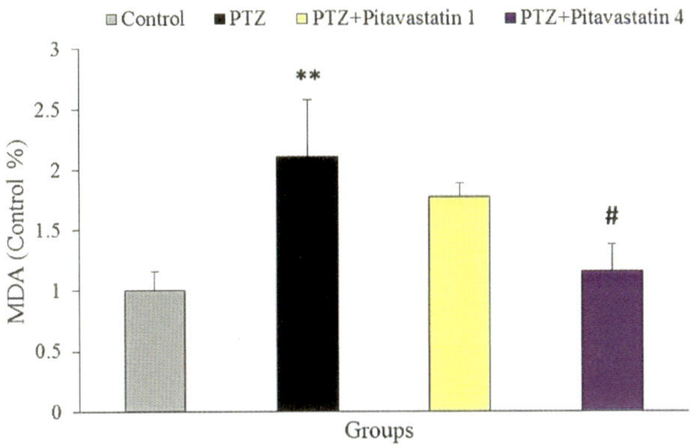

Figure 6. Relative content of brain MDA (Control %) at the end of experiment in groups of control, untreatment kindled group (PTZ) and kindled mice treated with 1 mg/kg (PTZ+Pitavastatin 1) and 4 mg/kg (PTZ+Pitavastatin 4) pitavastatin. The graph has been represented as the relative changes calculated by normalization to the data of control group. All values are presented as Mean±SEM.
** as significant difference compared to control ($P<0.01$)
[#] as significant difference compared to PTZ group ($P<0.05$)

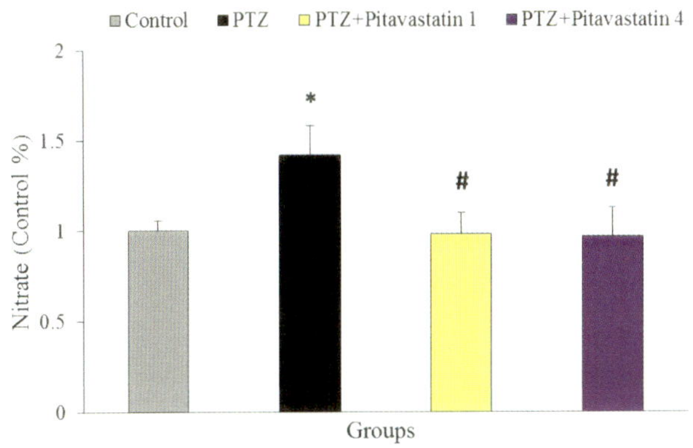

Figure 7. Relative content of brain nitrate (Control %) at the end of experiment in groups of control, untreatment kindled group (PTZ) and kindled mice treated with 1 mg/kg (PTZ+Pitavastatin 1) and 4 mg/kg (PTZ+Pitavastatin 4) pitavastatin. The graph has been represented as the relative changes calculated by normalization to the data of control group. All values are presented as Mean±SEM.
* as significant difference compared to control ($P<0.05$)
[#] as significant difference compared to PTZ group ($P<0.05$)

Discussion

Recently, many studies have reported the anticonvulsive effects of several statins such as atorvastatin and rosuvastatin.[15,19,20] In the present study, we showed that pitavastatin has anticonvulsive effects by improving the seizure behaviors such as increment of latency, reduction of durations and scores in PTZ kindling model of seizure. Treatment with pitavastatin did not noticeably enhance the activities of antioxidant enzymes (SOD and CAT) during seizures but pitavastatin considerably decreased the brain oxidative or nitrosative damage of kindled mice (reduction of brain MDA and nitrate). Likewise, pitavastatin in higher dose (4 mg/kg) was more effective compared to lower dose (1 mg/kg). Since free radicals play an important role in pathophysiology of seizure,[9,11] it is suggested that anticonvulsive effects of pitavastatin correlate with antioxidant effects of this compound.

The PTZ kindling model has been developed to study of the seizure in animal models. It has been identified that PTZ is a non-competitive antagonist of $GABA_A$ receptor and has convulsive effects after repetitive or single administration.[21] Our findings indicated that the injections of PTZ (65 mg/kg) were able to induced seizure in mice. The data of score as well as duration and latency confirmed the seizures in our study. These results are in agreement with the findings of other documented studies.[21,29] Several reports have also indicated that free radicals play a crucial role in pathogenesis of seizure behaviors of the PTZ-kindled animals.[7,8,12] The findings of current study are indicating that the contents of oxygen and nitrogen free radicals (brain MDA and nitrate) were considerably enhanced following kindling. These free radicals lead to cellular dysfunction by attacking the polyunsaturated sites of the biological membranes resulting into increased lipid peroxidation.[13,14] Also, it must be mentioned that brain is highly susceptible to oxidative stress because of high demand for oxygen and abundant polyunsaturated fatty acids. Our findings are indicating a significant reduction of the brain antioxidant enzymes following kindling because there was a considerable reduction in the activities of SOD and CAT. SOD is the main antioxidant enzyme of brain and CAT is an enzyme responsible for detoxification of H_2O_2 formed by the action of SOD.[30,31] Also, it must be mentioned that the ability of the antioxidant defense system of brain against ROS is feeble compared to other tissues, therefore brain cells are susceptible to more damages by free radicals.[31] Finally, it is suggested that weakening of brain antioxidant system and oxidative stress may play a crucial role in pathophysiology of seizure.

Many clinical and experimental findings have demonstrated the beneficial effects of statins on neurological diseases such as stroke and Alzheimer's disease.[16,30,32] Although there are limited studies indicating the anticonvulsive effects of statins,[18-20] there is no study about the anticonvulsive effects of pitavastatin. The findings of current study indicated that pitavastatin was able to increase the seizures latency and reduce the scores and durations of seizures. There was a progressive reduction in latency of PTZ-induced seizure at the next injections of PTZ, whereas pitavastatin particularly in higher dose (4 mg/kg) prevented this progressive reduction. These findings are indicating that pitavastatin like other statins has anticonvulsive effects. Pleiotropic effects of pitavastatin, including anti-oxidative stress and anti-inflammation properties as well as anti-apoptotic effects, have been proven by several recent studies.[16,33-35] It seems that these effects of pitavastatin be important in anticonvulsive effects of this compound like other statins. Reported, treatment with atorvastatin for seven days increases the latency of PTZ-induced seizure in mice.[18] Atorvastatin pretreatment has also reduced the hippocampal neural death and seizure activity of kainic acid-induced seizure.[17] Moreover, Seker *et al.* reported that rosuvastatin reduces epileptic form activity which was associated with improved blood-brain barrier integrity.[15]

Oxidative stress and mitochondrial dysfunction have been determined as a key factor in pathogenesis of many neurodegenerative diseases as well as epilepsy and seizure.[9,31] In the current study, pitavastatin considerably decreased the content of MDA, as a main index of ROS, particularly in higher dose (4 mg/kg). It has been reported that increment of free radicals and mitochondrial dysfunction are associated to initiation and progression of epilepsy.[8,12] Based on previous studies, ROS may lead to Ca^{2+}-dependent depolarization of mitochondrial membrane potential and ATP reduction, which can promote the processes of status epilepticus.[10] Since the antioxidant effects of pitavastatin has been confirmed in many pathological states of brain,[33,34] it is concluded that pitavastatin has anticonvulsive and antiepileptic properties through its power antioxidant effects. In the present study pitavastatin greatly decreased the content of nitrate, as a main index of nitric oxide (NO). NO has been implicated in the promoting of oxygen toxicity in brain. NO promotes the progression of epilepsy by induction of neural loss and reactive glial proliferation.[36] Moreover, high level of NO can react with superoxide anions resulting in peroxynitrite formation, which is a power inducer of cell death.[37] Therefore, it is suggested that pitavastatin modulates PTZ-induced seizure and improves seizure behaviors possibly by inhibition of the toxic effects of NO. However, more studies need to verify how pitavastatin reduce the brain NO in PTZ-induced seizure.

Our findings confirmed that the brain antioxidant enzymes such as SOD and CAT inactivate during seizure. SOD is an important antioxidant enzyme that quenches the superoxide anions in mitochondrial matrix.[10] Reported, reduction in SOD level during epileptogenesis may promote the neural death and brain damage.[38] Likewise, CAT is another antioxidant enzyme of brain, which can detoxify the H_2O_2 to form water and molecular oxygen.[31] Freitas *et al.* reported that CAT is an important antioxidant enzyme that plays protective role in hippocampus against status epilepticus.[39] In the current study, pitavastatin particularly in higher dose could enhance the activity of these enzymes in treated epileptic mice, whereas, the values of these enzymes (SOD and CAT) did not statistically differ compared to untreatment kindled mice. It is suggested that the intensity of seizures was great. Reported, other statins were able to increase the activities of antioxidant enzymes of brain such as SOD and CAT in many pathological states.[16,30,33] Therefore, other studies need to clarify the direct effects of pitavastatin on activities of the brain antioxidant enzymes during seizure.

Conclusion

In conclusion, the findings of present study suggest that chronic administration of pitavastatin is able to modulate the behaviors of seizures, which may be related to inhibition of the seizure-induced oxidative/nitrosative damage. It is concluded that treatment with pitavastatin may be helpful to prevent the seizure and seizure-induced brain damage beside the other anticonvulsant drugs.

Acknowledgments

The authors are cordially appreciating Mr. Mark Azad for providing the drugs and Mrs. Nahid Sarahian for helping in surgical protocols.

Ethical Issues

Not applicable.

Conflict of Interest

The authors declare no conflict of interests.

References

1. Kramer MA, Cash SS. Epilepsy as a disorder of cortical network organization. *Neuroscientist* 2012;18(4):360-72. doi: 10.1177/1073858411422754
2. Badawy RA, Harvey AS, Macdonell RA. Cortical hyperexcitability and epileptogenesis: Understanding the mechanisms of epilepsy - part 2. *J Clin Neurosci* 2009;16(4):485-500. doi: 10.1016/j.jocn.2008.10.001
3. Goldberg EM, Coulter DA. Mechanisms of epileptogenesis: A convergence on neural circuit dysfunction. *Nat Rev Neurosci* 2013;14(5):337-49. doi: 10.1038/nrn3482
4. Badawy RA, Harvey AS, Macdonell RA. Cortical hyperexcitability and epileptogenesis: Understanding the mechanisms of epilepsy - part 1. *J Clin Neurosci* 2009;16(3):355-65. doi: 10.1016/j.jocn.2008.08.026
5. Greenfield LJ, Jr. Molecular mechanisms of antiseizure drug activity at gabaa receptors. *Seizure* 2013;22(8):589-600. doi: 10.1016/j.seizure.2013.04.015
6. Perucca E, French J, Bialer M. Development of new antiepileptic drugs: Challenges, incentives, and recent advances. *Lancet Neurol* 2007;6(9):793-804. doi: 10.1016/S1474-4422(07)70215-6
7. Menon B, Ramalingam K, Kumar RV. Oxidative stress in patients with epilepsy is independent of antiepileptic drugs. *Seizure* 2012;21(10):780-4. doi: 10.1016/j.seizure.2012.09.003
8. Shin EJ, Jeong JH, Chung YH, Kim WK, Ko KH, Bach JH, et al. Role of oxidative stress in epileptic seizures. *Neurochem Int* 2011;59(2):122-37. doi: 10.1016/j.neuint.2011.03.025
9. Aguiar CC, Almeida AB, Araujo PV, de Abreu RN, Chaves EM, do Vale OC, et al. Oxidative stress and epilepsy: Literature review. *Oxid Med Cell Longev* 2012;2012:795259. doi: 10.1155/2012/795259
10. Rowley S, Patel M. Mitochondrial involvement and oxidative stress in temporal lobe epilepsy. *Free Radic Biol Med* 2013;62:121-31. doi: 10.1016/j.freeradbiomed.2013.02.002

11. Waldbaum S, Patel M. Mitochondrial dysfunction and oxidative stress: A contributing link to acquired epilepsy? *J Bioenerg Biomembr* 2010;42(6):449-55. doi: 10.1007/s10863-010-9320-9
12. Sudha K, Rao AV, Rao A. Oxidative stress and antioxidants in epilepsy. *Clin Chim Acta* 2001;303(1-2):19-24.
13. Liang LP, Jarrett SG, Patel M. Chelation of mitochondrial iron prevents seizure-induced mitochondrial dysfunction and neuronal injury. *J Neurosci* 2008;28(45):11550-6. doi: 10.1523/JNEUROSCI.3016-08.2008
14. Patel M. Mitochondrial dysfunction and oxidative stress: Cause and consequence of epileptic seizures. *Free Radic Biol Med* 2004;37(12):1951-62. doi: 10.1016/j.freeradbiomed.2004.08.021
15. Seker FB, Kilic U, Caglayan B, Ethemoglu MS, Caglayan AB, Ekimci N, et al. Hmg-coa reductase inhibitor rosuvastatin improves abnormal brain electrical activity via mechanisms involving enos. *Neuroscience* 2015;284:349-59. doi: 10.1016/j.neuroscience.2014.10.014
16. van der Most PJ, Dolga AM, Nijholt IM, Luiten PG, Eisel UL. Statins: Mechanisms of neuroprotection. *Prog Neurobiol* 2009;88(1):64-75. doi: 10.1016/j.pneurobio.2009.02.002
17. Lee JK, Won JS, Singh AK, Singh I. Statin inhibits kainic acid-induced seizure and associated inflammation and hippocampal cell death. *Neurosci Lett* 2008;440(3):260-4. doi: 10.1016/j.neulet.2008.05.112
18. Funck VR, de Oliveira CV, Pereira LM, Rambo LM, Ribeiro LR, Royes LF, et al. Differential effects of atorvastatin treatment and withdrawal on pentylenetetrazol-induced seizures. *Epilepsia* 2011;52(11):2094-104. doi: 10.1111/j.1528-1167.2011.03261.x
19. Rangel P, Cysneiros RM, Arida RM, de Albuquerque M, Colugnati DB, Scorza CA, et al. Lovastatin reduces neuronal cell death in hippocampal ca1 subfield after pilocarpine-induced status epilepticus: Preliminary results. *Arq Neuropsiquiatr* 2005;63(4):972-6. doi: /S0004-282X2005000600013
20. Xie C, Sun J, Qiao W, Lu D, Wei L, Na M, et al. Administration of simvastatin after kainic acid-induced status epilepticus restrains chronic temporal lobe epilepsy. *PLoS One* 2011;6(9):e24966. doi: 10.1371/journal.pone.0024966
21. Li B, Wang L, Sun Z, Zhou Y, Shao D, Zhao J, et al. The anticonvulsant effects of sr 57227 on pentylenetetrazole-induced seizure in mice. *PLoS One* 2014;9(4):e93158. doi: 10.1371/journal.pone.0093158
22. Zhu X, Shen K, Bai Y, Zhang A, Xia Z, Chao J, et al. Nadph oxidase activation is required for pentylenetetrazole kindling-induced hippocampal autophagy. *Free Radic Biol Med* 2016;94:230-42. doi: 10.1016/j.freeradbiomed.2016.03.004
23. Watanabe Y, Kaida Y, Fukuhara S, Takechi K, Uehara T, Kamei C. Participation of metabotropic glutamate receptors in pentetrazol-induced kindled seizure. *Epilepsia* 2011;52(1):140-50. doi: 10.1111/j.1528-1167.2010.02764.x
24. Vani JR, Mohammadi MT, Foroshani MS, Jafari M. Polyhydroxylated fullerene nanoparticles attenuate brain infarction and oxidative stress in rat model of ischemic stroke. *EXCLI J* 2016;15:378-90. doi: 10.17179/excli2016-309
25. Arjmand Abbassi Y, Mohammadi MT, Sarami Foroshani M, Raouf Sarshoori J. Captopril and valsartan may improve cognitive function through potentiation of the brain antioxidant defense system and attenuation of oxidative/nitrosative damage in stz-induced dementia in rat. *Adv Pharm Bull* 2016;6(4):531-9. doi: 10.15171/apb.2016.067
26. Darabi S, Mohammadi MT. Fullerenol nanoparticles decrease ischaemia-induced brain injury and oedema through inhibition of oxidative damage and aquaporin-1 expression in ischaemic stroke. *Brain Inj* 2017:1-9. doi: 10.1080/02699052.2017.1300835
27. Riahi S, Mohammadi MT, Sobhani V, Ababzadeh S. Chronic aerobic exercise decreases lectin-like low density lipoprotein (lox-1) receptor expression in heart of diabetic rat. *Iran Biomed J* 2016;20(1):26-32.
28. Bradford MM. A rapid and sensitive method for the quantitation of microgram quantities of protein utilizing the principle of protein-dye binding. *Anal Biochem* 1976;72:248-54.
29. Nassiri-Asl M, Zamansoltani F, Torabinejad B. Antiepileptic effects of quinine in the pentylenetetrazole model of seizure. *Seizure* 2009;18(2):129-32. doi: 10.1016/j.seizure.2008.08.002
30. Mohammadi MT, Amini R, Jahanbakhsh Z, Shekarforoush S. Effects of atorvastatin on the hypertension-induced oxidative stress in the rat brain. *Iran Biomed J* 2013;17(3):152-7.
31. Valko M, Leibfritz D, Moncol J, Cronin MT, Mazur M, Telser J. Free radicals and antioxidants in normal physiological functions and human disease. *Int J Biochem Cell Biol* 2007;39(1):44-84. doi: 10.1016/j.biocel.2006.07.001
32. Tu Q, Cao H, Zhong W, Ding B, Tang X. Atorvastatin protects against cerebral ischemia/reperfusion injury through anti-inflammatory and antioxidant effects. *Neural Regen Res* 2014;9(3):268-75. doi: 10.4103/1673-5374.128220
33. Kumagai R, Oki C, Muramatsu Y, Kurosaki R, Kato H, Araki T. Pitavastatin, a 3-hydroxy-3-methylglutaryl-coenzyme a (hmg-coa) reductase inhibitor, reduces hippocampal damage after transient cerebral ischemia in gerbils. *J Neural Transm (Vienna)* 2004;111(9):1103-20. doi: 10.1007/s00702-004-0150-y
34. Kurata T, Miyazaki K, Morimoto N, Kawai H, Ohta Y, Ikeda Y, et al. Atorvastatin and pitavastatin reduce

oxidative stress and improve ir/ldl-r signals in alzheimer's disease. *Neurol Res* 2013;35(2):193-205. doi: 10.1179/1743132812Y.0000000127

35. Kurata T, Miyazaki K, Kozuki M, Morimoto N, Ohta Y, Ikeda Y, et al. Atorvastatin and pitavastatin reduce senile plaques and inflammatory responses in a mouse model of alzheimer's disease. *Neurol Res* 2012;34(6):601-10. doi: 10.1179/1743132812Y.0000000054
36. Arhan E, Serdaroglu A, Ozturk B, Ozturk HS, Ozcelik A, Kurt N, et al. Effects of epilepsy and antiepileptic drugs on nitric oxide, lipid peroxidation and xanthine oxidase system in children with idiopathic epilepsy. *Seizure* 2011;20(2):138-42. doi: 10.1016/j.seizure.2010.11.003
37. Parathath SR, Parathath S, Tsirka SE. Nitric oxide mediates neurodegeneration and breakdown of the blood-brain barrier in tpa-dependent excitotoxic injury in mice. *J Cell Sci* 2006;119(Pt 2):339-49. doi: 10.1242/jcs.02734
38. Chen D, Lu Y, Yu W, Luo J, Xiao Z, Xiao F, et al. Clinical value of decreased superoxide dismutase 1 in patients with epilepsy. *Seizure* 2012;21(7):508-11. doi: 10.1016/j.seizure.2012.05.003
39. Freitas RM, Vasconcelos SM, Souza FC, Viana GS, Fonteles MM. Oxidative stress in the hippocampus after pilocarpine-induced status epilepticus in wistar rats. *FEBS J* 2005;272(6):1307-12. doi: 10.1111/j.1742-4658.2004.04537.x

The Effects of Cetirizine on P-glycoprotein Expression and Function *In vitro* and *In situ*

Mehran Mesgari Abbasi[1,2], Hadi Valizadeh[1], Hamed Hamishekar[1], Leila Mohammadnejad[3], Parvin Zakeri-Milani[4]*

[1] *Drug Applied Research Center, Tabriz University of Medical Sciences, Tabriz, Iran.*
[2] *Students Research Committee, Tabriz University of Medical Sciences, Tabriz, Iran.*
[3] *Immunology Research Center, Tabriz University of Medical Sciences, Tabriz, Iran.*
[4] *Liver and Gastrointestinal Diseases Research Center and Faculty of Pharmacy, Tabriz University of Medical Sciences, Tabriz, Iran.*

Keywords:
- Cetirizine
- Digoxin
- Intestinal permeability
- P-glycoprotein

Abstract

Purpose: P-glycoprotein (P-gp) plays a major role in oral absorption of drugs. Induction or inhibition of P-gp by drugs contributes to variability of its transport activity and often results in clinically relevant drug-drug interactions. The purpose of this study was to investigate the effect of cetirizine, a second generation H_1 antihistamine, on P-gp function and expression *in vitro* and *in situ*.

Methods: The *in-vitro* rhodamin-123 (Rho123) efflux assay in Caco-2 cells was used to study the effect of cetirizine on P-gp function. Western blot analysis was used for surveying the effect of cetirizine on expression of P-gp in Caco-2 cells. Rat *in situ* single-pass intestinal permeability technique was used to calculate the intestinal permeability of a known P-gp substrate (digoxin) in the presence of cetirizine. The amounts of digoxin and cetirizine in intestinal perfusion samples were analyzed using a HPLC method.

Results: The results showed significant increase in Rho123 uptake ($P < 0.05$) and also P-gp band intensity decrease in cetirizine-treated cells *in vitro*. Furthermore the intestinal permeability of digoxin was also increased significantly in the presence of cetirizine ($P < 0.01$).

Conclusion: Therefore it is concluded that cetirizine is a P-gp inhibitor and this should be considered in co administration of cetrizine with other P-gp substrate drugs. Further investigations are required to confirm our results and to determine the mechanism underlying P-gp inhibition by cetirizine.

Introduction

Currently, most drugs used in clinical practice are administered orally and must be adequately and consistently absorbed to achieve successful therapy. Appropriate regulation of drug delivery to the body, including intestinal absorption, hepatic metabolism, renal excretion, and transport into the tissues, is important to ensure suitable therapeutic efficacy. Maintaining appropriate serum concentration of drugs is also necessary to exert their beneficial effects and to prevent unexpected adverse effects, especially for drugs with narrow therapeutic index. Furthermore, the increasing potential of clinical drug–drug, herb–drug, and food-drug interactions resulted from developing new drugs and increasing wide-use of drugs and herbal drugs have been noticed. In addition to other mechanisms, membrane transporters are the most important factors involved in the mentioned interactions and they are major barriers limiting oral drug delivery.[1,2]

P-glycoprotein (P-gp) is the most important membrane transporter which is responsible for secreting (active efflux) passively diffused drugs and xenobiotics out of the cell.[2,3] P-gp is an ATP binding cassette protein and plays a major role in drug absorption and distribution due to its abundant expression on several barrier epithelia (including the epithelial cells of intestine, kidney, liver, brain, testis, adrenal gland, placenta, and bile canalicula) and its broad substrate specificity.[3] Some drugs, foods, and chemicals may be substrates of P-gp. The transport activity of P-gp can be induced or inhibited *in vivo* by a variety of drugs with different structures, such as verapamil, rifampicin, erythromycin, ketoconazole, and cyclosporine[4,5] which may affect the absorption of drugs themselves and the concomitantly used drugs. Induction (enhancing P-gp activity) or inhibition (impairing P-gp-mediated efflux) of P-gp by drugs or other xenobiotics contributes to variability of its transport activity and often results in clinically relevant interactions. Therefore, P-gp-related interactions have important clinical impacts

***Corresponding author:** Parvin Zakeri-Milani, Email: pzakeri@tbzmed.ac.ir and it is critical to understand which drugs are inducers or inhibitors of P-gp to minimize or avoid adverse interactions.[3,6]

Cetirizine, a member of the second generation H_1 antihistamines, is chemically known as (RS)-2-[2-[4-(4-chlorophenyl) phenylmethyl] piperazin-1-yl] ethoxy] acetic acid dihydrochloride (Figure 1). Cetirizine is a piperazine derivative and is marketed as a racemic mixture containing both levocetirizine and dextrocetirizine. It is a long-acting non-sedative antihistamine and an antagonist of H_1-receptor. Cetirizine di-hydrochloride is used for symptomatic treatment of allergic conditions including seasonal allergic rhinitis and chronic urticarial.[7-9]

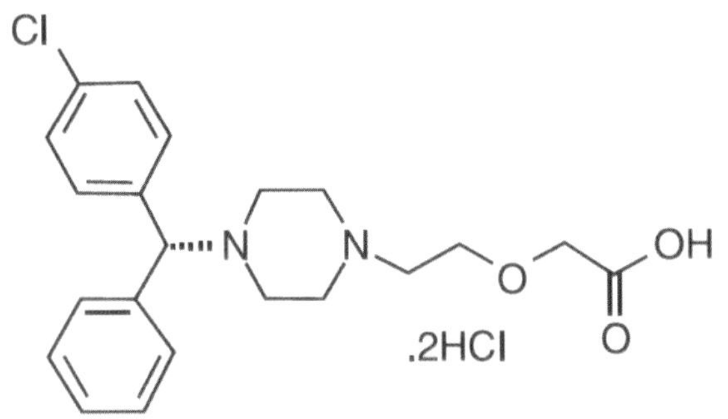

Figure 1. Chemical structure of cetirizine.[10]

Therefore the purpose of this study was to investigate the effect of cetirizine treatment on the P-gp function and its expression both *in vitro* and *in situ*. In addition, the potential role of digoxin, a typical substrate of P-gp, in intestinal effective permeability (P_{eff}) of cetirizine was also studied.

Materials and methods

Materials

Anti-P-gp mouse monoclonal antibody (ab80594) and rabbit polyclonal antibody (Ab) to beta actin (ab16039) were purchased from Abcam (Cambridge, UK). Horseradish peroxidase (HRP) conjugated anti-mouse Immunoglobulin (IgG) (AP8036) and anti-rabbit IgG (AP7181) were purchased from Razi Biotech (Karaj, Iran). Rhodamin-123 (Rho123), digoxin, verapamil, cetirizine, 3-(4,5-dime-thylthiazol-2-thiazolyl)-2,5-diphenyl-tetrazoliumbromide (MTT), penicillin-streptomycin, protease inhibitor cocktail and nonfat-dried milk bovine were purchased from Sigma–Aldrich (St. Louis, MO, USA). Dulbecco's modified eagle medium (DMEM), trypsin-EDTA (0.25%), fetal calf serum (FCS) were purchased from Gibco (Carlsbad, CA, USA). Tissue culture flasks and other disposable cell culture items were purchased from TPP Co. (Trasadingen, Switzerland). Enhanced chemiluminescence (ECL) western blotting detection kit, medical X-ray film, pre-stained protein ladder (10-250 kDa), and protein assay kit were purchased from Amersham (GE Healthcare, Chalfont St. Giles, UK), Fuji (Tokyo, Japan), Cinagen, and Pars Azmoon (Tehran, Iran), respectively. All other chemicals were purchased from Merck Co. (Darmstadt, Germany).

Cell Culture

Caco-2 cells were obtained from national cell bank of Iran (Pasteur Institute, Tehran, Iran) and were routinely cultured in Dulbecco's modified Eagle's medium (DMEM) containing 10% fetal bovine serum, 10,000 I.U./mL Penicillin, and 10,000 µg/mL Streptomycin. Cells were maintained in an incubator at 37°C with a humidified atmosphere of 5% CO_2 in a CO_2 incubator (Memmert, Schwabach, Germany). The culture medium was changed 2-3 times per week. After 2-3 weeks culture and differentiation of Caco-2 into intestinal-like cells, the cells were detached from the culture flask by addition of 0.25% trypsin-EDTA. Cells were then seeded at the needed density for performing the following tests.

Cytotoxicity study (MTT assay)

The MTT assay was used to determine the cytotoxicity of 0.2, 10, and 100 µM cetirizine. The Caco-2 cells were seeded into 96-well plates at a density of 15×10^3 cells per well. After 24 h, the medium was replaced with 200 µL per well of cetirizine different concentrations. After 24 h of incubation, MTT solution (2 mg/mL final concentration) was added to each well and incubated for 4 h at 37 °C in a CO_2 incubator. The MTT solution was removed and the resulting formazan crystals were solubilized with 200 µL/well of dimethyl-sulfoxide (DMSO) and 25 µL/well Sorensen buffer. The optical densities (ODs) were measured with an enzyme linked immune-sorbent assay (ELISA) plate reader (Statfax-2100, Awareness, Palm City, FL, USA) at 570 nm with background subtraction at 630 nm. The following formula was used for calculating percentage of cell viability.

$$\text{Cell viability \%} = \frac{\text{OD value of test}}{\text{OD value of control}} \times 100 \quad (1)$$

The mean ± standard deviation (SD) was calculated for each concentration and analyzed statistically.

Rho123 efflux assay

P-gp function study in Caco-2 cells was realized by the measurement of intracellular accumulation of Rho123, a well-known P-gp substrate, which is inversely proportional to P-gp activity. Caco-2 cells were seeded in 24-well plates and allowed to attach for 24 h. Then, the old medium was removed and cells were washed with PBS. New culture media containing 100 µM cetirizine and 300 µM verapamil, as P-gp inhibitor, were added to separate wells and left for another 24 h. After that, the old medium was removed and cells were washed three times with PBS. Rho123 solution [DMEM containing 10 mM HEPES (pH = 7.4) and 5 µM Rho123] was added and incubated for 3 h at 37°C, followed by three washes with ice-cold PBS (pH = 7.4). Cells were lysed in 1 %

Triton X-100 and centrifuged at 1500 g for 10 min (3-18k, Sigma). Supernatant was used to measure the Rh123 and the total protein contents. The cellular accumulation of Rho123 was determined quantitatively by fluorescence spectrophotometry (λ_{ex} = 485 nm, λ_{em} = 532 nm) (FP-750, Jasco, Japan) and normalized by the protein content of each sample determined by the protein assay kit (Pars Azmoon, Iran).[11-13]

Western blot

Caco-2 cells were seeded to a 6 well-plate in the density of 10^6 cells per well and treated for 48 h with the culture medium (as control), culture medium containing 0.2, 10, and 100 μM cetirizine, and 300 μM verapamil, as P-gp inhibitor. Then, solutions were removed and cells were washed with PBS, and incubated for 5 min with trypsin/EDTA 0.25 % in 37 °C. The detached cells were washed twice with PBS. Lysis buffer (Triton X-100 50 mM, NaCl 150 mM, EDTA 5 mM, 1 % protease inhibitor cocktail, tris-HCl, pH=7.4) was added and cell suspension was centrifuged at 1500 g for 5 min. Proteins were separated through sodium dodecyl sulfate-polyacrylamide 12.5 % running gel (SDS-PAGE) electrophoresis (80 V, 120 min). The gel was electro blotted to a poly-vinylidene di-fluoride (PVDF) membrane using a semi-dry western blotting system (Bio-Rad, Hercules, CA, USA). All membranes were blocked for nonspecific binding by incubation in 3% nonfat-dried milk for 1 h at room temperature and the membrane was washed 3 times with Tris buffered saline (TBS) with 0.1% Tween 20. Then, the membranes were incubated overnight with mouse monoclonal anti-P-gp antibody (1/1000 in TBS). After washing with TBS, the membrane was incubated with HRP-conjugated rabbit anti-mouse secondary antibody for 2 h. Membrane was washed and the proteins were then detected using an ECL kit. The proteins were visualized by exposing the membrane to a medical x-ray film (Fuji, Japan) for 5 min in a dark room and scanned using a bio-imaging analyzer (Bio-Rad, USA). β-actin was the internal standard, and was detected using rabbit polyclonal anti-β-actin as primary antibody and HRP-conjugated goat anti-rabbit IgG as secondary antibody. P-gp expression is presented as the ratio of P-gp band intensity to β -actin band intensity in the same blot run (P-gp/ β –actin).[14]

In situ single-pass intestinal permeability study

Animals

Male Sprague–Dawley rats (200–250 g) were supplied by Pasteur Institute of Iran. The animals were kept under 22 ± 2°C with a 12/12 light/dark cycle, and 55 – 60% relative humidity. Prior to experimentation, rats were fasted for 12-16 h (water *ad libitum*). All procedures were conducted in accordance with the humanity and animal ethic protocols. The animal study protocols were approved by the research ethical committee of Tabriz University of Medical Sciences (Ref No: TBZMED.REC.1394.378).

Single-pass intestinal perfusion (SPIP)

The animals were anesthetized with an intra-peritoneal injection of thiopantal sodium (60 mg/kg). A midline abdominal incision of 3-4 cm was made and approximately 10 cm of the jejunum segment of the intestine was isolated and cannulated at both ends with polypropylene tubes. The exposed segment was kept moist with body tempered saline. At first, the segment was rinsed with 37°C normal saline to wash and clear the segment, then PBS (pH = 7.4) containing 50 mg/l phenol red without drug (blank solution) was pumped through the segment at a constant flow rate of 0.2 ml/min (Q_{in}) through a volumetric infusion pump (Argus Medical AG, Switzerland). Blank perfused solution was collected at the outlet and used to prepare cetirizine and digoxin calibrator solutions and also for stability studies.[15,16] After reaching steady state, perfusates were quantitatively collected for every 10 min (2ml) lasting 90 min (9 samples). Water absorption and secretion and other changes during the perfusion may cause errors in the calculated permeability values, phenol red, therefore, was added at a concentration of 50 mg/L as a non-absorbable marker to correct the results. Digoxin (20 μM in blank solution), Verapamil as a typical P-gp inhibitor (in blank solution with digoxin 20 μM), and different concentrations of cetirizine (0.2, 10, and 100 μM in blank solution with digoxin 20 μM/L) were administrated as described above (n = 3) for each drug and each concentration).[15,16] At the end of procedure, the length of the segment was measured (cm) and the animal was euthanized. Samples were stored at -70°C (ultra-low temperature freezer, Jal Tajhiz Production, Karaj, Iran), until analysis. The concentrations of phenol red in perfused (outlet) samples were measured at 560 nm using an UV-VIS spectrophotometer (Ultra-spec 2000, Pharmacia, Pfizer, New York, NY, USA).[17] Digoxin and cetirizine amount in outlet samples were detected by HPLC method.

HPLC analysis of digoxin and cetirizine in intestinal perfused samples

The mobile phase for digoxin and cetirizine analysis was 35% (v/v) acetonitrile in water which was filtered through sintered glass filter P5 (1.0-1.6 μ, Winteg, Germany) and degassed in a sonicator. The mobile phase was pumped in isocratic mode at a flow rate of 2 ml/min at ambient temperature. UV detection was accomplished at 218 nm and samples of 20 μl were injected using Hamilton injector syringe (Hamilton, Switzerland) onto the column (Knauer- 15VE081ESJ - 150X4.6 mm with precolumn- Eurospher 100-5 C8, Berlin-Germany).[15] The high performance liquid chromatography (HPLC) system was composed of Smartline manager 5000, Smartline UV detector 2600, and Smartline pump 1000 (Knauer Advanced Scientific Instruments, Berlin, Germany). Figure 2 shows a representative HPLC chromatogram of analyzed samples.

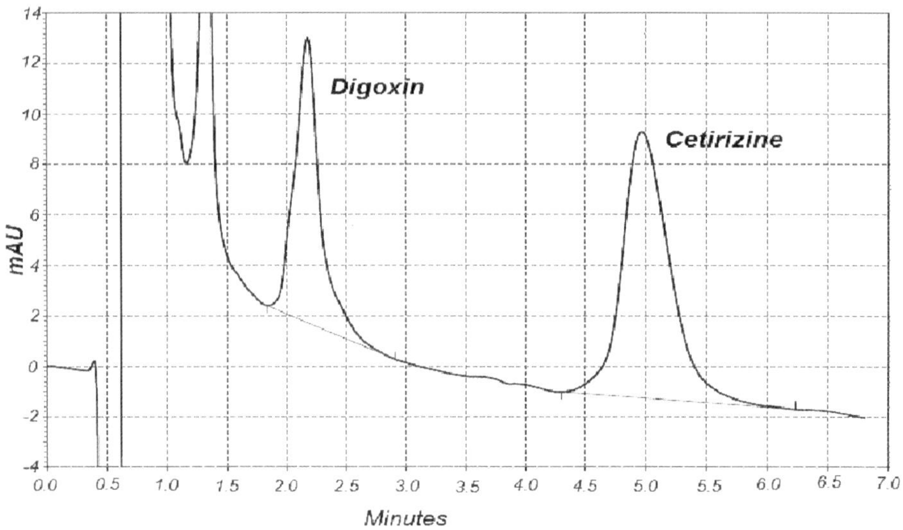

Figure 2. A representative HPLC chromatogram of cetirizine (10 μM) and digoxin (20 μM) in intestinal perfused sample.

Data analysis

P_{eff} values were calculated from the steady-state concentrations of compounds in the perfusate collected from the outlet tubing. Steady state was confirmed by the ratio of the outlet to inlet concentrations (corrected for water transport) versus time.[15-17] Corrected C_{out} (outlet concentration of the drug) was calculated from the following equation.[18]

$$C_{out\,(corr)} = C_{out} \times \frac{\text{Concentration of phenol red in } (CPR_{in})}{\text{Concentration of phenol red out } (CPR_{out})} \quad (2)$$

Where $C_{out\,(corr)}$ is corrected outlet concentration of the drug, C_{out} is outlet concentration of the drug, CPR_{in} is concentration of phenol red entering the intestinal segment and CPR_{out} is concentration of phenol red leaving the intestinal segment. Calculations were based on outlet perfusate steady state concentrations achieved after the selected time points. The steady-state intestinal P_{eff} was calculated according to following equation:

$$P_{eff} = \frac{-Q_{in} \times \ln (C_{out}/C_{in})}{2 \times 60 \pi r l} \quad (3)$$

P_{eff} represents effective permeability (cm/s), Q_{in} represents the perfusion rate (0.2 ml/min), C_{in} and C_{out} represent the concentrations of the test drug entering and leaving the segment respectively, r is the radius of the intestinal segment (0.18 cm), and l is the length of the intestinal segment (cm).

Statistical analysis

Data were presented as the mean ±SD. Statistical analyses were carried out using one-way analysis of variance (ANOVA) followed by Tukey's multiple comparison test and the differences between two groups were determined using the unpaired t-test. Statistical tests were performed with SPSS13.0 (SPSS Inc., Chicago, IL, USA), where $p < 0.05$ and $p < 0.01$ were considered to be statistically significant.

Results

Preliminary experiments showed that no considerable adsorption of compounds on the tubing and syringe took place and the stock and working standard solutions of cetirizine in water was stable during the experiments.[9]

Cytotoxicity study (MTT assay)

The cytotoxicity on cells was detected using MTT assay. Cetirizine, verapamil, and digoxin solutions showed no cytotoxicity on Caco-2 cells under the maximum dosage (100, 300, and 20 μM, respectively) (Figure 3).

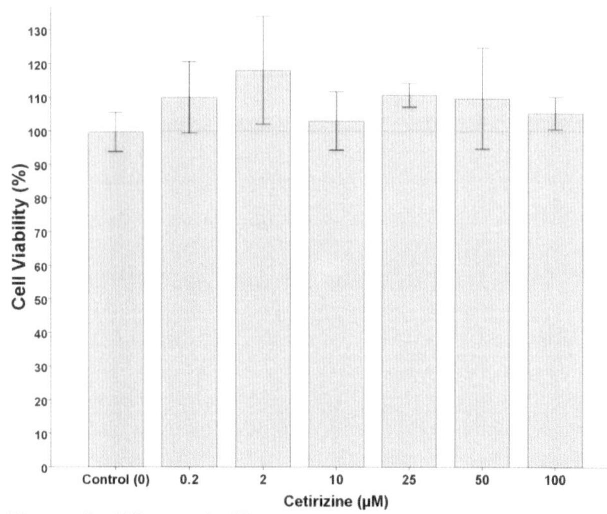

Figure 3. Effects of different concentrations of cetirizine on Caco-2 cells viability. Bars show mean ± SD of at least 3 measurements. * $p < 0.05$ was considered as significance level.

Rho123 efflux assay

To assess the impact of cetirizine treatment on the function of P-gp as an efflux pump *in vitro*, we examined the P-gp-mediated Rho123 transport in Caco-2 cells treated with cetirizine using verapamil as a P-gp inhibitor. As shown in Figure 4, 100 μM cetirizine significantly increased the intracellular accumulation of Rho123 in Caco-2 cells ($p < 0.05$). The mean intracellular concentration of Rho123 in control cells was 50.2 ± 6.0, while in cetirizine and verapamil treated cells were 88.8 ± 2.3 and 420.6 ± 25.4 pg/mg protein, respectively.

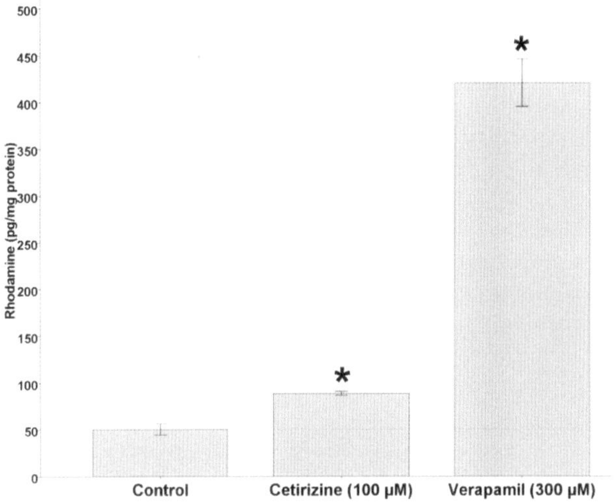

Figure 4. Effects of cetirizine and verapamil treatments on the intracellular accumulation of Rho123 in Caco-2 cells. Bars show mean ± SD of at least 4 measurements. * $p < 0.05$ was considered as significance level.

In situ single-pass intestinal permeability study

To further confirming the inhibitory effect of cetirizine on P-gp activity, the *in situ* experiments were conducted. For this purpose digoxin intestinal permeability, as a typical P-gp substrate, in jejunal segment of rats was determined. As shown in Figure 5, 0.2 μM cetirizine did not significantly increase the P_{eff} of digoxin relative to control group (digoxin alone) ($p > 0.05$), however the difference reached to significance level at higher concentrations (10 and 100 μM, $p < 0.01$). The P_{eff} values of digoxin (20 μM) in the absence and presence of verapamil, as a typical inhibitor, were 3.4 ± 0.8 and 8.9 ± 0.7 $\times 10^{-5}$cm/s, respectively. Whereas, the P_{eff} values of digoxin in the presence of 0.2, 10, and 100 μM cetirizine were found to be 4.4 ± 0.4, 6.8 ± 0.4, and 8.7 ± 1.0 $\times 10^{-5}$cm/s, respectively.

The concentration of cetirizine was also determined in intestinal perfused samples, and P_{eff} values of 10 and 100 μM cetirizine were also calculated. The results, illustrated in Figure 6, showed that by increasing the concentration of cetirizine from 10 to 100 μM, the P_{eff} value decreased from 6.7 ± 0.7 to 3.4 ± 0.4 $\times 10^{-5}$cm/s. The difference between two groups was statistically significant ($p = 0.02$).

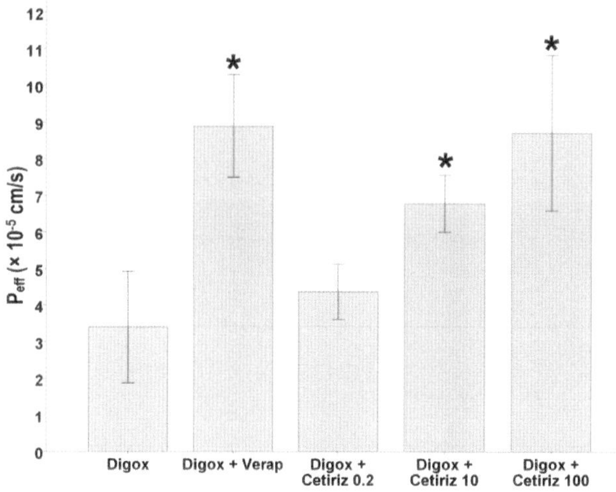

Figure 5. Effects of verapamil and 0.2, 10, and 100 μM cetirizine on the effective permeability (P_{eff}) of digoxin. Bars show mean ± SD of at least three measurements. * $p < 0.05$ was considered as significance level.

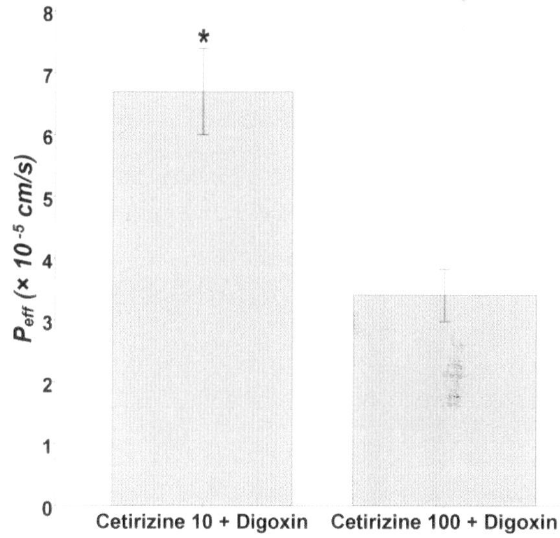

Figure 6. The effective permeability values of 10 and 100 μM cetirizine in the presence of 20 μM digoxin (n = 3). Bars show mean ± SD of at least three measurements. * $p < 0.05$ was considered as significance level.

Western Blotting

Immuno-blotting of Caco-2 cells were carried out using monoclonal antibody against P-gp, to further investigate the inhibitory effect of cetirizine treatment on P-gp activity after 48 h treating. The beta- actin protein expression was considered as internal immuno-blotting control. P-gp expression was presented as the ratio of P-gp band intensity to β -actin band intensity (P-gp/ β -actin) and were compared with verapamil and control bands in the same blot run.[14] Low density of immuno-blot bands of cetirizine treated cells compared with those of untreated cells (control), as shown in Figure 7, demonstrated low expression of P-gp.

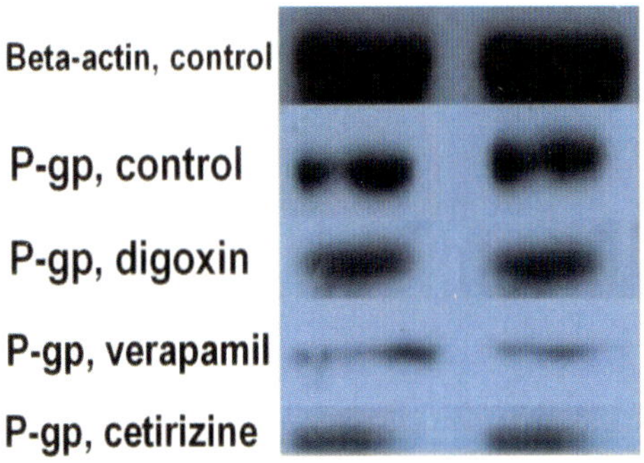

Figure 7. Western blot of P-gp and β- actin in 100 μM cetirizine and 300 μM verapamil treated, and control (non-treated) Caco-2 cells (bands of 2 samples of each are shown).

Discussion

In vitro and *in situ* results of the present study showed P-gp inhibition potential of cetirizine. The mean intracellular concentration of Rho123 in 100 μM cetirizine treated Caco-2 cells was 1.8 times the control cells and was statistically significant ($p < 0.05$) while it was 8.4 times in verapamil treated cells ($p < 0.01$). In SPIP study, P_{eff} of digoxin was increased to 1.3, 2, and 2.6 times the control in the presence of 0.2, 10, and 100 μM cetirizine, respectively. Although, the difference was not significant for 0.2 μM concentrations, it reached to a high significant level at 10 and 100 μM cetirizine ($p < 0.01$). The upward trend of P_{eff} of digoxin showed a dose-dependent P-gp inhibition effect of cetirizine, at least in the range of 0.2-100 μM concentrations. In our study, low density of P-gp immune-blot bands of cetirizine treated Caco-2 cells relative to non-treated cells showed down-regulation of P-gp expression by cetirizine.

P-gp inhibitors, as demonstrated by photo-affinity labeling, may exert their inhibitory effect by one of the following three mechanisms: (1) altering P-gp expression; (2) Disrupting the ATP hydrolysis; and (3) competition for a binding site or reversible inhibition.[19] It might be speculated that the P-gp inhibitory mechanisms of cetirizine are both altering P-gp expression and competition for P-gp binding sites. Western blotting results of present study confirm the idea. On the other hand, previous studies demonstrated P-gp substrate role of the cetirizine in mice blood-brain barrier (BBB),[20] 1b (mdr1a/b) knockout mice,[21] human MDR1-transfected Madin-Darby canine kidney cells,[21] and human Caco-2 cells[22] using monolayer efflux assay[20] and other *in vitro* and *in situ* assays. To the best of our knowledge, both digoxin and cetirizine are substrates of P-gp and competition for binding sites of P-gp molecules by them is suggested. As shown in Figure 5, by increasing the concentration of cetirizine from 0.2 to 100 μM, digoxin intestinal P_{eff} raised from 4.4 ± 0.4 to $8.7 \pm 1.0 \times 10^{-5}$cm/s, but P_{eff} of cetirizine decreased from 6.7 ± 0.7 to $3.4 \pm 0.4 \times 10^{-5}$cm/s; this may confirm the competition of two drugs for P-gp binding sites.

From the literature review, the physicochemical properties of cetirizine may help to suggest the P-gp inhibition effect of cetirizine. Ekins *et al.* focused on identifying functional groups of P-gp inhibitors active molecules in their study. The study was carried out with 27 inhibitors of digoxin transport in Caco-2 cells *in vitro*. They found that two hydrophobic groups along with a hydrogen-bond acceptor group and an aromatic core were required for P-gp inhibition.[23] The chemical structure of cetirizine was shown in Figure 1 ($C_{21}H_{27}Cl_3N_2O_3$) and it has one hydrogen bond donor, 5 hydrogen bond acceptors, and 8 rotatable bonds. Log octanol/water partition coefficients, log P and log D, of cetirizine are 4.48 and 1.04 (pH = 7.4), respectively. Polli *et al.* studied the influence of P-gp on the brain concentrations of cetirizine and hydroxyzine. They concluded that P-gp influences the brain concentration of cetirizine, as a P-gp substrate, but not hydroxyzine. They investigated and compared the physicochemical properties of cetirizine and hydroxyzine and suggested that the difference in the substrate activity is related to the log D_{oct} (pH = 7.4) values. The log D_{oct}, which is a measure of lipophilicity at pH = 7.4, for cetirizine was 1.04 compared with a value of 2.87 for hydroxyzine.[20] The carboxylic group of cetirizine can interact with the basic nitrogen via folded conformers due to the molecular structure of cetirizine. This can cause relatively high lipophilicity at physiological pH. Oral bioavailability of cetirizine is more than 70% and shows high intestinal absorption in human.[7,24]

P-gp activity undoubtedly plays an important role in limiting intestinal permeability of BCS class II–IV P-gp substrates (not for BCS class I compounds). The high P-gp expression levels in the intestine make the moderately absorbed P-gp substrates more susceptible to P-gp-mediated efflux. Inhibition of P-gp by inhibitors, like cetirizine, can move compounds of BCS class III and IV (for example, digoxin) to class I and II, respectively, by significantly increasing the permeability.[25] This may result in unexpected toxic effects of administrated drug(s). The unwanted drug-drug interactions may be reduced by considering the P-gp inhibitory effect or substrate activity of the concomitantly used drugs.

Conclusion

In conclusion, our results demonstrated that cetirizine treatment could down-regulate the function and expression of P-glycoprotein *in vitro* and *in situ* and its inhibition activity is dose-dependent. The P-gp inhibitory effect of cetirizine must be considered for predicting potential drug–drug interactions when the drug is administered concurrently with P-gp substrate drugs. However further investigations with larger sample sizes are required to approve the obtained results and also find out the exact P-gp inhibitory mechanisms of cetirizine.

Acknowledgments

We would like to thank the members of Drug Applied Research Center and Immunology Research Center of Tabriz University of Medical Sciences. This work was financially supported by Drug Applied Research Center of Tabriz University of Medical Sciences (Grant No. 91-123) and is a part of the PhD thesis of Dr. Mehran Mesgari Abbasi.

Ethical Issues

Not applicable.

Conflict of Interest

The authors report no conflicts of interest.

References

1. Kumar YS, Adukondalu D, Sathish D, Vishnu YV, Ramesh G, Latha AB, *et al.* P-glycoprotein- and cytochrome p-450-mediated herbal drug interactions. *Drug Metabol Drug Interact* 2010;25(1-4):3-16. doi: 10.1515/DMDI.2010.006
2. Kobori T, Harada S, Nakamoto K, Tokuyama S. Functional alterations of intestinal p-glycoprotein under diabetic conditions. *Biol Pharm Bull* 2013;36(9):1381-90. doi: 10.1248/bpb.b13-00369
3. Li Y, Huang L, Zeng X, Zhong G, Ying M, Huang M, *et al.* Down-regulation of P-gp expression and function after Mulberroside A treatment: potential role of protein kinase C and NF-kappa B. *Chem Biol Interact* 2014;213:44-50. doi: 10.1016/j.cbi.2014.02.004
4. Lin JH. Transporter-mediated drug interactions: Clinical implications and *in vitro* assessment. *Expert Opin Drug Metab Toxicol* 2007;3(1):81-92. doi: 10.1517/17425255.3.1.81
5. Horn JR, Hansten PD. Drug interactions with digoxin: The role of P-glycoprotein. *Pharm Times* 2004;2004:45-6.
6. Wessler JD, Grip LT, Mendell J, Giugliano RP. The P-glycoprotein transport system and cardiovascular drugs. *J Am Coll Cardiol* 2013;61(25):2495-502. doi: 10.1016/j.jacc.2013.02.058
7. Chen C. Physicochemical, pharmacological and pharmacokinetic properties of the zwitterionic antihistamines cetirizine and levocetirizine. *Curr Med Chem* 2008;15(21):2173-91. doi: 10.2174/092986708785747625
8. Bhatia NM, Ganbavale SK, Bhatia MS, More HN, Kokil SU. Rp-HPLC and spectrophotometric estimation of ambroxol hydrochloride and cetirizine hydrochloride in combined dosage form. *Indian J Pharm Sci* 2008;70(5):603-8. doi: 10.4103/0250-474X.45398
9. Souri E, Hatami A, Shabani Ravari N, Alvandifar F, Barazandeh Tehrani M. Validating a stability indicating HPLC method for kinetic study of cetirizine degradation in acidic and oxidative conditions. *Iran J Pham Res* 2013;12(2):287-94.
10. Yu H, Cornett C, Larsen J, Hansen SH. Reaction between drug substances and pharmaceutical excipients: Formation of esters between cetirizine and polyols. *J Pharm Biomed Anal* 2010;53(3):745-50. doi: 10.1016/j.jpba.2010.05.001
11. Zrieki A, Farinotti R, Buyse M. Cyclooxygenase-2 inhibitors prevent trinitrobenzene sulfonic acid-induced P-glycoprotein up-regulation *in vitro* and *in vivo*. *Eur J Pharmacol* 2010;636(1-3):189-97. doi: 10.1016/j.ejphar.2010.03.039
12. Zastre J, Jackson J, Bajwa M, Liggins R, Iqbal F, Burt H. Enhanced cellular accumulation of a P-glycoprotein substrate, rhodamine-123, by Caco-2 cells using low molecular weight methoxypolyethylene glycol-block-polycaprolactone diblock copolymers. *Eur J Pharm Biopharm* 2002;54(3):299-309. doi: 10.1016/S0939-6411(02)00119-4
13. Mohammadzadeh R, Baradaran B, Valizadeh H, Yousefi B, Zakeri-Milani P. Reduced ABCB1 expression and activity in the presence of acrylic copolymers. *Adv Pharm Bull* 2014;4(3):219-24. doi: 10.5681/apb.2014.032
14. Wang XD, Meng MX, Gao LB, Liu T, Xu Q, Zeng S. Permeation of astilbin and taxifolin in Caco-2 cell and their effects on the P-gp. *Int J Pharm* 2009;378(1-2):1-8. doi: 10.1016/j.ijpharm.2009.05.022
15. Patel JR, Barve KH. Intestinal permeability of lamivudine using single pass intestinal perfusion. *Indian J Pharm Sci* 2012;74(5):478-81. doi: 10.4103/0250-474X.108441
16. Zakeri-Milani P, Valizadeh H, Tajerzadeh H, Azarmi Y, Islambolchilar Z, Barzegar S, *et al.* Predicting human intestinal permeability using single-pass intestinal perfusion in rat. *J Pharm Pharm Sci* 2007;10(3):368-79.
17. Valizadeh H, Mehtari M, Zakeri-Milani P. Evidence for enhanced intestinal absorption of digoxin by P-glycoprotein inhibitors. *Trop J Pharm Res* 2012;11(6):939-45. doi: 10.4314/tjpr.v11i6.10
18. Prasad N, Bhasker S. Characterization of intestinal transport of vincristine in rats applying *in situ* single pass intestinal perfusion. *Pharmacologia* 2012;3(11):617-21. doi: 10.5567/pharmacologia.2012.617.621
19. Lopez D, Martinez-Luis S. Marine natural products with P-glycoprotein inhibitor properties. *Mar Drugs* 2014;12(1):525-46. doi: 10.3390/md12010525
20. Polli JW, Baughman TM, Humphreys JE, Jordan KH, Mote AL, Salisbury JA, *et al.* P-glycoprotein influences the brain concentrations of cetirizine (zyrtec), a second-generation non-sedating antihistamine. *J Pharm Sci* 2003;92(10):2082-9. doi: 10.1002/jps.10453
21. Chen C, Hanson E, Watson JW, Lee JS. P-glycoprotein limits the brain penetration of nonsedating but not sedating H1-antagonists. *Drug Metab Dispos* 2003;31(3):312-8. doi: 10.1124/dmd.31.3.312
22. Crowe A, Wright C. The impact of P-glycoprotein mediated efflux on absorption of 11 sedating and less-sedating antihistamines using Caco-2

monolayers. *Xenobiotica* 2012;42(6):538-49. doi: 10.3109/00498254.2011.643256

23. Ekins S, Kim RB, Leake BF, Dantzig AH, Schuetz EG, Lan LB, *et al.* Application of three-dimensional quantitative structure-activity relationships of P-glycoprotein inhibitors and substrates. *Mol Pharmacol* 2002;61(5):974-81. doi: 10.1124/mol.61.5.974
24. Zhang L, Cheng L, Hong J. The clinical use of cetirizine in the treatment of allergic rhinitis. *Pharmacol* 2013;92(1-2):14-25. doi: 10.1159/000351843
25. Varma MV, Panchagnula R. Prediction of *in vivo* intestinal absorption enhancement on P-glycoprotein inhibition, from rat *in situ* permeability. *J Pharm Sci* 2005;94(8):1694-704. doi: 10.1002/jps.20309

4

In vitro Cytotoxicity Effects of ^{197}Au/PAMAMG4 and ^{198}Au/PAMAMG4 Nanocomposites Against MCF7 and 4T1 Breast Cancer Cell Lines

Simin Janitabar-Darzi[1]*, Reza Rezaei[2], Kamal Yavari[1]

[1] *Radiopharmaceutical Research and Development Laboratory, Nuclear Science and Technology Research Institute, Tehran, Iran.*
[2] *Department of biochemistry, Faculty of Science, Zanjan University, Zanjan, Iran.*

Keywords:
- ^{198}Au/PAMAMG4
- 4T1
- MCF7
- C2C12
- Nanocompsite
- In vitro

Abstract

Purpose: Study on gold based therapeutic agents for cancer cells deracination has become under scrutiny in recent years owing to effective treatments are not available for rapidly progressive cancers. The aim of present study was to examine efficiency of radioactive ^{198}Au/PAMAMG4 and non-radioactive ^{197}Au/PAMAMG4 nancomposites against 4T1 and MCF7 breast cancer cell lines.

Methods: The PAMAMG4 dendrimer was treated with the gold anions and then, the mixture was chemically reduced by $NaBH_4$. Prepared ^{197}Au/PAMAMG4 was bombarded by thermal neutrons in the Tehran Research Reactor to ^{198}Au/PAMAMG4 be produced. Prepared nanocomposites were characterized by means of FT-IR, 1H NMR, Zeta-potential measurements, TEM and EDX analyses. The radionuclidic purity of the ^{198}Au/PAMAMG4 solution was determined using purity germanium (HPGe) spectroscopy and its stability in the presence of human serum was studied. In vitro studies were carried out to compare toxicity of PAMAMG4, ^{197}Au/PAMAMG4 and ^{198}Au/PAMAMG4 towards 4T1 and MCF7 cancerous cells and C2C12 normal cell lines.

Results: Characterization results exhibited that invitro agents, ^{197}Au/PAMAMG4 and ^{198}Au/PAMAMG4, were synthesized successfully. Cells viability after 24 h, 48 h, and 72 h incubation, using MTT assay showed that the toxicity of ^{198}Au/PAMAMG4 is significantly superior in comparison with ^{197}Au/PAMAMG4 and PAMAMG4. Furthermore, the toxicity of ^{198}Au/PAMAMG4 was higher on cancerous cells especially in higher level of concentrations after 72 hours ($P<0.05$).

Conclusion: In the current study, the preparation of ^{197}Au/PAMAMG4 and ^{198}Au/PAMAMG4 is described and the cytotoxic properties of them against the MCF7, 4T1 cancerous cells and C2C12 normal cells were evaluated using MTT assay.

Introduction

Gold nanoparticles (NPs) have recently received great technological and scientific interest due to their extensive applications in biology, catalysis, and nanotechnology.[1] Some polymer-based methods in order to preparation of AuNPs are reported up to now.[2-6] However, the dendrimer templating procedure for producing gold NPs is known as a powerful method to form organic-inorganic nanocomposites hybrid materials for medical and biological applications.[7,8] The dendrimers could stabilize the colloidal Au particles in aqueous solution at concentrations where unmodified colloids agglomerate. Additionally, the size of the colloids is a function of dendrimer generation.[8] As a new class of highly branched, monodispersed, and synthetic macromolecules, poly amidoamine (PAMAM) dendrimers have attracted a great deal of interest in the development of various biological applications.[9-14] The unique structural characteristics of PAMAM dendrimers allow one to design various dendrimer-metal nanocomposite.[14] Recently, applicability of PAMAM to deliver anticancer drugs and other bioactives is well-reported in the literatures, especially dendrimers belonging to the fourth (G4) and fifth (G5) generation of PAMAM class.[7-10,15-17] Poly amidoamine dendrimers contain a variety of functional groups capable of complexing metal cations, as well as interior voids in their structure capable of hosting small metal components and protecting them from further aggregation.[18]

The development of AuNP-based strategies for the eradication of cancer cells is important, because effective therapies are frequently not available for rapidly progressing cancers.[19] So far, many of the studies on AuNPs suggest that cancer cells are especially vulnerable to these particles. Thus, AuNP-based treatment can

***Corresponding author:** Simin Janitabar-Darzi, Email: sjanitabar@aeoi.org.ir destroy cancer cells, with minimal injury to healthy cells.[20]

Breast cancer, which is most resulted in metastasis, is the leading cause of cancer death in women with more than a million newly diagnosed cases annually worldwide.[21] 4T1 breast carcinoma is a highly malignant and poorly immunogenic marine tumor model that resembles advanced breast cancer in humans, and is refractory to most immune stimulation-based treatments.[19,22]

MCF7 is a breast cancer cell line isolated in 1970 from a 69-year-old Caucasian woman. MCF7 is the acronym of Michigan Cancer Foundation-7, referring to the institute in Detroit where the cell line was established in 1973 by Herbert Soule and co-workers.[23,24] Prior to MCF7, it was not possible for cancer researchers to obtain a mammary cell line that was capable of living longer than a few months.

Cytotoxicity assay is an appropriate method for screening new drugs within a short time in order to determine cell killing property of these chemical compounds regardless the mechanism of cell death. Usually in oncology research and clinical practices, in vitro testing is preferred prior to in vivo studies. MTT assay has been described as rapid, simple and reproducible method, widely used in the screening of anticancer drugs and to measure the cytotoxic properties.[25]

In the current study, the preparation of ^{197}Au/PAMAMG4 and ^{198}Au/PAMAMG4 is described and the cytotoxic properties of them against the MCF7, 4T1 cancerous cells and C2C12 normal cells were evaluated using MTT assay.

Materials and Methods

Materials

Materials used in this study included methanolic solution of PAMAMG4 dendrimer and MMT (3- (4,5-dimethylthiazolyl-2)-2,5-diphenyltetrazolium bromide) obtained from (Sigma-Aldrich, USA). Hydrogen tetracholoroaurate ($HAuCl_4$. $3H_2O$), sodium borohydride ($NaBH_4$), sodium hydroxide, DMSO (dimethyl sulfoxide) and Whatman paper were purchased from (Merck. Germany). RPMI medium 1640, DMEM medium, fetal bovine serum (FBS), gentamicin, streptomycin, penicillin G, trypsin, EDTA were obtained from (Gibco, USA). MCF7 human breast cancer cells, 4T1 mice breast adenocarcinoma cells, and C2C12 mice muscle normal cell were obtained from National Cell Bank of (Iran, Pasteur Institute, Tehran, Iran).

Synthesis and characterization of ^{197}Au/PAMAMG4 and ^{198}Au/PAMAMG4 nanohybrids

^{197}Au/PAMAMG4 was prepared by two consecutive stages: First, the complex between dendrimer and the gold anions was formed, then the complexed ions were chemically reduced by a reducing agent ($NaBH_4$).[26-28] Firstly 0.5μmol dendrimer was added to 5 mL of water with vigorously stirring. Then 5 mL of an aqueous solution of 0.5 μmol $HAuCl_4$ was added to the above solution. After stirring for further 45 min, procedure followed by addition of a basic aqueous solution of sodium borohydride (25 mM $NaBH_4$ in 0.3 M NaOH). The prepared light yellow solution turned to brown, indicating the formation of colloidal gold. The stirring process was continued for 1 h to complete the reaction. The reaction mixture was then dialyzed against PBS (3 times, 4L) and water (6 times, 4 L) for 1 day to remove the excess reactants. At this stage ^{197}Au/PAMAMG4 was prepared.

^{197}Au captures neutrons very efficiently because of its large cross section. ^{198}Au ($t_{1/2}$=2.69 days) decays dominantly by beta-radiation (99%, 0.96 MeV) and with a small gamma component (0.98%, 1.1 MeV).[29] Irradiation was performed at Tehran Research Reactor (TRR). Sample was irradiated in quartz vials for 2 hours, in core-face location, with a thermal neutron flux of $1 \times 10^{11} ncm^{-2}s^{-1}$. The radionuclidic purity of the prepared ^{198}Au/PAMAMG4 solution was determined for the presence of other radionuclides using purity germanium (HPGe) spectroscopy, through the detection of various interfering gamma emitting radionuclides. Final ^{198}Au/PAMAMG4 solution (88 μCi, 50 μL) was incubated in the presence of freshly prepared human serum (300 μL) (Purchased from Iranian Blood Transfusion Organization, Tehran, Iran) at 37°C for 7 days. The stability study of ^{198}Au/PAMAMG4 in final formulation was performing ITLC analysis using Whatman chromatography paper eluted with methanol: water (7:3) mixture.

Spectroscopic analyses of the samples were performed using a Fourier transform infrared (FT-IR) spectrometer (Perkin–Elmer 843). Zeta-potential measurements were performed using (Malvern, U.K) with a red diode laser at 633 nm. Proton NMR spectra were conducted on a nuclear magnetic resonance spectrometer (Bruker Avance III 400MHz, Germany) using commercially available D_2O as a solvent and Tetramethylsilane (TMS) as an internal standard. The morphology of prepared nanocomposites was studied by transmission electron microscopy (TEM, Philips-EM208S) and the content of Au in ^{198}Au/PAMAMG4 was determined by means of energy dispersive X-ray spectrometer (EDX, Oxford INCA, UK). EDX analysis was performed using lyophilized nanocopmosite sample without gold coating.

Cell culture and in vitro study

The MCF7 human breast cancer cells, 4T1 mice breast adenocarcinoma cells and C2C12 mice muscle normal cells were regularly cultured in RPMI 1640 medium and DMEM medium, respectively, supplemented with 10% FBS (Fetal bovine serum) and 1% penicillin-streptomycin at 37°C and 5% CO_2. The cytotoxicity of the PAMAMG4, ^{197}Au/PAMAMG4 and ^{198}Au/PAMAMG4 were investigated by an MTT cell viability assay. MCF7, 4T1 and C2C12 cells were seeded onto a 96-well plate at a density of 4×10^3 cells per well and cultivated in 100 μL of their mentioned medium under 37°C and 5% CO_2 for 24 h .[30] After that, the mediums were replaced with fresh RPMI and DMEM containing PAMAMG4, ^{197}Au/PAMAMG4 or ^{198}Au/PAMAMG4 with different concentrations ranging from 50 nM to 400 nM and the cells were incubated under 37 °C and 5% CO_2. The MTT assay was applied to study the cell viability after 24 h, 48 h and 72 h of drugs treatment. MTT (5.0 mg mL^{-1}, 20 μL) was added into each sample and the cells were incubated at 37 °C and 5% CO_2 for 4 h. Thereafter, the medium was removed and 150μL dimethylsulfoxide (DMSO) was added to dissolve the formazan crystals. The assays were performed according to the manufacturer's instructions using a Biochrom Scientific Anthos 2020 ELISA reader (Biochrom Scientific, U.K) at 570 nm.[31,32]

All the experiments were repeated at least three times. Results are presented as the mean ±SD. Statistical comparisons were carried out using a three and four way analysis of variance ANOVA with post hoc testing for comparison of Sidak tests. Pair-wise comparisons between treatments were made using independent sample t-test (IBM SPSS Statistic 23, Microsoft Excel). A p-Value of < 0.05 was considered statistically significant.

The changes of 4T1 cell morphology after treatment with the ^{197}Au/PAMAMG4 and ^{198}Au/PAMAMG4 nanocomposites was studied by microscopic visualization. The morphology of the cells was observed using an invert optical microscope (Nikon, Tokyo, Japan) under a magnification of 200×.

Results and Discussion

Characterization of ^{197}Au/PAMAMG4 and ^{198}Au/PAMAMG4 nanocomposite

Figure 1 shows a transmission infrared spectrum of ^{197}Au/PAMAMG4 and ^{198}Au/PAMAMG4 nanocomposites. The absorption peak at 3353cm^{-1} corresponded to N–H deformation vibration of tertiary amide, while the peak centered at 3287cm^{-1} was assigned to the N–H stretching vibration arising from its association. The next two peaks at 2944cm^{-1} and 2844cm^{-1} indicated unsymmetrical and symmetrical stretching vibration of methylene.[33] The amide band present at 1640cm^{-1} is characteristic of the dendrimer branches.[8] Also, N-H bending exhibits broad band at about 1640cm^{-1} for primary amine. The stretching vibration of C-N bonds is appeared at 1368cm^{-1}. The two peaks at 1132cm^{-1} and 1202cm^{-1} were related to the stretching vibrations of tertiary amine and primary amine, respectively. N-H out of plane bending occurs at 800$cm^{-1}$and the peak at 550cm^{-1} showed the bending vibration of tertiary amine.[34] Comparison of FTIR curve of non-active ^{197}Au/PAMAMG4 compound with radioactive ^{198}Au/PAMAMG4 exhibited that the N-H band present at 1640cm^{-1} is stronger at non-active complex. Furthermore, the intensity of the peak assigned at 1368cm^{-1} is increased in the radioactive complex. It could be due to the cleavage of some N-H bands of primary amines and production of some new tertiary amines as a result of polymerization of nanocomposite particles under described neutron bombarding condition. Partial cross-linking of the organic component (radiation polymerization) was also reported by Khan and co-workers.[30] Moreover, careful comparison of two curves reveals that neutron bombarding of ^{197}Au/PAMAMG4 induced a small shift in the stretching vibration of C-N bond of prepared ^{198}Au/PAMAMG4 to higher energy.

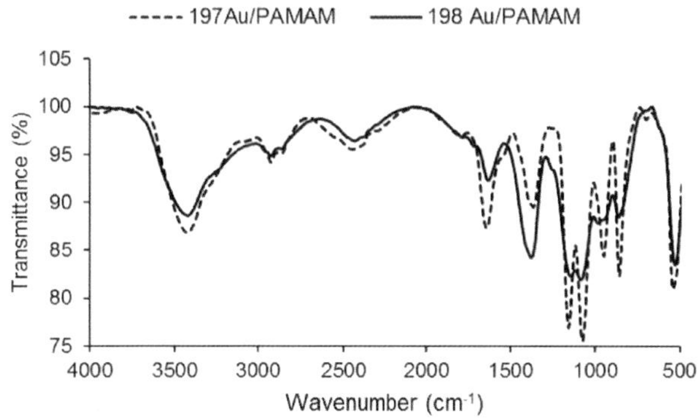

Figure 1. FT-IR spectrum of ^{197}Au/PAMAMG4 (dash curve) and ^{198}Au/PAMAMG4 (solid curve) nanocomposites.

^{1}H Nuclear Magnetic Resonance spectra of ^{197}Au/PAMAMG4 and ^{198}Au/PAMAMG4 nanocomposites are shown in Figure 2. Broadened peaks in the ^{1}H NMR spectrum of ^{198}Au/PAMAMG4 nanocomposite indicate partially of polimerization crosslinked PAMAMG4 during the neutron irradiation. The exact mechanism of polimerization is not known up to now. According to Tang and co-workers reports, the radical mechanisms and the local heat effects causing beta-alanine crosslinking, and in retro-Michael reaction may be responsible to take place a rearrangement of the molecular structure and finally polymerization.[35]

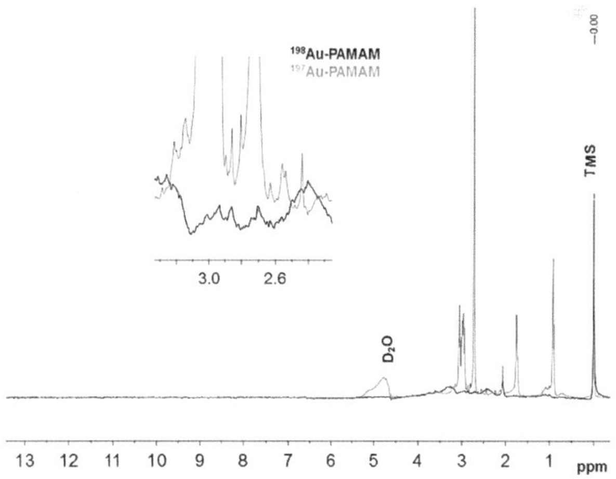

Figure 2. ^{1}H NMR spectra of ^{197}Au/PAMAMG4 and ^{198}Au/PAMAMG4 nanocomposites.

Zeta-potential measurements for ^{197}Au/PAMAMG4 and ^{198}Au/PAMAMG4 were also carried out to investigate the surface potential changes after the neutron irradiation. As shown in Figure 3, the negative potential of the ^{197}Au/PAMAMG4 (-23.9 mV) significantly changed after the neutron bombarding and producing of

^{198}Au/PAMAMG4 (-37.6 mV). Decreasing of surface positive charge could be related to involvement of primary amine terminal groups in the ensuing polymerization reactions during neutron bombardment.[29,36]

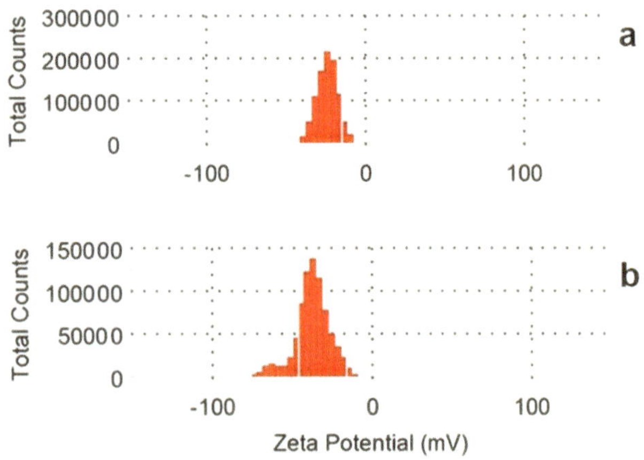

Figure 3. Zeta potential (ZP) of ^{197}Au/PAMAMG4 and ^{198}Au/PAMAMG4

Transmission electron microscopy analyses of nanoparticles were performed to understand the morphology and size of particles. TEM images (Figures 4a and b) show spherical shape for ^{197}Au/PAMAMG4 and ^{198}Au/PAMAMG4 compounds. Comparision of two pictures reveals that ^{198}Au/PAMAMG4 has larger particle size compared to ^{197}Au/PAMAMG4. This could be related to partial polymerization of PAMAMG4 due to neutron bombardment.[29]

The radionuclidic purity of the ^{198}Au/PAMAMG4 nanocomposie was checked by gamma-ray emission spectroscopy. Two main radioisotopes of gold have charming nuclear properties that make them desirable for imaging and therapy purposes. ^{198}Au has a moderate-energy beta maximum (0.96 keV) making it a good candidate for therapy, and a gamma emission (411 keV) that allows for in vivo tracking and dosimetry calculation. These properties led to the medical use of ^{198}Au as a brachytherapy agent for breast cancer. A second radioisotope, ^{199}Au, has a low-energy beta maximum and emits a 158keV gamma that is easily detected by SPECT camera.[37] Figure 5 shows the HPGe spectrum of the prepared compound. The prepared radioactive sample exhibited a characteristic gamma peak at 411KeV related to ^{198}Au ($t_{1/2}$ = 2.69 days), and there is no significant peak related to the ^{199}Au isotope in the HPGe spectrum.

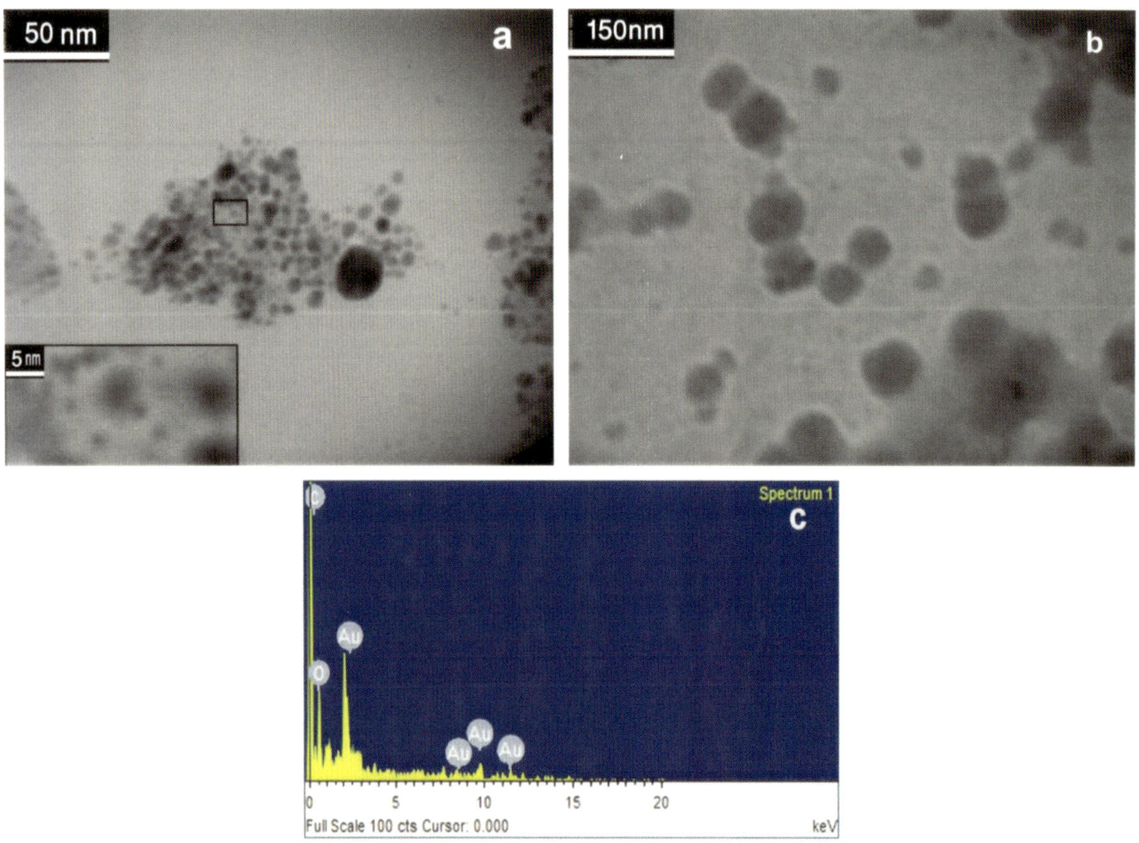

Figure 4. TEM images of ^{197}Au/PAMAMG4 (a) and ^{198}Au/PAMAMG4 nanocomposites(b), and EDX analysis of ^{198}Au/PAMAMG4 (C).

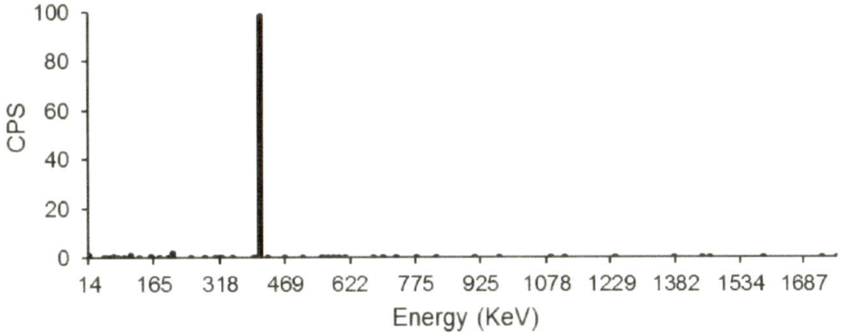

Figure 5. HPGe spectrum for 198Au/PAMAMG4 nanocomposite.

Figure 6 exhibits ITLC chromatogram of ^{198}Au/PAMAMG4 at pH=7.5. The ^{198}Au/PAMAMG4 complex in presence of human serum at 37 °C was found to be stable in final pharmaceutical sample and its radiochemical purity was calculated to be above 93.5% a week after the preparation by using Whatman 3 MM paper eluted with methanol: water (7:3) mixture.

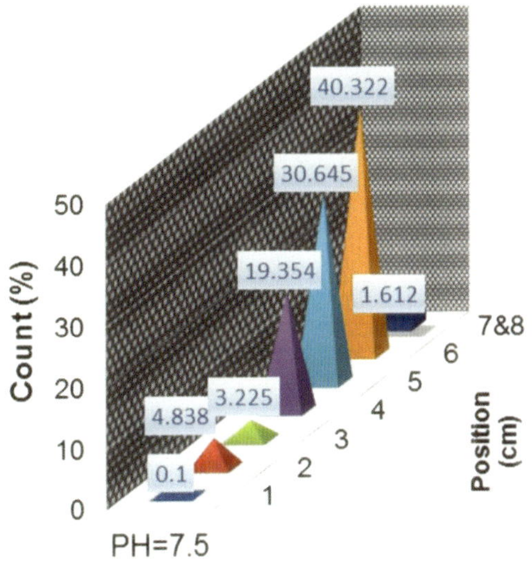

Figure 6. ITLC chromatogram of ^{198}Au/PAMAMG4 at pH=7.5 with methanol: water (7:3) mixture and using Whatman 3 MM.

Cytotoxicity of ^{197}Au/PAMAMG4 and ^{198}Au/PAMAMG4 nanocomposites

The cytotoxicity of the radioactive ^{198}Au/PAMAMG4 and non- radioactive ^{197}Au/PAMAMG4 against MCF7, 4T1 and C2C12 cells were assessed using the MTT assay. The MTT assay is based on the ability of a mitochondrial dehydrogenation enzyme in viable cells to cleave the tetrazolium rings of the pale yellow MTT and form formazan crystals with a purple color.[38] Therefore; the number of surviving cells is directly proportionate to the level of the formed formazan. Figures 7a, b and c reveal the cell viability of the cultured MCF7, 4T1 and C2C12 cells treated by 50, 100, 200 and 400 nM of PAMAMG4, ^{197}Au/PAMAMG4 and ^{198}Au/PAMAMG4 solutions. Control groups use only medium.

Assessing the effect of drugs including PAMAMG4, ^{197}Au/PAMAMG4 and ^{198}Au/PAMAMG4 on viability of three cell lines of MCF7, 4T1 and C2C12 in various concentrations after 24h incubation, based on the results of three way ANOVA showed a three way interactions of cell lines* drugs *concentrations as ($P<0.001$).

The result of all two ways interactions are as follow: cell lines* drugs ($P<0.001$), cell lines*concentrations ($P<0.001$), and drugs *concentrations ($P<0.001$), and for all main effects of cell lines, drugs and concentrations ($P<0.001$) is obtained. This means that the effect of PAMAMG4, ^{197}Au/PAMAMG4 and ^{198}Au/PAMAMG4 on viability of each of the cell lines varies as a function of the concentration of drugs.

Additionally considering the significance of the three ways interaction, the results of Sidak simultaneous post hoc tests showed the lowest amount of viability in MCF7 and 4T1*^{198}Au/PAMAMG4*concentration 400 (C400). In the other words, after 24 hours, treatment of MCF7 and 4T1 cell line with ^{198}Au/PAMAMG4 leads to lowest amount of viability in the highest level of concentration (Figure 7a).

To investigate how drugs affect on the viability of MCF7, 4T1 and C212 cell lines in various concentrations after 48 hours incubation, the results of three way ANOVA showed significant three way interactions of cell lines* drugs*concentrations with ($P < 0.001$).

For all two ways interactions cell lines* drugs, cell lines*concentrations and drugs*concentrations P is lower than 0.001. Also for all main effects of cell lines, drugs and concentrations P are lower than 0.001.

Furthermore, taking into account the significance of the three ways interaction, the results of Sidak post hoc tests showed the significant lower values of viability for MCF7 and 4T1*^{198}Au/PAMAMG4 *(C400,C200 and C100) and C2C12*^{198}Au/PAMAMG4*(C50) levels. The other levels of three factors were significantly in higher amounts of viability. Hence, after 48 hours, ^{198}Au/PAMAMG4 of MCF7 and 4T1 cell lines lead in lower amount of viability in the higher level of concentration (Figure 7b).

After 72 hours incubation, the results of three way ANOVA to study of the effect of drugs materials on viability of three cell lines of MCF7, 4T1 and C2C12 in various concentrations of drugs showed significant three ways interactions of cell lines* drugs *concentrations ($P < 0.001$), all two ways interactions of cell lines* drugs (P < 0.001), cell lines*concentrations (P < 0.001), and drugs *concentrations (P < 0.001) as well as for all main effects of cell lines, drugs and concentrations (P < 0.001). In the other words, the effects of drugs including PAMAMG4, ^{197}Au/PAMAMG4 and ^{198}Au/PAMAMG4 materials on the cell viability vary as a function of the cell lines for each concentration. Furthermore, pertaining to the significance of three ways interaction, based on the results of Sidak post hoc tests, lower values of viability were observed in MCF7 and 4T1*^{198}Au/PAMAMG4 *(C400 to 50 nM) levels, and other levels of the three factors had significantly higher amount of viability. As shown in Figure 7c, after 72 hours, the effect of ^{198}Au/PAMAMG4 towards 4T1 cell line results in the lowest amount of viability in higher level of concentration. To compare the changes in the viability during three time points of 24, 48 and 72 hours along with the effect of cell lines, drugs and concentrations, the findings of four way analysis of variance revealed the significant four ways interaction effect of times*cell lines* drugs*concentrations ($F(24,126)=7.42$, $P < 0.001$). It means that the changes of cell viability during three time points of 24, 48 and 72 hours varies for cell lines, each drug (PAMAMG4, ^{197}Au/PAMAMG4, and ^{198}Au/PAMAMG4) and within the levels of concentrations (C50 to C400). As can be seen the effect of cell lines, drugs (PAMAMG4, ^{197}Au/PAMAMG4 and ^{198}Au/PAMAMG4) and concentrations leads in significantly the lowest amount of viability after 72 hours based on the results obtained from the Sidak post hoc tests ($P < 0.05$).

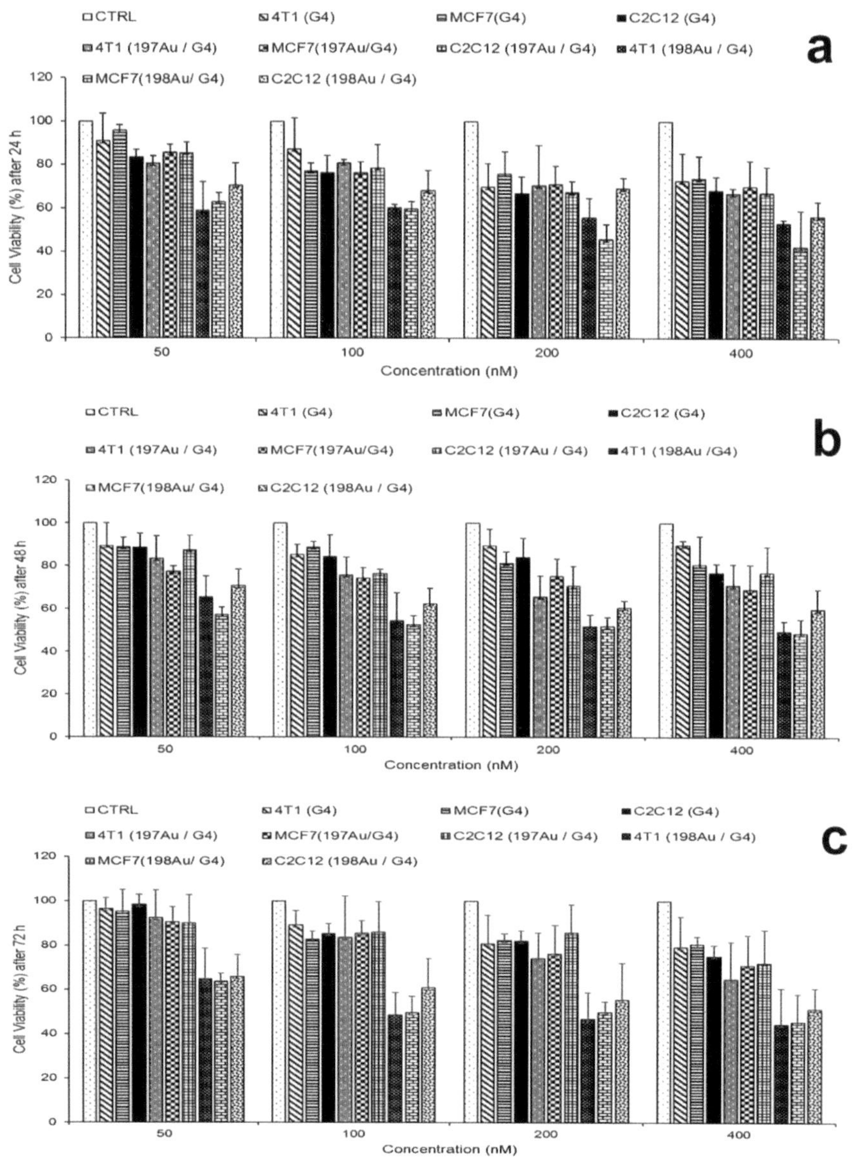

Figure 7. MTT-assay of the viability of MCF7, 4T1and C2C12 cells after treatment with different concentrations of PAMAMG4, ^{197}Au/PAMAMG4 and radioactive ^{198}Au/PAMAMG4 for 24, 48 and 72 h.

The cytotoxicity effects of the compounds towards the 4T1 cell line were further confirmed by microscopic visualization of changes of the cell morphology after treatment with the ^{197}Au/PAMAMG4 and ^{198}Au/PAMAMG4. It is reported that the treatment of cells with some test compounds induced morphological alterations such as retraction of cytoplasmatic expansions; detachment, formation of the round shaped cells as well as membrane blebs, all suggestive the induction of programmed cell death.[39]

Figure 8a shows the photomicrographs of the 4T1 cells, and Figures 8b and 8c reveal the photomicrographs of the 4T1 cells treated with ^{197}Au/PAMAMG4 and ^{198}Au/PAMAMG4, after 24 h, respectively. As shown in Figure 8b, minor morphological alterations are shown in the 4T1 cells treated with ^{197}Au/PAMAMG4 nanocomposite with concentration (400 nM) compared with the untreated cells. According to Figure 8b, the rounded and detached cells can be visualized in the cells treated with ^{197}Au/PAMAMG4 to some extent. In contrast, Figure 8c shows that a significant portion of the cells became rounded and non-adherent as a result of ^{198}Au/PAMAMG4 treatment. This phenomenon could be related to apoptosis of 4T1 cells due to ^{198}Au/PAMAMG4 (16.64 μCi) treatments. These results are consistent with the MTT assay data.

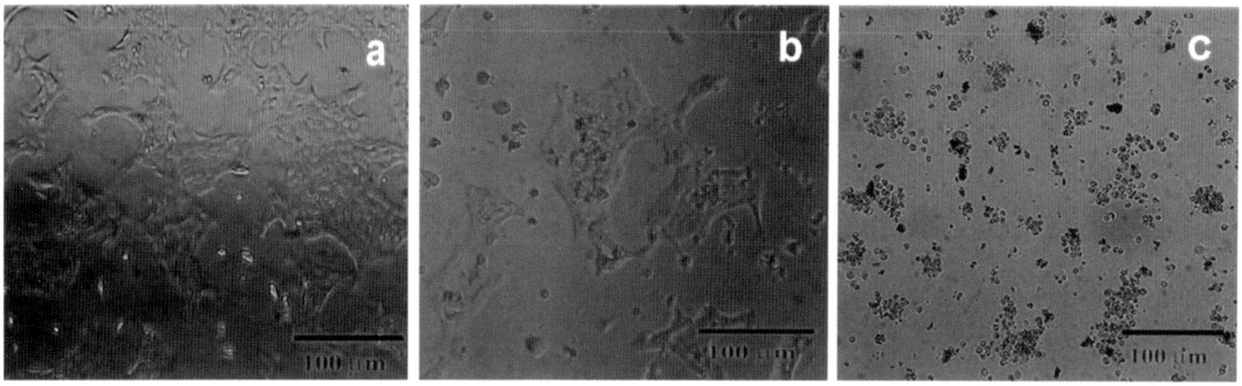

Figure 8. photomicrographs of the 4T1 cells (inverted microscopy, ×200) without treatment (a), and the 4T1 cells treated with ^{197}Au/PAMAMG4 (b) and ^{198}Au/PAMAMG4 (c).

Conclusion

In this study, radioactive ^{198}Au/PAMAMG4 nanocomposite was prepared successfully by neutron bombardment of synthesized non-radioactive ^{197}Au/PAMAMG4. ^{1}H NMR, FT-IR and TEM analyses reveals partially cross-linked polymerization of PAMAMG4 in the repared neutron bombarded sample (^{198}Au/PAMAMG4). In vitro anti-cancer assessments of radioactive ^{198}Au/PAMAMG4 mater and non-radioactive ^{197}Au/PAMAMG4 with regard to the MCF7, 4T1 and C2C12 cell lines were investigated. Analysis of variance followed by Sidak post-hoc test, shows that the toxicity of ^{198}Au/PAMAMG4 is significantly deferent from ^{197}Au/PAMAMG4 and PAMAMG4 on all of the three cell lines. The toxicity of ^{198}Au/PAMAMG4 is more on cancerous cells compared to normal cells especially in higher level of concentrations after 24, 48 and 72 hours ($P<0.05$). In conclusion, ^{198}Au/PAMAMG4 inhibited growth of MCF7 and 4T1 breast cancer cells in a dose- and time-dependent manner *in vitro*. Moreover, the effect of cell lines, drug types and concentrations of drugs leads to the lowest amount of viability after 72 h compared with 24 h and 48 h.

Acknowledgments

Support by Nuclear Science and Technology Research Institute of Atomic Energy Organization of Iran and Iran National Science Foundation (INSF) is greatly appreciated.

Ethical Issues

Not applicable.

Conflict of Interest

The authors declare no conflict of interests.

References

1. Shi X, Wang S, Sun H, Baker JR. Improved biocompatibility of surface functionalized dendrimer-entrapped gold nanoparticles. *Soft Matter* 2006;3(1):71-4. doi: 10.1039/B612972B
2. Mandal T, Dasgupta C, Maiti PK. Engineering gold nanoparticle interaction by PAMAM dendrimer. *J Phys Chem* C 2013;117(26):13627-36. doi: 10.1021/jp401218t
3. Zheng J, Petty JT, Dickson RM. High quantum yield blue emission from water-soluble Au8 nanodots. *J Am Chem Soc* 2003;125(26):7780-1. doi: 10.1021/ja035473v
4. Zheng L, Zhu J, Shen M, Chen X, Baker JR, Wang SH, et al. Targeted cancer cell inhibition using multifunctional dendrimer-entrapped gold nanoparticles. *Med Chem Commun* 2013;4(6):1001-5. doi: 10.1039/C3MD00050H
5. Li D, He Q, ui Y, Li J. Fabrication of pH-responsive nanocomposites of gold nanoparticles/poly (4-vinylpyridine). *Chem Mater* 2007;19(3):412-7. doi: 10.1021/cm062290+
6. Li D, He Q, Li J. Smart Core/Shell Nanocomposites: Intelligent Polymers Modified Gold Nanoparticles.

Adv Colloid Interface Sci 2009;149(1-2):28-38. doi: 10.1016/j.cis.2008.12.007
7. Zhou B, Zheng L, Peng C, Li D, Li J, Wen S, et al. Synthesis and characterization of PEGylated polyethylenimine-entrapped gold nanoparticles for blood pool and tumor CT imaging. ACS *Appl Mater Interfaces* 2014;6(19):17190-9. doi: 10.1021/am505006z
8. Garcia ME, Baker LA, Crooks RM. Preparation and characterization of dendrimer-gold colloid nanocomposites. *Anal Chem* 1999;71(1):256-8. doi: 10.1021/ac980588g
9. Peng C, Zheng L, Chen Q, Shen M, Guo R, Wang H, et al. PEGylated dendrimer-entrapped gold nanoparticles for in vivo blood pool and tumor imaging by computed tomography. *Biomaterials* 2012;33(4):1107-19. doi: 10.1016/j.biomaterials.2011.10.052
10. Wang Y, Guo R, Cao X, Shen M, Shi X. Encapsulation of 2-methoxyestradiol within multifunctional poly(amidoamine) dendrimers for targeted cancer therapy. *Biomaterials* 2011;32(12):3322-9. doi: 10.1016/j.biomaterials.2010.12.060
11. Zheng Y, Fu F, Zhang M, Shen M, Zhu M, Shi X. Multifunctional dendrimers modified with alpha-tocopheryl succinate for targeted cancer therapy. *Med Chem Commun* 2014;5(7):879-85. doi: 10.1039/C3MD00324H
12. Chen Q, Li K, Wen S, Liu H, Peng C, Cai H, et al. Targeted CT/MR dual mode imaging of tumors using multifunctional dendrimer-entrapped gold nanoparticles. *Biomaterials* 2013;34(21):5200-9. doi: 10.1016/j.biomaterials.2013.03.009
13. Wen S, Li K, Cai H, Chen Q, Shen M, Huang Y, et al. Multifunctional dendrimer-entrapped gold nanoparticles for dual mode CT/MR imaging applications. *Biomaterials* 2013;34(5):1570-80. doi: 10.1016/j.biomaterials.2012.11.010
14. Guo R, Wang H, Peng C, Shen M, Pan M, Cao X, et al. X-ray attenuation property of dendrimer-entrapped gold *nanoparticles. J Phys Chem C* 2009;114(1):50-6. doi: 10.1021/jp9078986
15. Grohn F, Bauer BJ, Akpalu YA, Jackson CL, Amis EJ. Dendrimer Templates for the Formation of Gold Nanoclusters. *Macromolecules* 2000;33(16):6042-50. doi: 10.1021/ma000149v
16. Zhang M, Guo R, Wang Y, Cao X, Shen M, Shi X. Multifunctional dendrimer/combretastatin A4 inclusion complexes enable in vitro targeted cancer therapy. *Int J Nanomedicine* 2011;6:2337-49. doi: 10.2147/IJN.S24705
17. Buczkowski A, Sekowski S, Grala A, Palecz D, Milowska K, Urbaniak P, et al. Interaction between PAMAM-NH(2) G4 dendrimer and 5-fluorouracil in aqueous solution. *Int J Pharm* 2011;408(1-2):266-70. doi: 10.1016/j.ijpharm.2011.02.014
18. Jain S, Hirst DG, Osullivan JM. Gold nanoparticles as novel agents for cancer therapy. *Br J Radiol* 2012;85(1010):101-13. doi: 10.1259/bjr/59448833
19. Ahmad MZ, Akhter S, Rahman Z, Akhter S, Anwar M, Mallik N, et al. Nanometric gold in cancer nanotechnology: current status and future prospect. *J Pharm Pharmacol* 2013;65(5):634-51. doi: 10.1111/jphp.12017
20. Jemal A, Thomas A, Murray T, Thun M. Cancer statistics, 2002. *CA Cancer J Clin* 2002;52(1):23-47.
21. Chen L, Huang TG, Meseck M, Mandeli J, Fallon J, Woo SL. Rejection of metastatic 4T1 breast cancer by attenuation of Treg cells in combination with immune stimulation. *Mol Ther* 2007;15(12):2194-202. doi: 10.1038/sj.mt.6300310
22. Nazarpoor Z, Khivantsev K, Kyriakidou E, Kubicki C, Ma S, Fanson PT, et al. Dendrimer-mediated synthesis of supported rhodium nanoparticles with controlled size: Effect of pH and dialysis. *J Colloid Interface Sci* 2013;398:22-32. doi: 10.1016/j.jcis.2013.02.005
23. Soule HD, Vazguez J, Long A, Albert S, Brennan M. A human cell line from a pleural effusion derived from a breast carcinoma. *J Natl Cancer Inst* 1973;51(5):1409-16.
24. Levenson AS, Jordan VC. MCF-7: The First Hormone-responsive Breast Cancer Cell Line. *Cancer Res* 1997;57(15):3071-8.
25. Alley MC, Scudiero DA, Monks A, Hursey ML, Czerwinski MJ, Fine DL, et al. Feasibility of drug screening with panels of human tumor cell lines using a microculture tetrazolium assay. *Cancer Res* 1988;48(3):589-601.
26. Divsar F, Nomani A, Chaloosi M, Haririan I. Synthesis and characterization of gold nanocomposites with modified and intact polyamidoamine dendrimers. *Microchim Acta* 2009; 165(3):421-6. doi: 10.1007/s00604-009-0156-0
27. Crooks RM, Zhao M, Sun L, Chechik V, Yeung LK. Dendrimer-encapsulated metal nanoparticles: synthesis, characterization, and applications to catalysis. *Acc Chem Res* 2001;34(3):181-90. doi: 10.1021/ar000110a
28. Pande S, Crooks RM. Analysis of poly(amidoamine) dendrimer structure by UV-Vis spectroscopy. *Langmuir* 2011;27(15):9609-13. doi: 10.1021/la201882
29. Khan MK, Minc LD, Nigavekar SS, Kariapper MST, Nair BM, Schipper M, et al. Fabrication of $\{^{198}Au^0\}$ radioactive composite nanodevices and their use for nanobrachytherapy. *Nanomed Nanotechnol Biol Med* 2008;4(1):57-69. doi: 10.1016/j.nano.2007.11.005
30. Nikzad S, Hashemi B, Hassan ZM, Mozdarani H. The Cell Survival of F10B16 Melanoma and 4T1 Breast Adenocarcinoma Irradiated to Gamma Radiation Using the MTT Assay Based on Two Different Calculation Methods. *J Biomed Phys Eng* 2013;3(2):29-36.

31. Kim WH, Chon CY, Moon YM, Kang JK, Park IS, Choi HJ. Effect of anticancer drugs and desferrioxamine in combination with radiation on Hepatoma cell lines. *Yonsei Med J* 1993;34(1):45-56. doi: 10.3349/ymj.1993.34.1.45
32. Price P, McMillan TJ. Use of the tetrazolium assay in measuring the response of human tumor cells to ionizing radiation. *Cancer Res* 1990;50(5):1392-6.
33. Wang P, Zhao XH, Wang ZY, Meng M, Li X, Ning Q. Generation 4 polyamidoamine dendrimers is a novel candidate of nano-carrier for gene delivery agents in breast cancer treatment. *Cancer Lett* 2010;298(1):34-49. doi: 10.1016/j.canlet.2010.06.001
34. Ji L, Zhang X. Ultrafine polyacrylonitrile/silica composite fibers via electrospinning. *Mater Lett* 2008;62(14):2161-4. doi: 10.1016/j.matlet.2007.11.051
35. Tang MX, Redemann CT, Szoka FC Jr. In vitro gene delivery by degraded polyamidoamine dendrimers. *Bioconjug Chem* 1996;7(6):703-14. doi: 10.1021/bc9600630
36. Chanda N, Kan P, Watkinson LD, Shukla R, Zambre A, Carmack TL, et al. Radioactive gold nanoparticles in cancer therapy: therapeutic efficacy studies of GA-198 AuNP nanoconstruct in prostate tumor-bearing mice. *Nanomedicine* 2010;6(2):201-9. doi: 10.1016/j.nano.2009.11.001
37. Cutler CS, Chanda N, Shukla R, Sisay N, Cantorias M, Zambre A, et al. Nanoparticles and phage display selected peptides for imaging and therapy of cancer. In: Baum RP, Rosch F, editors. Theranostics, Gallium-68, and Other Radionuclides. Springer Berlin Heidelberg; 2013. P. 133-47.
38. Prabaharan M, Grailer JJ, Pilla S, Steeber DA, Gong S. Folate-conjugated amphiphilic hyperbranched block copolymers based on Boltorn H40, poly(L-lactide) and poly(ethylene glycol) for tumor-targeted drug delivery. *Biomaterials* 2009;30(16):3009-19. doi: 10.1016/j.biomaterials.2009.02.011
39. Recio Despaigne AA, Da Silva JG, Da Costa PR, Dos Santos RG, Beraldo H. ROS-mediated cytotoxic effect of copper(II) hydrazone complexes against human glioma cells. *Molecules* 2014;19(11):17202-20. doi: 10.3390/molecules191117202

Optimization of Chitosan and Cellulose Acetate Phthalate Controlled Delivery of Methylprednisolone for Treatment of Inflammatory Bowel Disease

Swati Jagdale*, Apoorva Chandekar

Department of Pharmaceutics, MAEER's Maharashtra Institute of Pharmacy, MIT Campus, S. No. 124, Kothrud, Pune 411038, Savitribai Phule Pune University, India.

Keywords:
- Methylprednisolone
- Colon
- Targeting
- Press coated
- Tablet
- Chitosan

Abstract

Purpose: Inflammatory bowel disease (IBD) is a chronic, relapsing and often life-long disorder. The best way to tackle IBD is to develop a site targeted drug delivery. Methylprednisolone is a potent anti-inflammatory steroid. The relative potency of methylprednisolone to hydrocortisone is at least four is to one. The aim of the present research was to develop a colon targeted drug delivery for treatment of IBD.

Methods: Compression coated drug delivery system was designed and optimised. Core tablet contained drug, croscarmellose sodium (CCS-superdisintegrant), avicel (binder) and dicalcium phosphate (diluent). Design of experiment with 3^2 factorial design was applied for optimization of compression coated delivery. Chitosan and cellulose acetate phthalate were chosen as independent variables. Swelling index, hardness and % drug release were dependant variables.

Results: Core tablet (C5 batch) containing 2.15% CCS showed disintegration in less than 10sec. FTIR, UV and DSC study had shown absence of any significant physical and chemical interaction between drug and polymers. F8 was found to be optimised formulation. F8 contained 35% chitosan and 17.5% cellulose acetate phthalate. It showed drug release of 86.3% ± 6.1%, hardness 6.5 ± 1.5 and lag time 7 hrs. Simulated media drug release was 97.51 ± 8.6% with 7.5 hrs lag time. The results confirmed that the lag time was highly affected by the coating of the polymers as well as the concentration of the superdisintegrant used in core tablet.

Conclusion: *In-vitro* and *in-vivo* results confirmed a potential colon targeted drug therapy for treatment of IBD.

Introduction

Oral drug delivery is always the preferred form of delivery. The main problem with oral drug delivery is first pass metabolism. This becomes a major problem when drug needs to reach to the lower part of the gastrointestinal tract (GIT). To overcome this problem, targeted drug delivery systems are being developed. These formulations are designed to reach to the specific site to deliver drug.[1] Controlled delivery technology is divided in two subtypes as programmed and triggered release technology. Programmed release depends largely on the build-in program to release the drug rather than depending on interaction with the environment in a certain gastrointestinal segment (site specific target) or with a disease specific target. Examples of release profiles in this category are prolonged or delayed release. Triggered release technologies are the one where release is initiated upon interaction of the delivery system with a site specific target as pH, pressure or microbial flora. Since there is no influence of disease specific factors, this profile is often called site specific release.[2] In last few years the development of colon targeted drug delivery has received an increasing interest not only for a better treatment of specific local pathologies but also for the systemic therapy of both conventional and labile molecules. Colon targeted drug delivery system can be used to treat a number of diseases like colitis, Crohn's disease and colorectal cancer.[3] Especially those drugs that degrade in the hostile environment of the stomach and intestine can be protected from degradation and delivered directly to the colon. A large number of anti-asthmatics are delivered through this route.

Various approaches have been used in colon targeted drug delivery. Few include pH dependent system, time dependent system, pH and time dependent system and microbiologically triggered system. Newly developed techniques include pressure controlled drug delivery system, CODES ™ and osmotic controlled drug delivery system.[4,5] Pulsatile drug delivery systems are gaining a lot of interest now days. These systems are designed according to the circadian rhythm of the body. They

***Corresponding author:** Swati Jagdale, Emails: jagdaleswati@rediffmail.com ; swati.jagdale@mippune.edu deliver the drug at the specific time as per the pathophysiological need of the disease, resulting in improved patient compliance and therapeutic efficacy.[6,7] Literature survey has indicated that work has been carried out to target colon with delivery systems as time delayed capsule for diltiazem hydrochloride,[8] pulsatile delivery of theophylline,[9] flurbiprofen[10,11] and simvastatin,[12] piroxicam,[13] compression coating of 5-aminosalicylic acid matrix tablets,[14] fenoprofen calcium compressed coated tablets,[15] pH dependent delivery system of lercanidipine hydrochloride[16] etc.

Methylprednisolone is a potent anti-inflammatory steroid. It has greater anti-inflammatory potency than prednisolone. Even have fewer tendencies than prednisolone to induce sodium and water retention. The relative potency of methylprednisolone to hydrocortisone is at least four is to one. It belongs to BCS class II drug. Absolute bioavailability of methylprednisolone in normal healthy subjects is high i.e 82% to 89% after oral administration. The mean elimination half-life for methylprednisolone is in range of 1.8 to 5.2 hrs. Drug undergo high hepatic metabolism.[17-20] Literature study showed that dosage forms designed for methylprednisolone include freeze-dried product, immediate release (IR) tablet, immediate release capsule, microparticles in treatment of arthritis and pH sensitive hydrogels.[21,22] Commercially it is available as immediate release (IR) tablet. IR tablet has drawback of fluctuation to attain peak plasma concentration, variability in gastric emptying time, dose dumping, extensive first pass effect and low bioavailability. For colon diseases development of targeted drug delivery will release the drug at the site. This will minimize the side effects of the conventional dosage form and hence will improve the bioavailability and patient compliance. In the present research work methylprednisolone was chosen as a drug to target colon for treatment of IBD and colitis. The aim of the research was to give a site and time controlled drug delivery to colon. To achieve this aim, a compression coated drug delivery system containing chitosan and cellulose acetate phthalate was designed and optimized.

Materials and Methods

Methylprednisolone, chitosan, cellulose acetate phthalate (CAP), avicel, croscarmellose sodium (CCS), dicalcium phosphate (DCP), crospovidone, talc and magnesium stearate were purchased from Analab Fine chemicals, Mumbai.

Characterization of drug

Drug was characterized for melting point (melting point apparatus - LABIN), FTIR spectra (Varian 640 IR) in the wavelength region of 4000-400 cm^{-1} with diffusion reflectance principle and differential scanning calorimeter (DSC-60) at a temperature range of 50-300 °C with rate of 10 °C per minute in nitrogen atmosphere.

Solution of the drug in three different media (0.1N HCl, 7.4 pH phosphate buffer and 6.8 pH phosphate buffer) was scanned by UV-Visible spectrophotometer (UB Varian Carry 100) and λ_{max} was reported. Calibration curve in three media were recorded. The analytical method was validated for accuracy, inter-day and intra-day precision, linearity, limit of detection and limit of quantification. Stability of the drug was checked in all three dissolution media for duration of 24 hrs.

Drug-polymer interaction study

Drug alone, drug with polymers (chitosan and CAP) were mixed in 1:1 ratio. They were kept in stability chamber (Thermolab Scientific Equipments, 90/90/130 litres) for one month at accelerated stability conditions at 40 ± 2°C / 75 ± 5% RH. At the end of month, samples were analysed for FTIR, DSC and UV spectra.

Formulation of core and compression/press coated tablet

Core tablet were prepared using crospovidone as superdisintegrant in concentration of 1-5%. But those tablets lacked in hardness and had broken easily. Hence, crospovidone was replaced by croscarmellose sodium (CCS). Dicalcium phosphate (DCP) was used as diluent and avicel as binder. Tablets were compressed on Cadmac, Rimeck Minipress (8 station) machine using 6 mm round concave punch. Formulations were prepared with different concentration of CCS (1.5-8.5%) as shown in Table 1. Batch C5 was found to be most suitable formulation based on disintegration time and hardness.

Table 1. Formulation of core tablet

Ingredients (mg)	C1	C2	C3	C4	C5	C6
Methylprednisolone	8	8	8	8	8	8
Avicel ph 101	50	58	61	50	51	50
CCS	6	1	1	6	1.5	2
DCP	6	3	-	6	9.5	10

Total weight = 70 mg

Chitosan and CAP were chosen as polymer for outer coating of core tablet. Talc and magnesium stearate were added along with polymers as lubricant. DCP was dded as a diluent in the outer coat. At initial stage individual polymers were tried in different concentration. Individual polymer failed to maintain its integrity till it reaches to third media. Therefore for further study combination of polymer were tried. Chitosan was used in concentration range of 50-10 % and CAP in 10-50 %. To manufacture compression coated tablet direct compression method was used. 50% of coating mixture was first placed in the die cavity. Core tablet was then placed above this mixture. Then remaining quantity of coating mixture was added in die cavity to cover the core tablet. It was compressed on Cadmac, Rimeck Minipress compression machine (9 mm flat and plain punch) to obtain final weight of the tablet 200 mg with hardness 4-7 kg/cm^2.[2,23] Preliminary trials had shown that 40% chitosan and 20% CAP crossed first two media and enter intact in third media in the dissolution study.

Design of experiment (DOE)

3^2 factorial design was used as a tool to optimize the formula for coating polymer. In this design 3 levels and 2 factors were used. The factors were concentration of chitosan and concentration of CAP. The coded levels were +1, 0 and -1.[24,25] Factorial batch formulations were prepared as shown in Table 2. Manufacturing method is same as discussed above in compression/press coated tablet.[24,25]

Table 2. Formulation of compression coated tablet

Batch code	Chitosan (mg)	CAP (mg)	Talc (mg)	Mg. Stearate (mg)	Core Tablet (mg)	DCP (mg)
F1	80 (+1)	40 (+1)	1	1	70	8
F2	80 (+1)	35 (0)	1	1	70	13
F3	80 (+1)	30 (-1)	1	1	70	18
F4	75 (0)	40 (+1)	1	1	70	13
F5	75 (0)	35 (0)	1	1	70	18
F6	75 (0)	30 (-1)	1	1	70	23
F7	70 (-1)	40 (+1)	1	1	70	18
F8	70 (-1)	35 (0)	1	1	70	23
F9	70 (-1)	30 (-1)	1	1	70	28

Total weight = 200 mg; CAP: cellulose acetate phthalate; DCP: Dicalcium phosphate; Mg Stearate: Magnesium Stearate

Evaluation of core tablet:

Core tablet was evaluated for thickness (Vernier calliper), hardness (Monsanto hardness tester), friability (Roche friabilator -Veego), uniformity of content (UV-Visible spectrophotometer), weight variation (digital electronic balance) and disintegration time (digital tablet disintegration apparatus -Veego) at 37 ± 2°C in 900 ml phosphate buffer pH 6.8.

In- vitro dissolution study was carried out in 900 ml pH 6.8 phosphate buffer (PBS) at 37 ± 0.5°C in USP dissolution apparatus type II (Electro Lab, Model TDT-08L). Rotation speed was maintained at 50 rpm. Samples from this solution were withdrawn at time interval and analysed at λ max.

Compression /Press coated tablet

Evaluation of powder flow properties was carried out by measuring angle of repose (fixed funnel method), bulk density and tapped density (digital bulk density apparatus - Bio Techno Lab, Make Lab HOSP).Compressibility index and Hausner's ratio was calculated.

Evaluation of coated tablet for tablet thickness, friability, drug content, weight variation and hardness were carried out in similar manner as mention in evaluation of the core tablet.

To determine swelling index for tablet, it was immersed in a flask of USP dissolution test apparatus containing 250 ml of medium at 37°C (for first 2 hrs in pH 1.2 HCl, next 3 hrs in pH 7.4 PBS and lastly in pH 6.8 PBS for 3 hrs). At specific time interval, the swollen tablets were withdrawn from the medium and weighed. Light blotting with a filter paper was used for removal of excess surface water. Study was performed in three replicates. The swelling behavior of the coated tablet was calculated using Eq.1

$$SI = [W_t - W_0] / W_0 \times 100 \qquad \text{Equation 1}$$

Where, SI is swelling index of the tablet, W_t is the weight of tablet after appropriate time interval t in respective media and W_0 is the initial weight of dry tablet.

For *in- vitro* dissolution study the tablets were placed in USP dissolution apparatus type II. To simulate the pH changes along the GI tract, three dissolution media were used. Recent studies with sensitive and reliable equipment contradict the traditional view and provide evidence of a decrease in pH at the gastrointestinal region between the ileum and the colon. Apparently the colon has a lower pH value (6.5) than that of the small intestine (7.0–7.8).[9] Radio telemetry showed highest pH (7.5 ± 0.5) in the terminal ileum. On entry into the colon, the pH drops to 6.4 ± 0.6. The pH in the mid colon is 6.6 ± 0.8 and in the left colon 7.0 ± 0.7.There is fall in pH on entry into the colon due to the presence of short chain fatty acids arising from bacterial fermentation of polysaccharides.[4] Considering these reported references in present study first media used was pH 1.2 HCl for 2 hrs (average gastric emptying time is about 2 hrs). Second media was pH 7.4 phosphate buffer solution for next 3 hrs (average small intestinal transit time is about 3 hrs). Lastly the study was carried out in third media i.e. pH 6.8 phosphate buffer solution (colon) until the tablet burst.[4,8,9,16] Samples were collected till 8 hrs at specific time interval and analysed by UV spectrophotometer. Percent drug release was calculated.

For dissolution study in simulated media F7 and F8 batches chosen. Simulated media were based on sequential pH change method as gastric fluid pH 5, intestinal fluid pH 5.8 and colonic fluid pH 7. The composition of the media was prepared and used in present study was as reported by Marques et al.[26]

Stability study was carried for the optimized batch F8 at long term (30°C ± 2°C/65% RH ± 5% RH) and accelerated conditions (40±2°C/75±5% RH) over a period of three months according to ICH guidelines in stability chamber (Thermo Lab Scientific Equipments). At the end of three months and in between time intervals for long term stability study, tablets were withdrawn from the stability chamber and examined for physical evaluation and drug content.

Statistical analysis of data

In-vitro release kinetics was carried by PCP DISSO.v2.08

Similarity factor was calculated using BIT software. Similarity study was carried out in between marketed tablet of methylprednisolone (Medrol 8 mg, Pfizer Italia) and optimized formulation F8.

Design expert software version 9.0 was used to obtain ANOVA analysis and response surface graphs for factorial design.

In-vivo X-ray imaging placebo study

In-vivo X-ray imaging placebo study was performed on three healthy human volunteers using X-ray generating unit. Optimized batch F8 was evaluated. Methylprednisolone was replaced with radio opaque agent, barium sulphate. The core tablet contained barium sulphate (8 mg), CCS (1.5 mg), Avicel (51 mg) and DCP (9.5 mg). For coated tablet chitosan (70 mg), CAP (35 mg), DCP (23 mg), talc (1 mg) and magnesium stearate (1 mg) were used. The study was carried out as per World Medical Association guidelines and Helsinki ethical principle. The aim was only to check the position of optimized formulation in body. The study does not involve any blood or any other kind of sampling. Informed consent of human volunteer was taken before participation. The study was carried out under supervision of expert radiologist and physician. For placebo study volunteers aged between 24-26 years and weighing 55-60 Kg were selected. Each volunteer after an overnight fasting was ingested with tablet orally with 200 ml water. The volunteers were served with breakfast at 2 hrs and lunch at 4 hrs after the administration of the tablet. The tablets were visualized using X-ray technique. Abdominal radiographs were taken after 1, 2 and 5 hrs in all volunteers.[27,28]

Results and Discussion

Characterization of drug

Melting point of drug was obtained at 231° C which was matching with the reported literature data [18].This proved purity of drug. FTIR spectra (Figure 1A) showed sharp peaks at 1450 cm^{-1} and 1375 cm^{-1} indicating CH_3 (bend), peak at 1680-1600 cm^{-1} indicated C=C (alkenes), peak at 1300-1000 cm^{-1} indicated C-O (alcohol), at 1725-1705 cm^{-1} indicated C=O (ketone), broad absorption near 3400-3300 cm^{-1} indicated O-H (alcohol). All these peaks indicated presence of drug in pure form matching with standard values reported in the literature.[29]

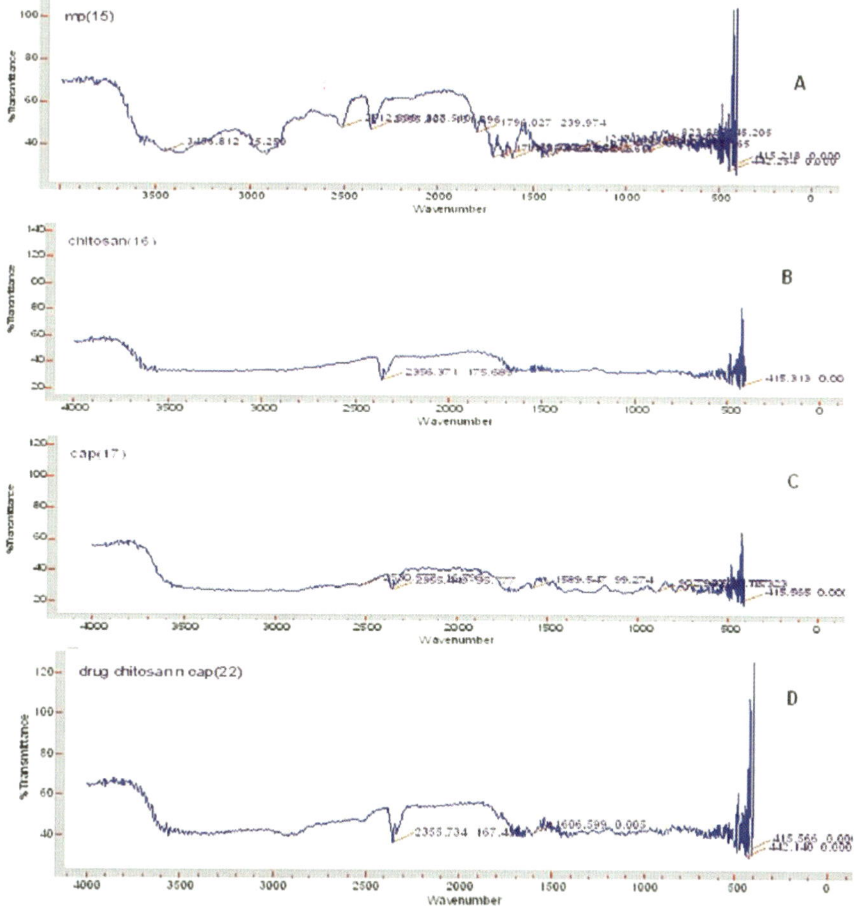

Figure 1. FTIR spectra for (A) Methylprednisolone, (B) chitosan, (C) CAP and (D) Formulation

The DSC graph for methylprednisolone (Figure 2A) showed sharp peaks at 117.4°C, 177.38° C and 216.9°C. UV spectroscopic study showed λ max at 246.13 nm. It was found that the drug follows Beer-Lambert's law. For accuracy study, percent recovery for 80% was 98.92%, for 100% it was 99.36% and for 120% it was 99.19%. From the data obtained from interday as well as intraday study, the method was found to be precise. The drug solution was found to be linear in the range on 5-25μg/mL. LOD and LOQ were found to be 0.157μg/mL and 0.549μg/mL respectively.

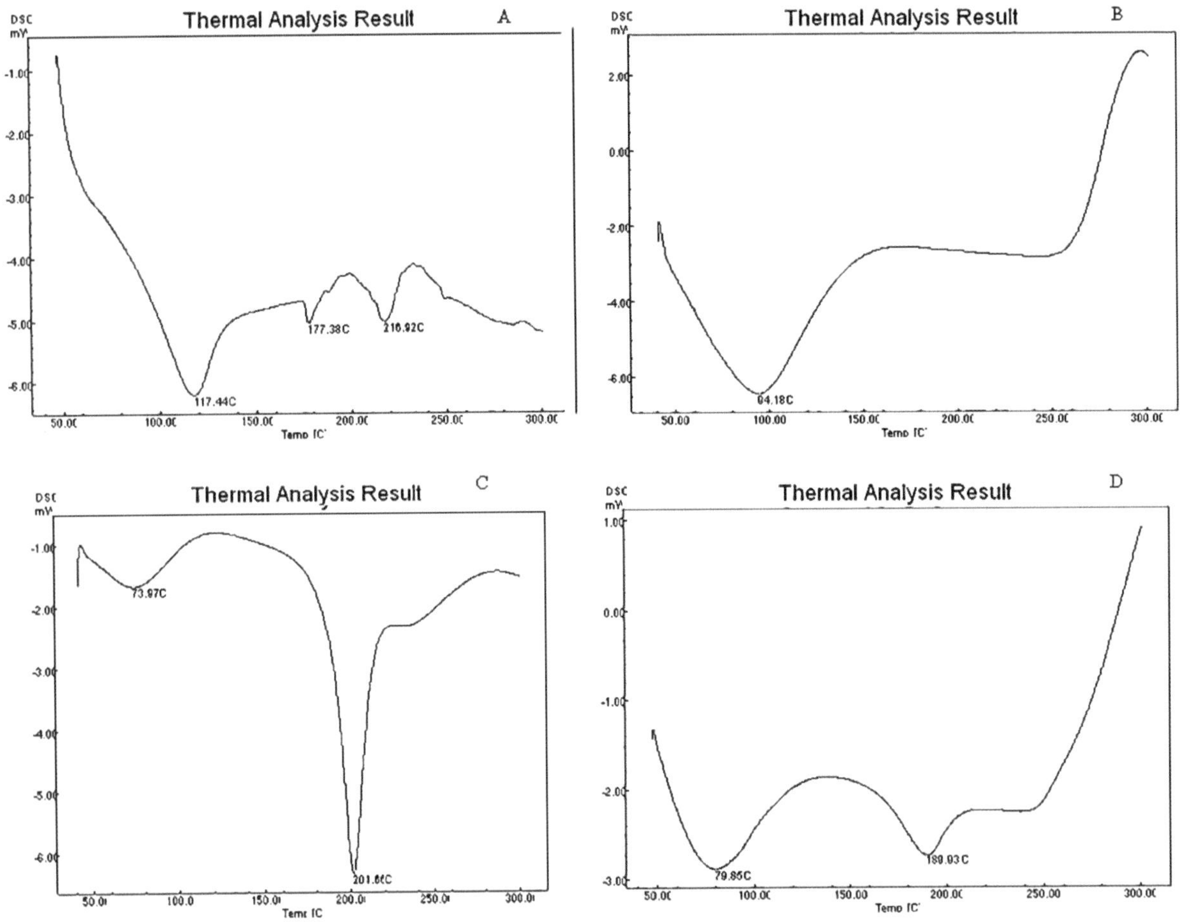

Figure 2. DSC graph of (A) Methylprednisolone, (B) chitosan, (C) CAP and (D) Formulation.

Drug- polymer interaction study

As shown in Figure 1A, FTIR spectra of drug showed peaks at 1450 cm^{-1} and 1375 cm^{-1}, 1680-1600 cm^{-1}, 1300-1000 cm^{-1}, 1725-1705 cm^{-1} and broad absorption near 3400-3300 cm^{-1}. Chitosan (Figure 1B) showed peak at 2356 cm^{-1} and 415 cm^{-1}. CAP (Figure 1C) showed peak at 415 cm^{-1},2350 cm^{-1}, 2355 cm^{-1}, 1589 cm^{-1},902 cm^{-1} and 796 cm^{-1}. Formulation (Figure 1D) showed peaks at 415 cm^{-1},1600 cm^{-1} and 2355 cm^{-1}. Few peaks of drug as well as polymer may have merge due to polymer interlinking and engulfing of drug in matrix. As the major peak for drug and polymer remains unchanged it can be said that there was no significant physical and chemical interaction between drug and polymer.

DSC graph of pure methylprednisolone (Figure 2A) showed peaks at 117°, 177° and 216°C. Chitosan (Figure 2B) showed peak at 94° C while CAP (Figure 2C) showed peaks at 73° and 201°C . Formulation F8 (Figure 2D) on the other hand showed peaks at 79° and 189° C. Some peaks of CAP and methylprednisolone did not shift significantly while the remaining peak of CAP, methylprednisolone and chitosan were not present. The shift in the peak can be explained mainly due to polymer interlinking and engulfing of the drug in the polymer matrix.

UV spectra had shown that λ_{max} for the drug remained same with polymer as well as in the formulation. As there was no shift or change in λ_{max}, it indicated absence of any kind of physical and chemical interaction between drug with polymer and excipients.

Formulation of core and coated tablet

In manufacturing for core tablet crospovidone was used as superdisintegrant at initial stage but the batches failed to meet disintegration criteria. Hence croscarmellose sodium was used. Also, lactose was used as diluent in earlier trial but the tablets did not have enough hardness, Hence, it was replaced by DCP. C5 was found to be most suitable batch with croscarmellose sodium as superdisintegrant which was used further for compression coating.

Preliminary trial batches for coated tablet had shown hardness in the range of 4.5-7 kg/cm^2. Individual polymers were tried but those tablets broke even before reaching the second media. The concentration of the polymers were varied in 50 -10% of chitosan and 50 -10% of CAP. It was observed that tablet containing higher concentration of chitosan did not disintegrate after 24 hrs. Whereas tablet containing higher concentration of CAP did not had enough hardness to hold the tablet till it reaches to third media. The tablet containing 40% chitosan and 20% CAP was found to be suitable as it reached to third media.

Core tablet C5 showed thickness in the range of 2 ± 0.01mm, hardness 1.5 ± 0.02kg/cm^2, diameter 6 ± 0.1mm, friability 0.47 ± 0.1%, uniformity of content 99.26 ± 4.3%, uniformity of weight 70 ± 0.2 mg, disintegration time 5 ± 3 sec and percent drug release 99.62 ± 5.6%.

Design of experiment

The powder blend for all batches had shown angle of repose in range of 25-30°, bulk and tap density 0.48-0.69, compressibility index 11-20% and Hausner's ratio 1.13-1.20. All these results showed good flow properties for the powder blend as reported in literature.[30]

For F1 to F9 batches, hardness was found in the range of 5- 6.5 kg/cm^2, weight variation 199-202 mg, friability 0.37 - 0.52%, drug content 97- 99%, thickness was around 0.2 mm and diameter was around 9 mm. Summary for all evaluation parameters is as shown in Table 3.

Table 3. Post-compression parameters evaluation for coated tablet

Batch code	Hardness (kg/ cm^2)	Weight variation	Friability (%)	Drug Content (%)	Thickness (mm)	Diameter (mm)
F1	5.5 ± 1.4	200.1 ± 1.2	0.52 ± 0.01	98.57 ± 1.2	0.2 ± 1.6	9 ± 1.3
F2	5 ± 1.3	200.5 ± 1.6	0.49 ± 1.1	97.06 ± 1.6	0.2 ± 1.1	9 ± 1.5
F3	5 ± 1.2	201.4 ± 1.5	0.46 ± 1.2	98.97 ± 1.9	0.2 ± 1.2	9 ± 1.6
F4	5.5 ± 1.4	199.3 ± 1.6	0.42 ± 1.3	98.50 ± 1.6	0.2 ± 1.6	9 ± 1.5
F5	6 ± 1.5	199.7 ± 1.2	0.37 ± 1.5	98.43 ± 1.7	0.2 ± 1.7	9 ± 1.9
F6	5.5 ± 1.0	199.8 ± 1.8	0.47 ± 1.4	97.93 ± 1.3	0.2 ± 1.4	9 ± 1.8
F7	6 ± 1.3	200.2 ± 1.6	0.41 ± 1.8	99.4 ± 1.4	0.2 ± 1.8	9 ± 1.3
F8	6.5 ± 1.5	200.2 ± 1.7	0.38 ± 1.6	99.25 ± 1.6	0.2 ± 1.6	9 ± 1.2
F9	5.5 ± 1.4	202.3 ± 1	0.39 ± 1.2	98.06 ± 1.2	0.2 ± 1.2	9 ± 1.1

Polymers played a major role in the swelling property of the tablet. Chitosan and CAP are both hygroscopic polymers. On entering the media, both polymers had shown swelling property. Direct relation was found between swelling index and lag time. The swelling pattern for batches can be seen in Figure 3. The tablet having maximum swelling index had shown highest lag time. The swelling capacity of CAP played a major role in swelling index of tablet. The tablet containing higher concentrations of CAP had shown maximum swelling as compare to low concentration. Those tablets with low concentration of CAP had broken at faster rate. F1 and F8 batches showed maximum swelling whereas F6 had broken in half an hour only. Swelling capacity of polymer HPMC had shown similar role for reported work of diltiazem, lercanidipine and flurbiprofen.[8,11,16,25]

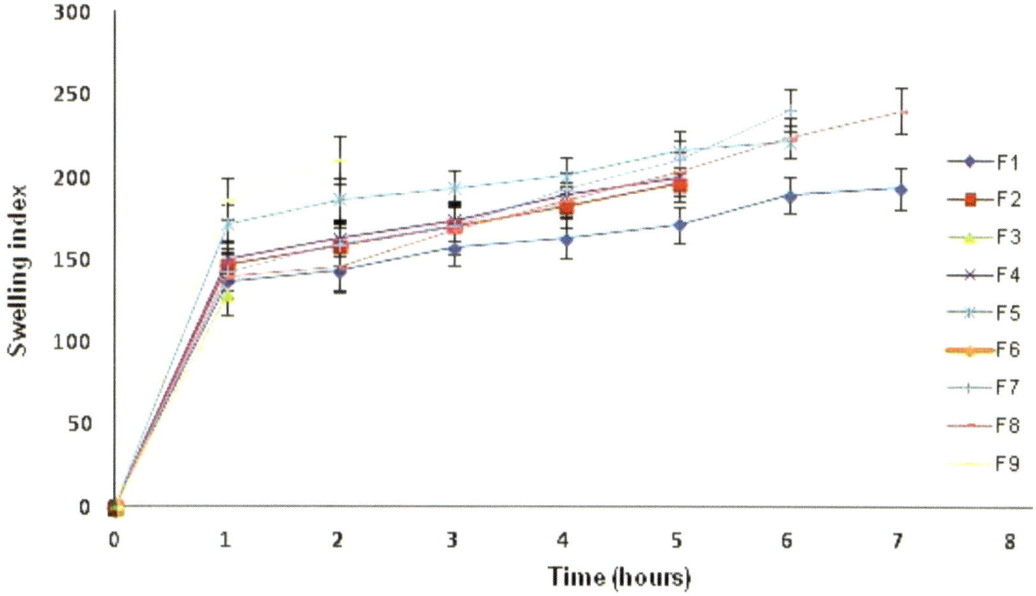

Figure 3. Swelling indices for F1-F9 batches

From *in-vitro* dissolution study, it was observed that both the polymer starts swelling after coming in contact with the media. After reaching their maximum swelling capacity, the outer layer of the tablet contacting polymers get rupture which allow core tablet to come outside .Since the core tablet contains superdisintegrant, it immediately broke down and released the drug in outer media. It can be seen (Figure 4a) that F6 and F9 disintegrated before the time it can reach to third media that is colon (before 5 hrs). F6 and F9 contain low concentration of CAP. This indicated that the concentration of CAP played an important role in bypassing first two media. *In-vitro* dissolution study proved that minimum 17.5% CAP was required in the tablet so as to reach to the colon. Batches F7 and F8 showed the maximum drug release (≥ 90%) in 7-8 hrs.[25,31]

Batches F7 and F8 were studied in simulated media. Batch F8 (35% chitosan and 17.5% CAP) showed maximum drug release of around 97.51 ± 5.6% (Figure 4b). After 3 months for batch F8, evaluation parameters were as thickness (0.2 ± 0.04 mm), diameter (9 ± 0.5 mm), hardness (6 ± 1.4 kg/cm^2), weight variation (199.54 ± 1.6 mg), friability (0.34 ± 1.1%), percent drug release (85.43 ± 5.9%) and percent drug content (98.16 ± 1.9%). There was no significant change in the values before and after indicating the stability of the formulation.

Batch F8 showed zero order release. It indicated that the dosage form releases same amount of drug in a given unit of time.[32]

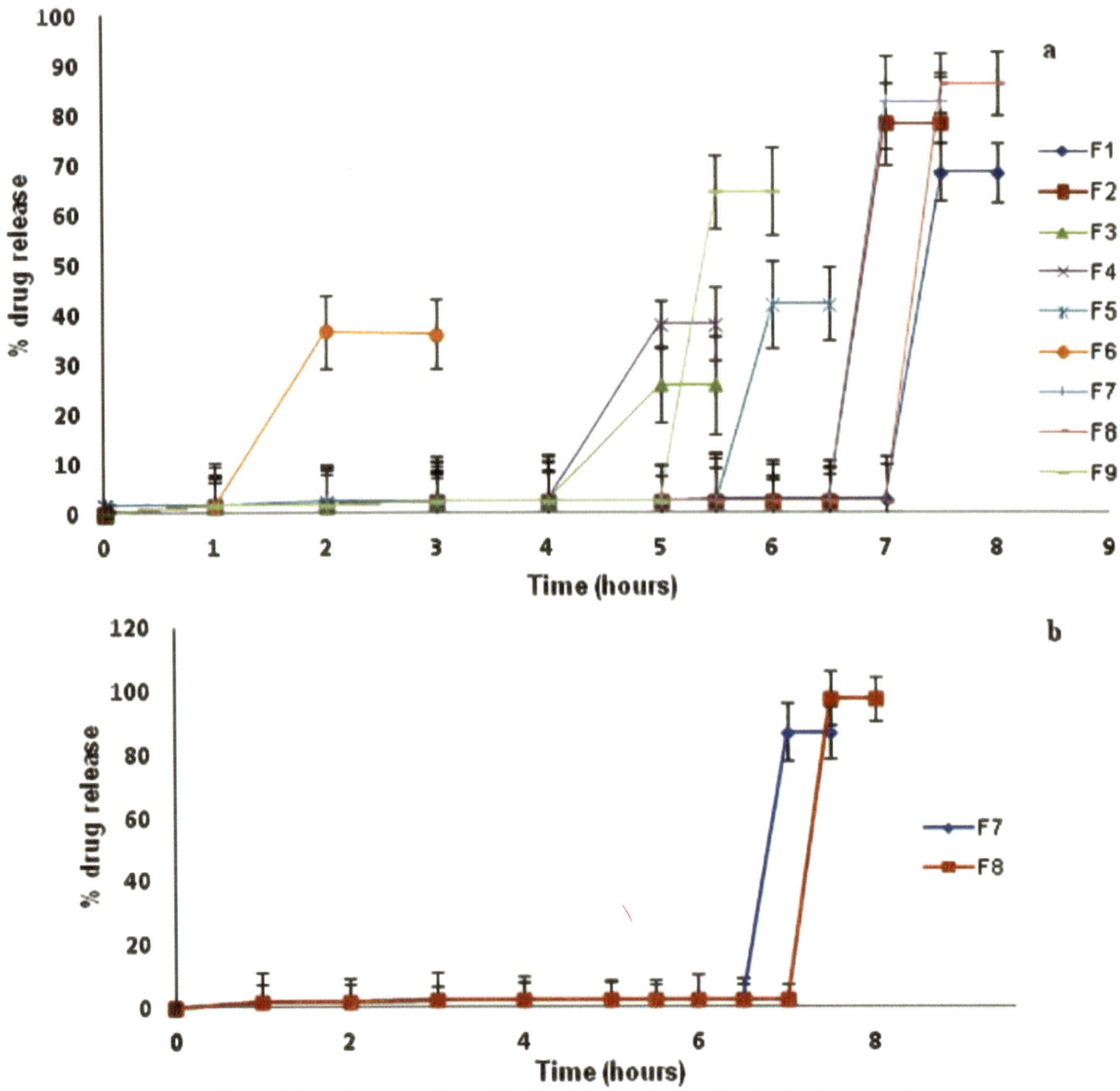

Figure 4. Dissolution profile **a:** F1-F9 batches; **b:** F7 and F8 in simulated media

Response surface plots

Response surface plots were used to determine the effect of independent variables on the dependent variables. Independent variables were concentrations of both the polymers whereas dependent variables were swelling index, hardness and percent drug release. Response surface plots were derived from design expert software version 9.0.3.1. It was seen that swelling index was most significant between 3-5 hrs whereas percent drug release and hardness were not found to be that significant factors.

Equation for swelling index at 3 hrs:

$$\text{Swelling index} = +184.89 - 2.17A + 83.33B - 3.25AB \quad \text{Equation 2}$$

Equation for swelling index at 5 hrs:

$$\text{Swelling index} = +210.67 - 7.83A + 97.00B - 10.00AB \quad \text{Equation 3}$$

Where, A = chitosan and B = CAP

ANOVA results indicated that swelling index was the only significant factor. This indicated that change of media played an important role for swelling of the tablet. The media was changed first after 2 hrs and then after 5 hrs. Thus, when the tablet was in the second media the swelling was most dominant. When the tablet reached to the third media the swelling got continued but it did not have that much significant effect as compared with first two media.

Response surface and contour plots of the respective responses were generated as shown in Figure 5. Table 4a indicates the ANOVA data.[33]

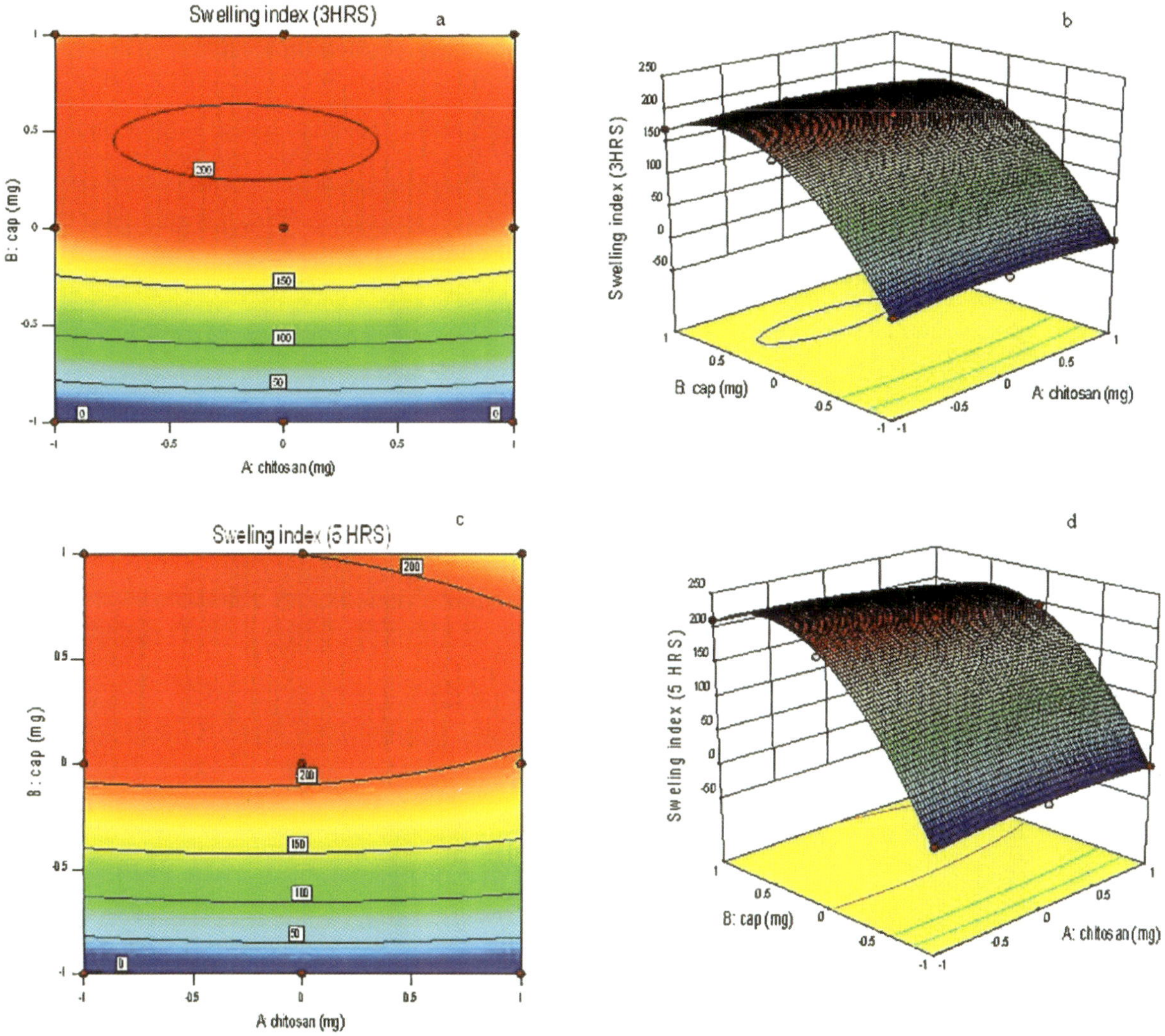

Figure 5. **a, c**: Contour plot showing the influence of chitosan and CAP on swelling index at 3 hrs and at 5 hrs
b, d: Response surface plot showing the relationship between various levels of chitosan and CAP at 3 hrs and at 5 hrs

Table 4a. ANOVA results

Response model	Sum of squares	df	Means square	F value	P value	R^2	Adequate precision
Swelling index at 3 hrs	59769.36	5	11953.87	186.59	0.0006	0.9968	29.009
Swelling index at 5 hrs	80694.67	5	16138.93	328.62	0.0003	0.9982	37.691

From Eq. 2; for swelling index at 3 hrs, it was found that CAP showed positive effect on swelling index. Chitosan showed significantly less effect on swelling index as compared to CAP. The p-value for swelling index at 3 hrs was found to be 0.0006 which was less than 0.0500.This indicated that the model was highly significant.

From Eq. 3; for swelling index at 5 hrs, it was found that again CAP showed positive effect while chitosan showed negative effect. The difference in the values between 3 and 5 hrs was not much large.

Predicted optimized batch by design expert was F8 batch. Predicted results as shown in Table 4b indicated validation of design expert software.

Table 4b. Validation Data

Composition			Predicted value		Observed value		Standard deviation		SEM (Std. error of mean)	
Polymer	Coded value	Actual value (mg)	SI at 3 hrs (%)	SI at 5 hrs (%)	SI at 3 hrs (%)	SI at 5 hrs (%)	SI at 3 hrs	SI at 5 hrs	SI at 3hrs (%)	SI at 5hrs (%)
Chitosan	-1	70	176.22	210	167.9	203.4	8.00405	7.00793	5.96587	5.2234
CAP	0	35								

The similarity factor (f_2) obtained was 14. The value indicated that marketed formulation (immediate release) and the designed formulation were not similar in their release pattern. As the design dosage form was to be targeted to colon, this gave indication that the designed can reach to the colon.[34]

In-vivo X-ray imaging (placebo) study

Radiographs of human volunteers were taken after a specified time interval. *In - vivo* X-ray imaging placebo study for colon targeted delivery of methylprednisolone in human volunteers had shown that the tablet did not float in stomach. The tablet even did not break down in stomach and small intestine. Tablet remains intact. Tablet also did not adhere to any part of the gastrointestinal tract i.e. stomach and small intestine. From Figure 6 it can be seen that the tablet can be located in the ascending part of colon after 5hrs of ingestion. This indicated that the optimized formulation in body will have the capacity to pass stomach and small intestine and enter in third media which is colon. This gave a positive assurance that the optimized delivery will give targeted drug delivery to colon.[35]

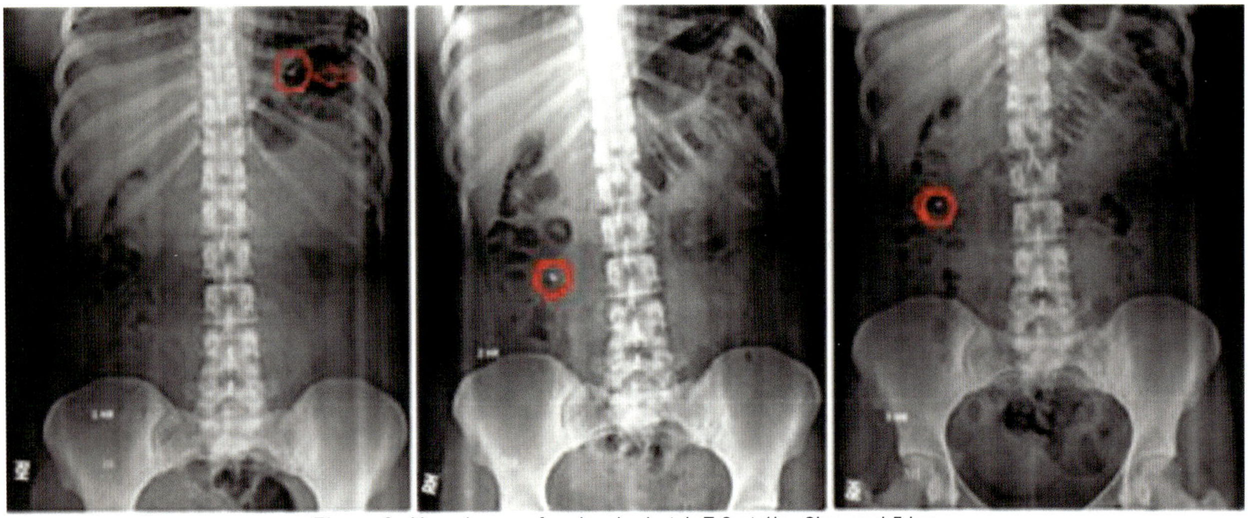

Figure 6. X-ray images for placebo batch F 8 at 1hr, 2hrs and 5 hrs

Conclusion

An attempt had been made to optimize a colon targeted drug delivery containing polymer chitosan and cellulose acetate phthalate. The main objective was to avoid first pass metabolism of the drug and to give a therapy for colon diseases. Direct compression technique was used for compression coated delivery. Design of experiment was applied for optimization of coating layer. F8 was the optimized batch. ANOVA results indicated that swelling index was the most significant factor in controlling the lag time and hence release of drug. CAP played most important role in swelling. *In-vitro* as well as *in –vivo* study indicated presence of delivery in third media indicating protection of the drug from being released in the upper region of GI system, i.e. stomach and small intestine. Thus F8 formulation can act as potential for treatment of colon diseases that can achieve maximum therapeutic efficacy.

Acknowledgments

The authors are thankful to Savitribai Phule Pune University, Maharashtra, India for providing financial assistance under Board of College and University Development *(BCUD)* Project Grant for the present research work. The authors are thankful to SKN General Hospital and Medical College, Narhe, Pune, for providing facility to carry *In-vivo* x-ray imaging (placebo) study. Authors are also thankful to Dr. B. S. Kuchekar, Principal and management of MAEER's Maharashtra Institute of Pharmacy, Pune for providing all the facilities to carry out the research work.

Ethical Issues

The study was carried out as per World Medical Association guidelines and Helsinki ethical principle.

Conflict of Interest

The authors declare no conflict of interests.

References

1. Chourasia MK, Jain SK. Pharmaceutical approaches to colon targeted drug delivery systems. *J Pharm Pharm Sci* 2003;6(1):33-66.
2. Basit AW. Advances in colonic drug delivery. *Drugs* 2005;65(14):1991-2007.
3. Ng SC, Kamm MA. Review article: New drug formulations, chemical entities and therapeutic approaches for the management of ulcerative colitis. *Aliment Pharmacol Ther* 2008;28(7):815-29. doi: 10.1111/j.1365-2036.2008.03800.x
4. Prasanth VV, Jayaprakash R, Mathew ST. Colon specific drug delivery systems: a review on various pharmaceutical approaches. *J Appl Pharm Sci* 2012;02(01):163-9
5. Philip AK, Philip B. Colon targeted drug delivery systems: A review on primary and novel approaches. *Oman Med J* 2010;25(2):79-87. doi: 10.5001/omj.2010.24
6. Qureshi AM, Momin M, Rathod S, Dev A, Kute C. Colon targeted drug delivery system: A review on current approaches. *Ind J Pharm Biol Res* 2013;1(4):130-47.
7. Lin SY, Kawashima Y. Current status and approaches to developing press-coated chronodelivery drug systems. *J Control Release* 2012;157(3):331-53. doi: 10.1016/j.jconrel.2011.09.065
8. Kamalakkannan V, Kumaran KSG. Time delayed capsule device for chronopharmaceutical drug delivery system of diltiazem hydrochloride formulation and evaluation. *Res J Pharm Bio Chem Sci* 2014;5(1):707-28
9. Mastiholimath VS, Dandagi PM, Jain SS, Gadad AP, Kulkarni AR. Time and ph dependent colon specific, pulsatile delivery of theophylline for nocturnal asthma. *Int J Pharm* 2007;328(1):49-56. doi: 10.1016/j.ijpharm.2006.07.045
10. Vemula SK, Bontha VK. Flurbiprofen pulsatile colon-specific delivery: formulation and evaluation of double-compression coated tablets. *J Pharm Anal Insight* 2016;1.1. doi: 10.16966/2471-8122.104
11. Vemula SK, Bontha VK. Colon targeted guar gum compression coated tablets of flurbiprofen: Formulation, development, and pharmacokinetics. *Biomed Res Int* 2013;2013:287919. doi: 10.1155/2013/287919
12. Sukanya M, Kishore VS. Design and development of chronopharmaceutical drug delivery of Simvastatin. *J Chem Pharm Res* 2012;4(6):3195-200
13. Bandari S, Sanka K, Jukanti R, Reddy Veerareddy P. Formulation and *in vitro* evaluation of pulsatile colon drug delivery system of piroxicam using 32 factorial design. *Der Pharm Lett* 2010;2(4):177-88
14. Das M, Ghosh L. Evaluation of polymers for compression coating oaminosalicylic acid matrix tablets for colon targeting. *Int J Pharm Sci* 2013;5(3):122-5
15. Potu A, Pasunooti S, Veerareddy P, Burra S. Formulation and evaluation of fenoprofen calcium compressed coated tablets for colon specific drug delivery. *Asian J Pharm Clin Res* 2011;4(2):88-95
16. Goudanavar P, Pani RV, Hiremath D, Fattepur S. Design and evaluation of time and pH dependent delivery systems of lercanidipine hydrochloride for chronomodulated therapy. *Studia Universitatis* 2014;24(3):333-49.
17. Notes on data of the drug methylprednisolone by drug bank, http://www.drugbank.ca/drugs/DB00959 Accessed on 03 July 2015.
18. Government of India, Ministry of health and welfare. Indian Pharmacopoeia, Vol. I,II. New Delhi: Controller of Publications; 2014.
19. Notes on drug, drug interactions and drug dosage forms. Current index of medical specialties (CIMS), http://www.mims.com/india/drug/search?q=methylprednisolone. Accessed on 03 July 2015.
20. Barar FSK. Essentials of Pharmacotherapeutics. 5th ed. Delhi: S. Chand & Company Ltd; 2000.
21. Tobar-Grande B, Godoy R, Bustos P, von Plessing C, Fattal E, Tsapis N, et al. Development of biodegradable methylprednisolone microparticles for treatment of articular pathology using a spray-drying technique. *Int J Nanomedicine* 2013;8:2065-76. doi: 10.2147/IJN.S39327
22. Joshi GB, Hemant KSY, Singh MN, Shivakumar HG. Development of pH sensitive hydrogel for intestinal delivery of methylprednisolone using novel chitosan derivative. *Int J Pharm Pharma Sci* 2011;3(1):200-3
23. Sinha VR, Kumria R. Coating polymers for colon specific drug delivery: A comparative in vitro evaluation. *Acta Pharm* 2003;53(1):41-7.
24. Shah N, Patel M, Shah T, Amin A. Design, development and optimization of colon targeted drug delivery system for Crohn's disease. *J Pharm Educ Res* 2011;2(1):42-9.
25. Jagdale S, Chandekar A. Site targeted press coated delivery of methylprednisolone using eudragit rs 100 and chitosan for treatment of colitis. *Recent Pat Antiinfect Drug Discov* 2016;11(1):32-43.
26. Marques MRC, Loebenberg R, Almukainzi M. Simulated biological fluids with possible application in dissolution testing. *Dissolut Technol* 2011:15-28. doi: 10.14227/DT180311P15
27. Sinha VR, Mittal BR, Kumria R. In vivo evaluation of time and site of disintegration of polysaccharide tablet prepared for colon-specific drug delivery. *Int J Pharm* 2005;289(1-2):79-85. doi: 10.1016/j.ijpharm.2004.10.019
28. International Ethical Guidelines for Biomedical Research Involving Human subjects, Council for

International organizations of Medical Sciences in Collaboration with the World Health Organization, Geneva, 2002. Available from: http://www.cioms.ch/publications/layout_guide2002.pdf (accessed on 03 rd July 2015)
29. Pavia DL, Lampman GM, Kriz GS, Vyvyan JA. Introduction to spectroscopy. 5th ed. India: Cengage Learning India Private Limited; 2015.
30. Aulton ME. Aulton's Pharmaceutics-The design and manufacture of medicine. 2nd ed. Hungary: Churchill Livingstone Elsevier; 2008.
31. Hude RU, Jagdale SC. Optimization of time controlled 6-mercaptopurine delivery for site-specific targeting to colon diseases. *Curr Drug Deliv* 2016;13(4):534-44.
32. Dash S, Murthy PN, Nath L, Chowdhury P. Kinetic modeling on drug release from controlled drug delivery systems. *Acta Pol Pharm* 2010;67(3):217-23.
33. Jagdale SC, Patil S, Kuchekar BS. Application of design of experiment for floating drug delivery of tapentadol hydrochloride. *Comput Math Methods Med* 2013;2013:625729. doi: 10.1155/2013/625729
34. Sadaphal KP, Thakare VM, Gandhi BR, Tekade BW. Formulation and evaluation of pulsatile drug delivery system for chronobiological disorder: asthma. *Int J Drug Deliv* 2011;3(11):348-56
35. Ghimire M, McInnes FJ, Watson DG, Mullen AB, Stevens HN. In-vitro/in-vivo correlation of pulsatile drug release from press-coated tablet formulations: A pharmacoscintigraphic study in the beagle dog. *Eur J Pharm Biopharm* 2007;67(2):515-23. doi: 10.1016/j.ejpb.2007.03.002

The Effect of Particle Size on the Deposition of Solid Lipid Nanoparticles in Different Skin Layers

Zahra Mardhiah Adib[1], Saeed Ghanbarzadeh[2], Maryam Kouhsoltani[3], Ahmad Yari Khosroshahi[4], Hamed Hamishehkar[5]*

[1] Research Center for Pharmaceutical Nanotechnology and Students' Research Committee, Tabriz University of Medical Sciences, Tabriz, Iran.

[2] Zanjan Pharmaceutical Nanotechnology Research Center, Department of Pharmaceutics, Faculty of Pharmacy, Zanjan University of Medical Sciences, Zanjan, Iran.

[3] Department of Oral and Maxillofacial Pathology, Faculty of Dentistry, Tabriz University of Medical Sciences, Tabriz, Iran.

[4] Biotechnology Research Center and Faculty of Pharmacy, Tabriz University of Medical Sciences, Tabriz, Iran.

[5] Drug Applied Research Center, Tabriz University of Medical Sciences, Tabriz, Iran.

Keywords:
- Solid lipid nanoparticle
- SLN
- Topical drug delivery
- Skin penetration
- Rhodamine B

Abstract

Purpose: In the present study the effect of particle size, as a substantial parameters in skin penetration, on the deposition depth and rate of SLNs in different layers of skin was explored.

Methods: SLNs in different particle size ranges (80, 333 and 971 nm) made of Precirol as solid lipid were prepared using hot melt homogenization technique and pigmented by Rhodamine B to be able to be tracked in the skin under inspection of fluorescent microscopy. After 0.5 h, 3 h, 6 h and 24 h of SLNs administration on rat skin, animals were sacrificed and exercised skins were sliced by a freeze microtome. SLNs were monitored in the skin structure under fluorescence microscope.

Results: The size of SLNs played a crucial role in the penetration to deep skin layers. The sub100 nm size range of SLNs showed the most promising skin penetration rate and depth mainly via hair follicles.

Conclusion: The results of the present study indicated that the selection of an appropriate size of particles may be a valuable factor impacting the therapeutic outcomes of dermal drug administration.

Introduction

Treating skin diseases topically has many advantages: it is a non-aggressive and easy way to deliver drug, it has fewer systemic side effects compared with parenteral or oral drug delivery routes, it is possible to use high drug concentrations on the skin, the frequency of application is reduced, especially for drugs with a short half-life, drug input is terminated at initial administration time points by removing the drug, and patient compliance is improved.[1,2] The horny layer, or stratum corneum (SC), of the skin is the main barrier for drug delivery since only a small percentage of the applied drug can penetrate.[3] To overcome low uptake rates, nano particulate systems are developed. Lipid based nanopraticles not only enhance skin absorption but also can allow drug targeting to the skin layers. Solid lipid nanoparticles (SLNs) are one of the main subclasses of lipid based nanocarriers which attracted major attention in dermal drug delivery.[4] SLNs are colloidal carriers developed in 1991 as an alternative to traditional colloidal carriers, such as emulsions, liposomes, and polymeric micro- and nanoparticles, to overcome their drawbacks by protecting the incorporated drug against degradation and providing size stability during storage time, biocompatibility and biodegradability, respectively.[5] Additionally, SLNs show many other advantages, such as control and target drug release, easy scale up, enhanced bioavailability of entrapped bioactive compounds, composition of physiological compounds or toxicologically-acceptable compounds, and avoidance of organic solvents.[6,7] During the past few years, SLNs have been used for the topical application of various drugs, such as anti-inflammatory and antifungal drugs, isotretinoin, podophyllotoxin, vitamin A, and many others. SLNs also represent a promising carrier system for cosmetic active ingredients because of their numerous advantages over existing conventional formulations.[8-11] There are different approaches to modulating the penetration of active ingredients into the skin. In general, increased penetration is desirable in cases of pharmaceutical purposes, either accumulation of drug in the upper skin layer for local treatment or to achieve permeation of the skin leading to systemic

***Corresponding author:** Hamed Hamishehkar, Email: Hamishehkarh@tbzmed.ac.ir absorption. However, for cosmetic actives, penetration only to a limited degree is desired to prevent any pharmaceutical effects. Therefore, depending on the purpose of the topical formulation, different requirements might be fulfilled by dermal formulations.[12-14] The degree to which active ingredients penetrate the skin from topically-applied formulations depends on many factors, e.g., the physicochemical properties of the active compound, the physical state of the SC, and the nature of the carrier (e.g., polarity of the solvent and particle size). It is assumed that a decrease in particle size will cause an increase in the amount of drug found in the deeper skin strata. The number of studies investigating how particle size on its own affects delivery and absorption of a drug substance into the skin is insufficient, and the results are controversial.[15-18] The current study investigated and compared the influence of particle size on penetration depth of SLNs into different skin layers.

Materials and Methods

Materials

Precirol® ATO5 was purchased from Gattefossé Company (Lyon, France). Span® 80 was obtained from BDH Laboratory (Cambridge, England). Poloxamer® 407 was supplied from *Sigma*-Aldrich Company (Darmstadt, *Germany*). Rhodamine B was obtained from Merck Chemicals Company (Darmstadt, Germany). Chloroform (Dae-Junge, Korea), methanol (Caledon, Canada) and diethyl ether (KianKaveh Pharmaceutical and Chemical Company, Tehran, Iran) were used as received. All chemicals were pharmaceutical grade and used without further modification. All solutions were prepared with deionized water.

Preparations of Rhodamine B-loaded SLN

SLNs were prepared by the hot melt homogenization method. The primary goal in the first step of SLN production is to prepare a nanoemulsion from molten solid lipid. Briefly, 2 g of solid lipid, Precirol was melted at about 70 °C and Span® 80, as an oil phase surfactant, was added to the melted lipid phase. Subsequently, Rhodamine B was dissolved in water and added dropwise into the oil phase under stirring at different stirring rates by homogenizer (DIAX 900, Heidolph, Germany) for different time to prepare SLNs in different sizes (Table 1). Finally, aqueous phase (Poloxamer 3% w/v) was dropped into the oil phase, keeping the temperature at 70 °C under homogenization to prepare an oil in water nanoemulsion. Rhodamine B-loaded SLNs (0.004 %) were obtained by allowing the hot nanoemulsion to cool down at room temperature.[4] The Rhodamine B aqueous solution (Poloxamer 3% w/v) in the same concentration of SLNs formulation dispersion was used as control. Formulations was used for skin penetration experiments within one month after preparation since our experiments showed size stability of SLNs at least for one month.

Table 1. Particle size distribution parameters of prepared solid lipid nanoparticles

Formulation	Modal D (nm)	MVD* (nm)	$D_{10\%}$**(nm)	$D_{50\%}$**(nm)	$D_{90\%}$** (nm)
SLN 1	77	77	53	77	117
SLN 2	330	329	231	330	455
SLN 3	962	932	588	962	1628

*MVD: Mean Volume Diameter

**$D_{10\%}$, $D_{50\%}$ and $D_{90\%}$ are the equivalent volume diameter at 10%, 50% and 90% cumulative volume, respectively.

Characterization of Rhodamine B-loaded SLN

Particle size was analyzed by laser diffraction method using particle size analyzer (SALD 2101, Shimadzu, Japan) which provides information about the mean diameter of the bulk population based on the volume mean diameter (VMD). Prior to measurement, SLN formulation samples were diluted with double-distilled water. Each sample was measured in triplicate. Zeta potential of prepared SLN formulations were analyzed by a Malvern zeta analyzer (Nano ZS, Malvern, UK).[19,20] The loading capacity percent (LC%) was expressed as the percentage of entrapped Rhodamine B to the lipid. The amount of loaded Rhodamine B was determined by first separation of the un-entrapped Rhodamine B by centrifugation method using of Amicon® Ultra-15 with molecular weight cutoff of 100 kDa (Millipore, Germany) tube. The formulation was added to the upper chamber of the Amicon® tube and then the tube was centrifuged (Sigma 3K30, Germany) at 5000 rpm for 5 minutes and then the concentration of free Rhodamine B in the lower chamber of Amicon® tube was measured using UV/Visible spectrophotometer (Shimadzu-1601, Japan) (λ_{max} = 260 nm, linear in the range of 2-30 µg/mL with R2=0.998) and mathematically calculated according to the following equation:

$$LC(\%) = \frac{W_{(Encapsulated\ drug)}}{W_{(Total\ lipid)}} \times 100$$

$W_{(Encapsulated\ drug)}$ is the amount of loaded Rhodamine B and $W_{(Total\ lipid)}$ is the amount of used lipid in the preparation process. The formulations in the upper chamber of Amicon® tube were rinsed five times by aqueous solution to eliminate unloaded Rhodamine B. These rinsed formulations were used for the rest experiments.[21,22]

In vivo skin penetration study

Male Wistar rats (weighing 200–250 g) were obtained from Pasteur Institute (Tehran, Iran), housed in animal facilities of the Drug Applied Research Center (Tabriz University of Medical Science) and used for skin permeation and drug deposition studies. All animal experiments were conducted according to the Guide for Care and Use of Laboratory Animals of Tabriz University of Medical Sciences, Tabriz-Iran (National Institutes of Health Publication No 85-23, revised 1985). The abdominal full thickness skin was carefully and mildy shaved using an electric razor in a way to avoid stratum corneum damage. 200 μL of the each formulations with different size was applied on the skin surface and after 0.5, 3, 6 and 24 h exposure, rats were sacrified with excess ether inhalation and the exposed skin was cut into 1.5×1.5 cm^2 pieces and rinsed with distilled water. Each set of experiments was performed in triplicate. Aqueous solution of Rhodamine B was also used as control. Skins were cut into vertical slices with 20 μm thickness by a freeze microtome and slices were stored at 4 °C and analyzed within 24 h. The skin slices were investigated under both normal light and fluorescence microscopes. The images were taken from normal light and fluorescence microscope of the same area and the dye distribution in the skin was evaluated qualitatively.[4]

Results and Discussion

Rhodamine B was properly loaded into SLN formulations in LC percentages ranging 45% to 56%. 56%. Rhodamine B in higher and lower amounts than the previously investigated dose (0.004%) were prepared and applied to the skin. The concentrated formulations illustrated much more color intensity than the diluted ones which did not provide sufficient color strength to allow nanoparticle tracking (data not shown). The mean particle size of lipid nanoparticles usually depends on several factors, such as type and concentration of lipid surfactants and the viscosity in lipid phases.[4] To avoid interfering with other effective parameters in skin penetration, the total amounts of lipid phase and surfactant were kept constant. The speed of homogenizer and the process time were changed to provide three SLN formulations with distinctly different submicron particle sizes. Table 1 illustrates the size characteristics of Rhodamine B-loaded SLN formulations. Figure 1 indicates that the fabricated SLN formulations had distinct size ranges which allowed for an accurate investigation of the impact of different submicron sizes on the skin penetration of SLNs.

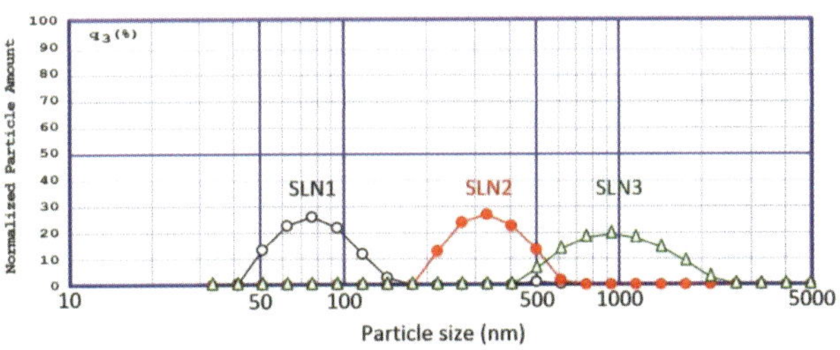

Figure 1. Particle size distribution pattern of SLN1, SLN2 and SLN3 formulations.

Figure 2 shows the skin penetration capability of Rhodamine B solely in the solution state 0.5, 3, 6, and 24 h after administration onto the skin. The results indicated that, although the physicochemical characteristics of Rhodamine B (MW of 422 and Log P of 1.95) are suitable for skin penetration (MW<500 and Log P 1-4),[23,24] no evidence of skin penetration by Rhodamin B was observed even after 6 and 24 h (Figure 2). A minor penetration of Rhodamine B solution may have occurred because of close contact with superficial junctions of the SC and furrows between the corneocytes islands and hair follicles, allowing the superficial spreading of active agents.[11,25]

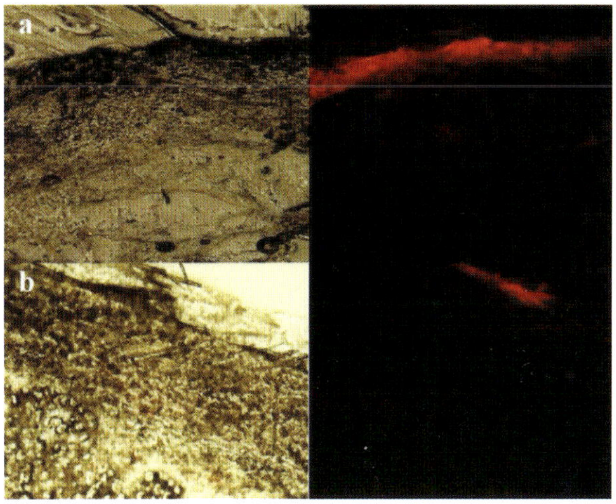

Figure 2. Fluorescence and normal light microscopes images of Rhodamin B solution 6 h (a) and (b) 24 h after application on rat skin.

Figures 3, 4, and 5 show the normal light and fluorescence imaging microscopies of formulations SLN1, SLN2, and SLN3, respectively. To evaluate the rate of penetration, the distribution pattern of Rhodamine B was explored 0.5, 3, 6, and 24 h after the SLN formulation was administered onto the skin. The impact of SLN size on skin penetration was assessed by the results reported in Figures 3-5. The comparison of Figures 3a-5a indicated that only SLN1 could pass SC mainly through hair follicles (shown by circles in Figure 3a). Therefore, the sub-100 nm size range is crucial for the onset of action in dermal drug delivery. One characteristic that makes nanoparticles interesting for topical application is their tendency to diffuse and accumulate in hair follicles. The particles can aggregate in the follicular opening and penetrate along the follicular dug when applied onto the skin surface.[26,27] It has been shown that nanoparticles preferentially permeate into the follicles, but not the SC, enabling high accumulation within the follicular reservoir.[17,28] Correspondingly, the comparison of Figures 3c, d - 5c, d indicated that larger SLN particles (SLN2 and SLN3) could not penetrate into deep layers of skin even after 6 and 24 h. Only the SLN in the mid-size range (SLN2) could penetrate the upper skin layers (Figure 4b). SLN1 could penetrate into lower skin layers after 24 h (Figure 3d) as depicted by arrows. Figures 3b and 3d illustrate that hair follicles provided the most important and dominant penetration route of SLNs.

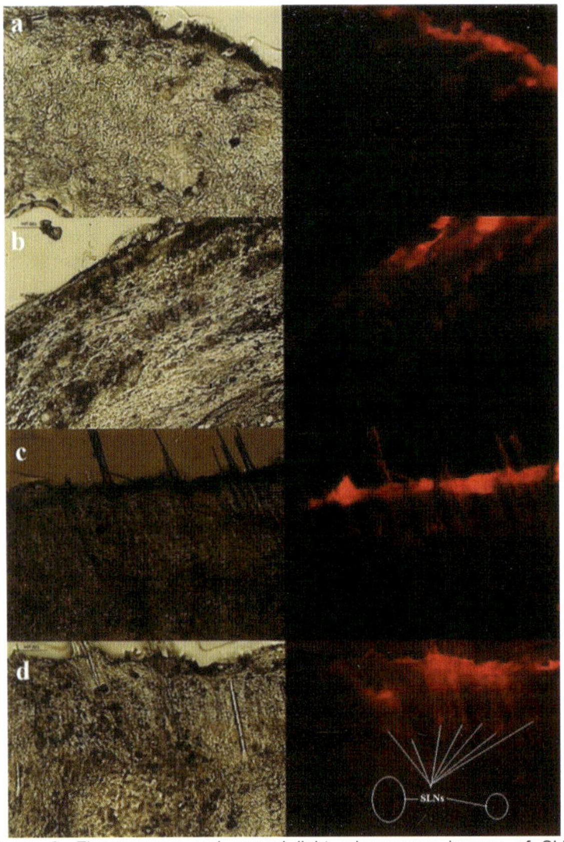

Figure 3. Fluorescence and normal light microscopes images of SLN1 formulation 0.5 h (a), 3 h (b), 6 h (c) and (d) 24 h after application on rat skin.

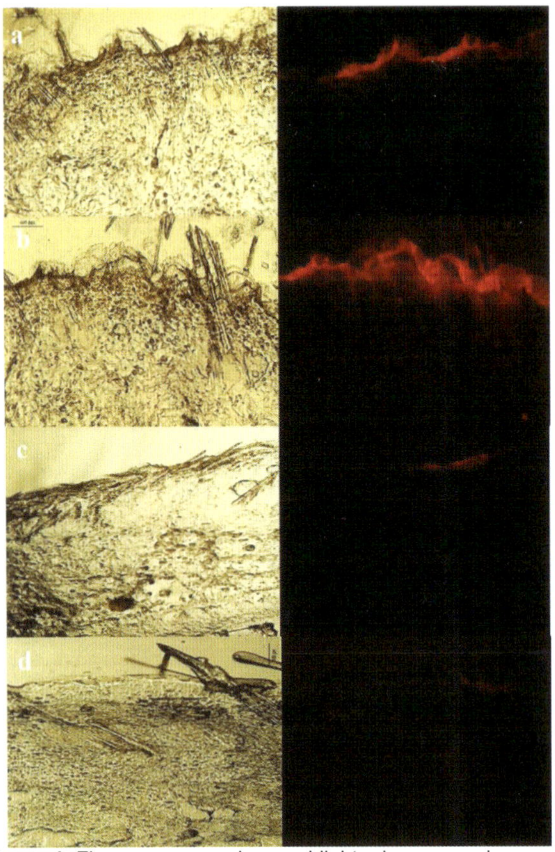

Figure 4. Fluorescence and normal light microscopes images of SLN2 formulation 0.5 h (a), 3 h (b), 6 h (c) and (d) 24 h after application on rat skin.

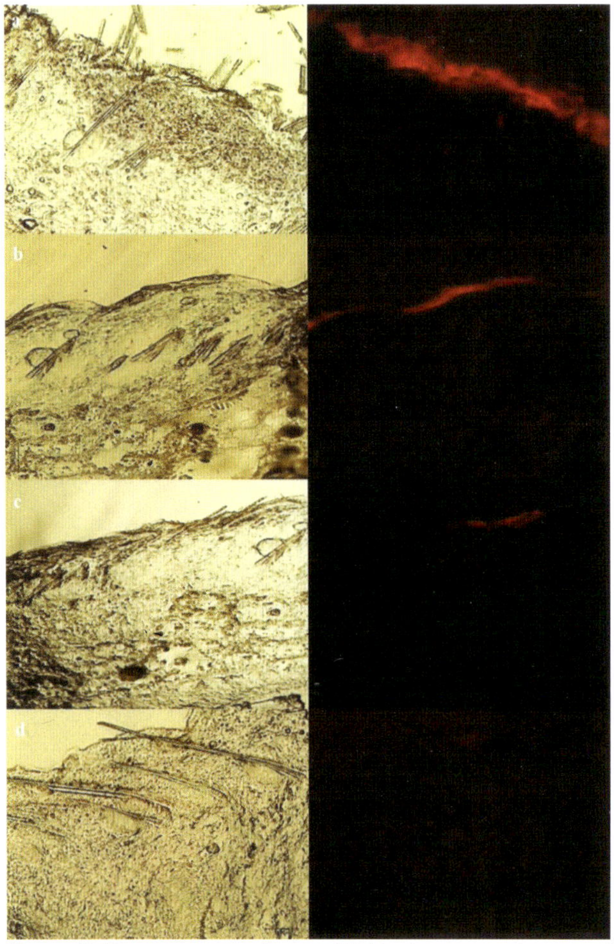

Figure 5. Fluorescence and normal light microscopes images of SLN3 formulation 0.5 h (a), 3 h (b), 6 h (c) and (d) 24 h after application on rat skin.

It has been reported that SLNs approximately 260 nm in size were able to penetrate into the deeper layers of the skin and preferentially accumulate in hair follicles.[16] Other studies have also reported that hair follicles serve as long-term reservoirs for topically-applied drug substances, storing them for up to 10 days, which is ten times longer than the reservoir of the SC.[29] The findings of the current study showed that sizes under 100 nm are in the appropriate size range for deep skin penetration. This result contradicts the report of Patzelt et al., which showed that reductions in particle size (643 nm, 470 nm, 300 nm, 122 nm) led to a significant reduction in particle penetration depth.[30] In support of the current findings, Abddel Mottaleb et al. reported results indicating that the follicular penetration of nanoparticles increases following a decrease in size.[31]

Conclusion

Skin is a widely-used route of delivery for various local and systemic drugs. It provides a natural physical barrier against particle penetration, but there are opportunities to deliver therapeutic nanoparticles. Most drug delivery particle technologies are based on lipid carriers, i.e. SLNs. It has already been shown for various drugs that topical formulations containing lipid nanoparticles can enhance penetration into the skin, thus increasing treatment efficiency, target the epidermis, and reduce systemic absorption and side effects. In the present study, the HMH method was used to prepare Rhodamine B-loaded SLNs with identical compositions and different submicron sizes. The findings concluded that sub-100 nm SLNs can efficiently penetrate into deep layers of skin mostly via hair follicles. In conclusion, nanoparticle size appears to be of major relevance for the enhancement of depth and rate of skin penetration by substances. The suitable mechanism for skin targeting still needs further study. Furthermore, a better understanding of how lipid nanoparticles modify drug penetration into the skin, how lipid particles interact with the lipids of the stratum corneum, and finally how they affect drug penetration is necessary.

Acknowledgments
The authors would like to thank Drug Applied Research Center, Tabriz University of Medical Sciences for financial support. This article is based on a thesis submitted for Pharm D degree (No. 3773) in Faculty of Pharmacy, Tabriz University of Medical Sciences.

Ethical Issues
Not applicable.

Conflict of Interest
The authors report no conflicts of interest.

References
1. Ghanbarzadeh S, Arami S. Formulation and evaluation of piroxicam transferosomal gel: An approach for penetration enhancement. *J Drug Deliv Sci Technol* 2013;23(6):587-90. doi:10.1016/S1773-2247(13)50089-X
2. Ghanbarzadeh S, Khorrami A, Arami S. Preparation of optimized naproxen nano liposomes using response surface methodology. *J Pharm Invest* 2014;44(1):33-9. doi: 10.1007/s40005-013-0098-8
3. Hamishehkar H, Shokri J, Fallahi S, Jahangiri A, Ghanbarzadeh S, Kouhsoltani M. Histopathological evaluation of caffeine-loaded solid lipid nanoparticles in efficient treatment of cellulite. *Drug Dev Ind Pharm* 2015;41(10):1640-6. doi: 10.3109/03639045.2014.980426
4. Hamishehkar H, Ghanbarzadeh S, Sepehran S, Javadzadeh Y, Adib ZM, Kouhsoltani M. Histological assessment of follicular delivery of flutamide by solid lipid nanoparticles: Potential tool for the treatment of androgenic alopecia. *Drug Dev Ind Pharm* 2015:1-8. doi: 10.3109/03639045.2015.1062896
5. Ezzati Nazhad Dolatabadi J, Valizadeh H, Hamishehkar H. Solid lipid nanoparticles as efficient drug and gene delivery systems: Recent breakthroughs. *Adv pharm Bull* 2015;5(2):151-9. doi: 10.15171/apb.2015.022
6. Muller RH, Mader K, Gohla S. Solid lipid nanoparticles (sln) for controlled drug delivery - a review of the state of the art. *Eur J Pharm Biopharm* 2000;50(1):161-77.
7. Pardeike J, Hommoss A, Muller RH. Lipid nanoparticles (sln, nlc) in cosmetic and pharmaceutical dermal products. *Int J Pharm* 2009;366(1-2):170-84. doi: 10.1016/j.ijpharm.2008.10.003
8. Mandawgade SD, Patravale VB. Development of slns from natural lipids: Application to topical delivery of tretinoin. *Int J Pharm* 2008;363(1-2):132-8. doi: 10.1016/j.ijpharm.2008.06.028
9. Kuchler S, Herrmann W, Panek-Minkin G, Blaschke T, Zoschke C, Kramer KD, et al. Sln for topical application in skin diseases--characterization of drug-carrier and carrier-target interactions. *Int J Pharm* 2010;390(2):225-33. doi: 10.1016/j.ijpharm.2010.02.004
10. Jenning V, Schafer-Korting M, Gohla S. Vitamin a-loaded solid lipid nanoparticles for topical use: Drug release properties. *J Control Release* 2000;66(2-3):115-26.
11. Schafer-Korting M, Mehnert W, Korting HC. Lipid nanoparticles for improved topical application of drugs for skin diseases. *Adv Drug Deliv Rev* 2007;59(6):427-43. doi: 10.1016/j.addr.2007.04.006
12. Prausnitz MR, Langer R. Transdermal drug delivery. *Nat Biotechnol* 2008;26(11):1261-8. doi: 10.1038/nbt.1504
13. Schreier H, Bouwstra J. Liposomes and niosomes as topical drug carriers: Dermal and transdermal drug delivery. *J Controlled Release* 1994;30(1):1-15. doi: 10.1016/0168-3659(94)90039-6
14. Ghanbarzadeh S, Khorrami A, Arami S. Nonionic surfactant-based vesicular system for transdermal drug delivery. *Drug Deliv* 2015;22(8):1071-7. doi: 10.3109/10717544.2013.873837
15. Verma DD, Verma S, Blume G, Fahr A. Particle size of liposomes influences dermal delivery of substances into skin. *Int J Pharm* 2003;258(1-2):141-51.
16. Jenning V, Gysler A, Schafer-Korting M, Gohla SH. Vitamin a loaded solid lipid nanoparticles for topical use: Occlusive properties and drug targeting to the upper skin. *Eur J Pharm Biopharm* 2000;49(3):211-8.
17. Lademann J, Richter H, Teichmann A, Otberg N, Blume-Peytavi U, Luengo J, et al. Nanoparticles--an efficient carrier for drug delivery into the hair follicles. *Eur J Pharm Biopharm* 2007;66(2):159-64. doi: 10.1016/j.ejpb.2006.10.019
18. Gamer AO, Leibold E, van Ravenzwaay B. The in vitro absorption of microfine zinc oxide and titanium dioxide through porcine skin. *Toxicol In Vitro* 2006;20(3):301-7. doi: 10.1016/j.tiv.2005.08.008
19. Ghaderi S, Ghanbarzadeh S, Mohammadhassani Z, Hamishehkar H. Formulation of gammaoryzanol-loaded nanoparticles for potential application in

fortifying food products. *Adv Pharm Bull* 2014;4(Suppl 2):549-54. doi: 10.5681/apb.2014.081
20. Ghanbarzadeh S, Arami S, Pourmoazzen Z, Khorrami A. Improvement of the antiproliferative effect of rapamycin on tumor cell lines by poly (monomethylitaconate)-based ph-sensitive, plasma stable liposomes. *Colloids Surf B Biointerfaces* 2014;115:323-30. doi: 10.1016/j.colsurfb.2013.12.024
21. Ghaderi S, Ghanbarzadeh S, Hamishehkar H. Evaluation of different methods for preparing nanoparticle containing gammaoryzanol for potential use in food fortification. *Pharm Sci* 2015;20:130-4.
22. Rasaee S, Ghanbarzadeh S, Mohammadi M, Hamishehkar H. Nano phytosomes of quercetin: A promising formulation for fortification of food products with antioxidants. *Pharm Sci* 2014;20(3):96-101.
23. Kang L, Yap CW, Lim PF, Chen YZ, Ho PC, Chan YW, et al. Formulation development of transdermal dosage forms: Quantitative structure-activity relationship model for predicting activities of terpenes that enhance drug penetration through human skin. *J Control Release* 2007;120(3):211-9. doi: 10.1016/j.jconrel.2007.05.006
24. Cronin MT, Dearden JC, Moss GP, Murray-Dickson G. Investigation of the mechanism of flux across human skin in vitro by quantitative structure-permeability relationships. *Eur J Pharm Sci* 1999;7(4):325-30.
25. Fang CL, Aljuffali IA, Li YC, Fang JY. Delivery and targeting of nanoparticles into hair follicles. *Ther Deliv* 2014;5(9):991-1006. doi: 10.4155/tde.14.61
26. Dokka S, Cooper SR, Kelly S, Hardee GE, Karras JG. Dermal delivery of topically applied oligonucleotides via follicular transport in mouse skin. *J Invest Dermatol* 2005;124(5):971-5. doi: 10.1111/j.0022-202X.2005.23672.x
27. Otberg N, Teichmann A, Rasuljev U, Sinkgraven R, Sterry W, Lademann J. Follicular penetration of topically applied caffeine via a shampoo formulation. *Skin Pharmacol Physiol* 2007;20(4):195-8. doi: 10.1159/000101389
28. Teichmann A, Jacobi U, Ossadnik M, Richter H, Koch S, Sterry W, et al. Differential stripping: Determination of the amount of topically applied substances penetrated into the hair follicles. *J Invest Dermatol* 2005;125(2):264-9. doi: 10.1111/j.0022-202X.2005.23779.x
29. Lademann J, Richter H, Schaefer UF, Blume-Peytavi U, Teichmann A, Otberg N, et al. Hair follicles - a long-term reservoir for drug delivery. *Skin Pharmacol Physiol* 2006;19(4):232-6. doi: 10.1159/000093119
30. Patzelt A, Richter H, Knorr F, Schafer U, Lehr CM, Dahne L, et al. Selective follicular targeting by modification of the particle sizes. *J Control Release* 2011;150(1):45-8. doi: 10.1016/j.jconrel.2010.11.015
31. Abdel-Mottaleb MM, Mortada ND, El-Shamy AA, Awad GA. Physically cross-linked polyvinyl alcohol for the topical delivery of fluconazole. *Drug Dev Ind Pharm* 2009;35(3):311-20. doi: 10.1080/03639040802325893

Evaluating Adherence of Health-Care Team to Standard Guideline of Colistin Use at Intensive Care Units of a Referral Hospital in Shiraz, Southwest of Iran

Afsaneh Vazin, Iman Karimzadeh*, Atiyeh Zand, Nazafarin Hatami-Mazinani, Dena Firouzabadi

Department of Clinical Pharmacy, Faculty of Pharmacy, Shiraz University of Medical Sciences, Shiraz, Iran.

Keywords:
- Colistin guideline
- Adherence
- Clinical Pharmacist
- Intensive care unit

Abstract

Purpose: To evaluate colistin use according to global standard drug consumption in intensive care units of a referral hospital in Shiraz, Iran

Methods: A prospective, interventional study was performed during an 11 month period on 100 patients admitted to ICUs of a teaching hospital being treated with colistin for at least 3 subsequent doses. Required demographic, clinical, and paraclinical data were gathered by a pharmacist. Fifteen indexes were considered to evaluate colistin use. A clinical pharmacist reviewed indication and dose of colistin at the time of prescribing this agent.

Results: In our study population, pneumonia (69%) was the main indication of colistin. In 87% of patients, colistin administration was based on microbiological laboratory evidence. Continuation of therapy was inappropriate in 5% of cases. By the intervention of the clinical pharmacist, colistin was discontinued in all patients in whom empirical therapy was continued incorrectly. None of the patients received loading dose of colistin. The maintenance dose, dose interval, and duration of treatment of colistin were appropriate in 76%, 71%, and 100% of patients, respectively. For none of the patients, the pharmacokinetic dosing method was used. In all patients, serum creatinine and WBC count were evaluated on daily basis. The sum indexes of colistin use were relevant to standard guidelines in 67.33% of the cases.

Conclusion: The results of this study highlight the necessity of the pharmaceutical care team participation in all stages of treatment with antibiotics. After pharmacist interventions, some criteria of colistin utilization were corrected and brought closer to standard values.

Introduction

Acinetobacter is a non-fermentative gram negative coccobacilli with high capability for colonization in human body.[1] *Acinetobacter baumannii* is an invasive and resistant microorganism existing in immunosuppressed patients such as Intensive Care Unit (ICU) patients on mechanical ventilation.[2] *A. baumannii* infection has become a clinical concern due to its ability to produce wide spectrum antibiotic resistance, either intrinsic or acquired.[3]

Colistin was derived from a microorganism named *Bacillus polymyxa*, a Colistinus subspecies. It was first used to treat patients infected with gram negative microorganisms in 1959.[4-6] The most important adverse effects of colistin, when given intravenously, are renal and neurological toxicities.[7] In some patients, allergic reactions, gastrointestinal events, and pulmonary toxicities have been also reported.[8] Later, by the introduction of more available and less toxic antibiotics such as aminoglycosides, the rate of colistin usage was decreased. Unfortunately, by the increase in the prevalence of multiple drug-resistant (MDR) hospital-acquired infections, use of colistin has been risen once again.[9]

Adverse effects, drug resistance, the outburst of MDR organisms, and serious pressure on limited medication costs are the major complications of antibiotic misuse.[10,11] Drug use evaluations (DUE) are administrative approaches to both improve the pattern of use and reduce the cost of medications. Programs evaluating the use of drugs are structural, innovative and progressive in which they determine a drug's pattern of consumption in different situations and diseases and its goal is to reduce inappropriate medication administration, enhancing medication effectiveness, and reducing medication costs.[12,13]

To the best of our knowledge, no study has been done on the DUE of colistin so far. For the first time, we decided to evaluate colistin use pattern according to global standards in the ICUs of a referral hospital in Iran. Beside that, interventions of a clinical pharmacist in detecting and correcting inappropriate dose and indication of colistin in the same settings were also studied.

***Corresponding author:** Iman Karimzadeh, Email: karimzadee@sums.ac.ir

Materials and Methods

Study setting

A prospective, interventional study was performed during an 11 month period from December 2014 to September 2015 on patients admitted to 4 internal, general, central, and emergency ICUs of Nemazee hospital, a general multispecialty, referral, tertiary health-care setting, affiliated to Shiraz University of Medical Sciences, Shiraz, Iran. The Institutional Review Board and the Medical Ethics Committee of the hospital approved the study.

Study population

All patients being treated with colistin that received at least 3 subsequent doses of the antibiotic were included in this study. Patients received less than three doses of colistin, due to any reason such as ward transfer, hospital discharge, or death were excluded from the study.

Data collection

Data gathering was done by a general pharmacist under the supervision of a senior clinical pharmacy attending. Demographic data including age, sex, height, and total body weight were collected and the patient's ideal body weight was calculated accordingly. The patient's medical history, diagnosis, reason for patient's referral to the ward, final diagnosis, pre-existing medical conditions, and whether the patient's infection was acquired from community or hospital, were all recorded. Laboratory data consisting microbiological culture, hematologic parameters including white blood cell (WBC), biochemical data including blood urea nitrogen (BUN), serum creatinine, and immunologic factors (procalcitonin, c-reactive protein [CRP]) were also recorded before and during the course of colistin treatment. To evaluate colistin use compared to available guidelines and recommendations, fifteen indexes were taken into account. Each index was scored as either 0 or 1.

These items were as follow: 1) indication, 2) preparation and dilution, 3) administration route, 4) duration of each infusion, 5) administration of loading dose, 6) daily dose, 7) administration intervals, 8) duration of treatment according to isolated pathogen, 9) evaluation of the microbiological culture before prescription, 10) evaluation of microbiological culture 48-72 hours after administration, 11) considering the patient's BUN and creatinine before prescribing, 12) monitoring serum creatinine level periodically during the treatment, 13) reducing the dose or discontinuation in patients who developed colistin nephrotoxicity (defined by a rise in serum creatinine of more than 0.3 mg/dl within 48 hours or a 1.5 folds increase compared to baseline values within 7 days, or a decrease in urine volume to less than 0.5 ml/kg/h for more than 6 hours), 14) re-evaluation of dosing if needed (in cases of change in serum creatinine or partial clinical response), and 15) the presence of a moderate or major interaction between colistin and other co-administered medications identified by the Lexi-Interact online version. In addition to the above indexes, the patients were also monitored for probable adverse effects of colistin.[14]

Concurrent with the screening phase of the study, the drug and therapeutic committee of the hospital was committed a clinical pharmacist to review and verify colistin orders regarding indication and dose in the studied ICUs at the time of initiating this agent. In the case of unnecessary indication or inappropriate dose, the clinical pharmacist gave his corrective suggestions.

Statistical analyses

Continuous and categorical variables were expressed as mean ± standard deviation (SD) and percentage, respectively. Descriptive analyses were carried out by the Statistical Package for the Social Sciences (SPSS) version 20 software (IBM company, New York, NY, United States).

Results

During the study period, a total of 126 patients were primarily screened. Among them, 100 were eligible to be included in the study. Forty three percent, 21%, 19%, 17% of the study populations were admitted to the internal, general, central, and emergency ICUs, respectively. The causes of patient drop out from the study were as follows: death (71%), transfer to other wards (23%), and early discontinuation of colistin (11%). Demographic data of patients have been demonstrated in Table 1. Their mean ± SD age was 56.70 ± 18.18 years. Sixty four percent of the cohort was male.

Table1. Demographic and clinical characteristics of the study population (n = 100)

Demographic and clinical data		Value
Age (year)	Mean ± SD	56.70 ± 18.18
	Range	22-96
	Sex, Male/Female ratio	64/36
Weight (Kg)	Mean ± SD	68.05 ± 12.61
	Range	45-95
Height (Cm)	Mean ± SD	167.36 ± 8.76
	Range	150-190
Ideal body weight (Kg)	Mean ± SD	62.4 ± 9.78
	Range	45.5-84
Infection, n (%)	Pneumonia	69 (69)
	Sepsis	14 (14)
	Wound infection	9 (9)
	Urinary tract infection	5(5)
	Pericarditis	3 (3)
Infection type, n (%)	Community acquired	3 (3)
	Hospital acquired	97 (97)

Colistin indication for each patient has been listed in Table 2. Ventilator associated pneumonia (69%) was the most common indication of colistin followed by sepsis (14%), and skin/soft tissue infection (9%). Regarding source of infection, 97% were categorized as hospital acquired. Colistin treatment in 87% cases was based on the microbiological culture data (definite therapy) and the remaining (13%) were classified as an empiric. Considering the involved organism, most (78%) cases were *Acinetobacter* spp. followed by *Klebsiella* spp. (16%) and *Pseudomonas* spp. or *Escherichia coli* (6%).

Table 2. Colistin indications in the study population (n = 100)

Indication	N (%)
Pneumonia	69 (69)
Sepsis	14 (14)
Skin/soft tissue infection	9 (9)
Urinary tract infection	5 (5)
Peritonitis	3 (3)

Colistin was administered as an intravenous infusion in all patients. Its route of administration was correct in 100% of patients. In 39% of the cases, the methods of preparation and dilution were correct. Duration of infusion was correct in 65% of patients and in the remaining 35%, it was less than 30 minutes. The mean ± SD duration of colistin therapy was 15.61 ± 11.55 days. Treatment duration of colistin ranged between 2 and 21 days. The administration time interval and duration of treatment were correct in 71% and 84% of patients, respectively.

The pharmacokinetic dosing method was used for no patients. Seventy six percent of the administered doses at the beginning of the treatment were appropriate. Among inappropriate initial doses, 22% and 2% were lower and higher than those recommended, respectively. Loading dose was not administered for any of the patients during the study period. Colistin maintenance dose was appropriate in 76% of cases during the treatment course. In 13% of patients in whom colistin was started empirically, continuation of therapy was inappropriate in 5% of cases. Colistin was discontinued in all these patients after the clinical pharmacist's intervention. Among cases of definite therapy, the isolated pathogen was sensitive to other antibiotics rather than colistin (7%). In most of the patients (94%), no data regarding microbiological culture had been provided 48-72 hours after initiating therapy with colistin. The acceptance rates of physicians about clinical pharmacist interventions regarding colistin indication and dose were 100% and 89%, respectively.

In all patients, WBC count was done daily from the first to last day of colistin treatment. At the first day of colistin administration, WBC count of 57% of the study population was more than 10,000/μl. In contrast, only 31% of the cohort had WBC counts above 10,000/μl at the end of colistin treatment. Microbiological culture and decision making accordingly were done for 61% of the patients. In more than half (54%) and one-third (36%) of the cohort, CRP and body temperature were considered as indexes of colistin treatment response. Other factors such as serum procalcitonin were also taken into account in 9% of the cases.

In all patients, serum creatinine was evaluated on daily basis. In 91% of the patients, the first dose of colistin was adjusted according to the patient's serum creatinine and BUN. In 45% of the patients who developed nephrotoxicity, no action was taken; However in the remaining 55%, the time intervals of colistin administration were increased. For 39% of the patients, re-evaluation of colistin dose had to be made according to relevant serum creatinine. But no dose adjustment had been done for 51% of these patients. According to the fact that our study population was all critically ill patients with poor conditions and on the other hand, they were received sedative medications, evaluating the neurologic toxic effects of colistin was not feasible. Allergic reactions to colistin were not seen in any patient.

In 29% of the patients, a level D potential drug interaction (according to Lexi-Interact definition) with colistin was identified. These drug-drug interactions have been brought in Table 3. No drug interaction level X was identified.

Table 3. Type, probable mechanism, severity, and frequency of moderate and major potential drug interactions of colistin with co-administered medications in the study population (n = 100)

Drug-drug interaction	Probable mechanism	Severity	Percentage
Colistin + Vancomycin	Vancomycin may enhance the nephrotoxic effects of colistin	Moderate	51.7
Colistin + Amphotericin B	Amphotericin B may enhance the nephrotoxic effects of colistin	Moderate	31
Colistin + Aminoglycosides	Aminoglycosides may enhance the nephrotoxic effects of colistin	Moderate	24.1
Colistin + Atracurium	Atracurium may enhance the neurotoxic effects of colistin	Moderate	3.4

Table 4 has summarized the 15 studied indexes of colistin use in our cohort. The mean ± SD score of colistin use indexes in the study population was 10.1 ±1.72. In other words, the sum indexes of colistin use were in accordance to standard guidelines in 67.33% of the cases.

Table 4. Fifteen indexes of colistin use in the study population (n = 100)

No	Index	Appropriate/Performed, percent	Inappropriate/Not performed, percent
1	Indication	88	12
2	Method of preparation and dilution	39	61
3	Administration route	100	0
4	Duration of each infusion	65	35
5	Administration of a loading dose	0	100
6	Maintenance daily dose	76	24
7	Administration time interval	71	29
8	Duration of treatment	84	16
9	Evaluation of the microbiological culture before prescription	87	13
10	Evaluation of microbiological culture 48-72 hours after administration	6	94
11	Considering the patient's renal function before prescribing	91	9
12	Monitoring serum creatinine level periodically during the treatment	100	0
13	Reducing the dose or discontinuation in patients who developed colistin nephrotoxicity	55	45
14	Re-evaluation of dosing if needed	39	51
15	Considering moderate or major interaction between colistin and other co-administered	29	71

Discussion

Due to the fact that antibiotic resistance has become an important issue worldwide and awareness regarding incorrect and excessive antibiotic use in hospitals has become more, most antibiotic stewardship programs have aimed towards limiting the use of these medications. Limiting the use of certain groups of antibiotics can help to achieve this goal.[15] Results of a study in the United States showed that limiting the use of antibiotics has been considered in 56% of the newly published guidelines and also in 81% of medical teaching centers.[9] On the other hand, decreasing hospital acquired infections can lead to less antibiotic use such as colistin, and also reduction in the rate of resistant or MDR microorganisms.

In this study, we evaluated colistin use pattern in 4 ICUs of a referral hospital in Shiraz. Considering the fact that a high percentage of infections originate from hospitals, it is mandatory to implement better policies to prevent hospital acquired infections. The rate of carbapenem resistant *A. baumannii* isolates in Shiraz hospitals is concerning that necessitates taking special measures.[16]

Low rates of colistin-resistant *Acinetobacter* spp. have been reported in Iran.[17] For instance, 1% of *Acinetobacter* spp. isolates were resistant to colistin at Hamedan in 2011-2012, 11.6% at Isfahan in 2011-2012, and 12% at Tehran in 2009-2010. However, more recent studies from other parts of Iran like Tehran, Ahvaz, and Kermanshah have demonstrated that the susceptibility of *Acinetobacter* spp. to colistin has been 100%.[18-22] Similar data have been reported from at least two surveys in Nemazee hospital within 2008-2009 and 2013.[16,23] Therefore, colistin in combination with other appropriate antibiotics can be considered as the last antibacterial drug in the treatment of MDR infections caused by gram negative pathogens in our center.

In our study population, pneumonia was the main indication (about 69% of the cases) of colistin. In 87% of patients, colistin administration was based on microbiological evidence. In contrast, colistin was prescribed empirically in only 13% of the cases. This issue can be justified partially by exploiting carbapenem discs for determining the antimicrobial susceptibilities of *Acinetobacter spp.* according to the last Clinical and Laboratory Standard Institute (CLSI) guideline. This led physicians to choose other antibiotics rather than colistin as their first choice. This action was started from the winter of 2014 in the microbiological laboratory of Nemazee hospital.

By the intervention of pharmaceutical care unit, colistin was discontinued in all patients in whom empirical therapy was continued incorrectly. In a prospective cohort study done by Reina *et al.* on colistin in 2005, 185 patients admitted at the ICU for more than 48 hours and had either *Acinetobacter spp.* or *Pseudomonas aeruginosa* infections, were included. The population was divided into two groups and for 55 of them, colistin and for the remaining 130 individuals, other antibiotics were prescribed. It was demonstrated that inappropriate empirical therapy with colistin was much more common than that with other antibiotics (100% versus 8%, respectively). Interestingly, the cure rate on the 6th day of admission and also death rate were similar in both groups.[24]

A number of studies have demonstrated that physicians have a tendency towards empirical prescription of broad spectrum antibiotics. However, some of these empirical prescriptions have been for the treatment of serious and life-threatening infections. Also in patients with poor condition, use of a great number of broad spectrum antibiotics for a prolonged duration has been implicated.[25] On the other hand, in 7% of our patients that microbiological culture had been done before starting treatment, colistin was prescribed inappropriately and the culture results indicated that patients were sensitive to more available and less toxic antibiotics. In all such cases, colistin was replaced with other appropriate antibiotics such as carbapenems after the clinical pharmacist intervention.

Similar to other antibacterial agents, obtaining a second microbiological culture 48 to 72 hours after the start of colistin therapy has been recommended to evaluate patient response to the treatment. This was done for only 6% of our patients. However, noting that ventilator associated pneumonia (69%) was the most common indication of colistin in our cohort. Obtaining a second microbiological culture 48 to 72 hours after the start of colistin therapy is crucial for evaluating response to treatment in only certain infections such as sepsis.

In our study, colistin was administered only as an intravenous infusion. Duration of colistin infusion has been stated to be at least 30 minutes according to manufacturer package insert. In 65% of our study population, this duration was correct. Reconstitution and dilution of colistin was not done based on reference standards in 61% of cases. Therefore, the concentration of the resulting solution was lower than that was mentioned elsewhere. This medication is commonly available as two parenteral formulations worldwide. European and US products have expressed doses as sodium colisthimetate and colistin base, respectively. Eighty milligram of sodium colisthimetate is almost equivalent to 30 mg of colistin base activity.[26] According to the drug information provided by the United States manufacturers, the recommended maximum daily dose is 10,000,000 IU (800 mg) based on sodium colistimetate that is about two times the maximum dose recommended by the European manufacturers (6,000,000 IU or 480 mg). Unfortunately, most physicians are not aware of such differences and usually use data provided by the United States that recommends dosing according to colistin base. This can lead to the prescription of either higher or lower doses of colistin required and each can lead to toxicity or failure in treatment of the patient, respectively.

Routine monitoring of either serum or plasma concentration of colistin has not been well established yet; however according to drug information provided by the manufacturer, especially in cases in whom treatment failure or toxicity is probable, specifically in neonates and patients with cystic fibrosis, therapeutic drug monitoring (TDM) can be beneficial. Colistin serum concentration was not determined in any of our study population. Since there is the possibility of delayed action of colistin, microbial resistance, treatment failure and rise in mortality, a loading dose of 9,000,000-12,000,000 IU has been suggested.[27] Nevertheless, none of our patients was given the loading dose of colistin. This may be partially due to lack of knowledge of physicians regarding the possibility of administering the loading dose. Another reason might be their concern over developing colistin nephrotoxicity. Lack of sufficient medication available in the Iranian pharmaceutical market can be another reason for this finding in our study.

During the study, nephrotoxicity developed in 31% of the patients. Different definitions have been used for determining colistin nephrotoxicity, but in recent studies as ours, RIFLE criteria have been mostly used.[27,28] In this study, we found out that about two-thirds of the patients that developed nephrotoxicity while being treated with colistin also received other nephrotoxic agents, mainly vancomycin. Incidence of colistin nephrotoxicity was reported to be ranged from zero to 54%. These variations can be due to different criteria used for the definition of nephrotoxicity, different study populations, different clinical status of patients, and the presence of risk factors for nephrotoxicity such as co-administration of nephrotoxic agents.[26]

It has been recommended that serum creatinine should be evaluated regularly during colistin treatment. Similarly, it was done for our cohort. It seems that in the current study setting, serum creatinine was evaluated daily as a routine practice of the wards for all patients received colistin without considering its changing trend. In some cases, colistin nephrotoxicity may appear even after the discontinuation of therapy, but it seems unlikely that this would be the reason for daily serum creatinine monitoring after stopping colistin.

The time interval of colistin administration was increased in about 55% of the patients who developed nephrotoxicity. According to treatment protocols, in the case of rise in patient's serum creatinine during therapy, either dose adjustment or discontinuation of therapy can be considered. Colistin pharmacokinetics has inter-individual and intra-individual variations and therefore requires individualized dosing. Considering this issue, colistin dose adjustment was needed for 39% of our patients. However, it was not performed for 51% of them. This may be due to fact that no attention was paid by the clinicians to dosing concepts according to pharmacokinetic of colistin.

In prescribing antibiotics, different factors such as the selection of the correct dose, correct administration, and the interval between doses are important and some issues such as obtaining culture before antibiotic administration, adverse drug events, TDM, laboratory data, the correct time to give the antibiotic and duration of therapy are other substantial factors that have to be considered.[15] In our cohort, the sum indexes of colistin use were relevant to standard guidelines in 67.33% of the cases. However, this score is not the actual as well as comprehensive index of colistin utilization in our population because scoring all the mentioned indexes for the whole patients was not feasible. In summary, the most important weak points in administering colistin in our cohort were as follows: not administering loading dose, incorrect method of reconstitution and dilution, and lack of dose adjustment in certain conditions. In contrast, positive points of colistin utilization in the study population were the correct route of administration and duration of infusion, serum creatinine monitoring on a daily basis, appropriate indications, obtaining microbiological data before starting therapy, and correct dose as well as interval of administration. Because of relatively small sample size, statistical analyses were not possible and selection of larger sample size can lead to better and more reliable results. The acceptance rate of clinical pharmacist's intervention by physicians was 100% regarding colistin indication. However, regarding dose and time interval of administration with the acceptance rate of 89%, less attention was paid to the clinical pharmacist's comments. This could be due to lack of clinical pharmacist's follow up after the intervention. Therefore, the persistent and regular attendance of pharmacists in daily rounds of the ward can reduce medication errors in the pharmacotherapy processes. Interestingly, the acceptance rate of clinical pharmacist interventions in the current survey was within the range reported from both European (73-89%) and American (85-99%) studies.[29]

Conclusion

Our data demonstrated that different indexes of colistin use were in accordance to standard guidelines in 67.33% of the cases. In addition, after clinical pharmacist interventions, some criteria of colistin utilization regarding dose and indication were corrected and brought closer to standard values. In health-care settings, not enough attention is usually paid to pharmacokinetics of the medication and also its preparation and dilution and also in our case, ignoring loading dose administration especially in critically ill patients. Active and reciprocal collaboration of pharmacists with physicians can help towards improving pattern of use and can hopefully motivate the healthcare group in establishing better policies for antibiotic use.

Acknowledgments

This research was performed by Atieh Zand in partial fulfillment of the requirements for certification as a pharmacist. The present paper was adopted from the proposal number 93-01-05-8461 approved by vice-chancellor for research affairs of Shiraz University of Medical Sciences.

Ethical Issues

The Institutional Review Board and the Medical Ethics Committee of the hospital approved the study.

Conflict of Interest

The authors declare no conflict of interests.

References

1. Obeidat N, Jawdat F, Al-Bakri AG, Shehabi AA. Major biologic characteristics of acinetobacter baumannii isolates from hospital environmental and patients' respiratory tract sources. *Am J Infect Control* 2014;42(4):401-4. doi: 10.1016/j.ajic.2013.10.010
2. Perez F, Hujer AM, Hujer KM, Decker BK, Rather PN, Bonomo RA. Global challenge of multidrug-resistant acinetobacter baumannii. *Antimicrob Agents Chemother* 2007;51(10):3471-84. doi: 10.1128/AAC.01464-06
3. Karageorgopoulos DE, Falagas ME. Current control and treatment of multidrug-resistant acinetobacter baumannii infections. *Lancet Infect Dis* 2008;8(12):751-62. doi: 10.1016/S1473-3099(08)70279-2
4. Koyama Y, Kurosasa A, Tsuchiya A, Takakuta K. A new antibiotic 'colistin'produced by spore-forming soil bacteria. *J Antibiot (Tokyo)* 1950;3:457-8.
5. Kumazawa J, Yagisawa M. The history of antibiotics: The japanese story. *J Infect Chemother* 2002;8(2):125-33. doi: 10.1007/s101560200022
6. Grayson ML, M Crowe SM, McCarthy JS, Mills J, Johan W Mouton JW, et al. *The Use of Antibiotics.* 5th ed. London: Heinemann; 1997.
7. Colistin: An overview. Available from: https://www.uptodate.com/contents/search. Accessed November 3, 2016.
8. Charles F, Lora L, Morton P. Drug Information Handbook, w/International Trade Names Index. Hudson, Ohio: Lexi-Comp; 2011.
9. Shahbazi F, Dashti-Khavidaki S. Colistin: Efficacy and safety in different populations. *Expert Rev Clin Pharmacol* 2015;8(4):423-48. doi: 10.1586/17512433.2015.1053390
10. Arda B, Sipahi OR, Yamazhan T, Tasbakan M, Pullukcu H, Tunger A, et al. Short-term effect of antibiotic control policy on the usage patterns and cost of antimicrobials, mortality, nosocomial infection rates and antibacterial resistance. *J Infect* 2007;55(1):41-8. doi: 10.1016/j.jinf.2007.02.014
11. Garau J. Impact of antibiotic restrictions: The ethical perspective. *Clin Microbiol Infect* 2006;12 Suppl 5:16-24. doi: 10.1111/j.1469-0691.2006.01527.x
12. Sang-Cheol B. Drug utilization review: economical aspect. *J Korean Med Assoc* 2004;47(2):156-60. doi: 10.5124/jkma.2004.47.2.156
13. World Health Organization. Introduction to drug utilization research. 2003. Available from: http//:apps.who.int/medicinedocs/en/d/Js4876e. Accessed November 3, 2014.
14. Dijkmans AC, Wilms EB, Kamerling IM, Birkhoff W, Ortiz-Zacarias NV, van Nieuwkoop C, et al. Colistin: Revival of an old polymyxin antibiotic. *Ther Drug Monit* 2015;37(4):419-27. doi: 10.1097/FTD.0000000000000172
15. Doron S, Davidson LE. Antimicrobial stewardship. *Mayo Clin Proc* 2011;86(11):1113-23. doi: 10.4065/mcp.2011.0358
16. Kooti S, Motamedifar M, Sarvari J. Antibiotic resistance profile and distribution of oxacillinase genes among clinical isolates of acinetobacter

baumannii in shiraz teaching hospitals, 2012 - 2013. *Jundishapur J Microbiol* 2015;8(8):e20215. doi: 10.5812/jjm.20215v2
17. Karimzadeh I, Sadeghimanesh N, Mirzaee M, Sagheb MM. Evaluating the resistance pattern of gramnegative bacteria during three years at the nephrology ward of a referral hospital in southwest of Iran. *J Nephropathol* 2017;6(3):210-9. doi: 10.15171/jnp.2017.35
18. Safari M, Saidijam M, Bahador A, Jafari R, Alikhani MY. High prevalence of multidrug resistance and metallo-beta-lactamase (mbetal) producing acinetobacter baumannii isolated from patients in icu wards, hamadan, iran. *J Res Health Sci* 2013;13(2):162-7.
19. Shahcheraghi F, Abbasalipour M, Feizabadi M, Ebrahimipour G, Akbari N. Isolation and genetic characterization of metallo-beta-lactamase and carbapenamase producing strains of acinetobacter baumannii from patients at tehran hospitals. *Iran J Microbiol* 2011;3(2):68-74.
20. Karmostaji A, Peerayeh SN, Salmanian AH. Distribution of OXA-type class D β-lactamase genes among nosocomial multi drug resistant Acinetobacter baumannii isolated in Tehran hospitals. *Jundishapur J Microbiol* 2013;6(5):e8219. doi: 10.5812/jjm.8219
21. Shoja S, Moosavian M, Peymani A, Tabatabaiefar MA, Rostami S, Ebrahimi N. Genotyping of carbapenem resistant acinetobacter baumannii isolated from tracheal tube discharge of hospitalized patients in intensive care units, ahvaz, iran. *Iran J Microbiol* 2013;5(4):315-22.
22. Mohajeri P, Farahani A, Feizabadi MM, Ketabi H, Abiri R, Najafi F. Antimicrobial susceptibility profiling and genomic diversity of acinetobacter baumannii isolates: A study in western iran. *Iran J Microbiol* 2013;5(3):195-202.
23. Japoni A, Vazin A, Davarpanah MA, Afkhami Ardakani M, Alborzi A, Japoni S, et al. Ventilator-associated pneumonia in iranian intensive care units. *J Infect Dev Ctries* 2011;5(4):286-93.
24. Reina R, Estenssoro E, Saenz G, Canales HS, Gonzalvo R, Vidal G, et al. Safety and efficacy of colistin in acinetobacter and pseudomonas infections: A prospective cohort study. *Intensive Care Med* 2005;31(8):1058-65. doi: 10.1007/s00134-005-2691-4
25. Cuthbertson BH, Thompson M, Sherry A, Wright MM, Bellingan GJ, Intensive Care S. Antibiotic-treated infections in intensive care patients in the uk. *Anaesthesia* 2004;59(9):885-90. doi: 10.1111/j.1365-2044.2004.03742.x
26. Garonzik SM, Li J, Thamlikitkul V, Paterson DL, Shoham S, Jacob J, et al. Population pharmacokinetics of colistin methanesulfonate and formed colistin in critically ill patients from a multicenter study provide dosing suggestions for various categories of patients. *Antimicrob Agents Chemother* 2011;55(7):3284-94. doi: 10.1128/AAC.01733-10
27. Dalfino L, Puntillo F, Mosca A, Monno R, Spada ML, Coppolecchia S, et al. High-dose, extended-interval colistin administration in critically ill patients: Is this the right dosing strategy? A preliminary study. *Clin Infect Dis* 2012;54(12):1720-6. doi: 10.1093/cid/cis286
28. Ordooei Javan A, Shokouhi S, Sahraei Z. A review on colistin nephrotoxicity. *Eur J Clin Pharmacol* 2015;71(7):801-10. doi: 10.1007/s00228-015-1865-4
29. Khalili H, Karimzadeh I, Mirzabeigi P, Dashti-Khavidaki S. Evaluation of clinical pharmacist's interventions in an infectious diseases ward and impact on patient's direct medication cost. *Eur J Intern Med* 2013;24(3):227-33. doi: 10.1016/j.ejim.2012.11.014

Pharmacokinetic Parameters and Over-Responsiveness of Iranian Population to Propranolol

Ebrahim Salehifar[1]*, Shima Ebrahim[2], Mohammad-Reza Shiran[3], Fatemeh Faramarzi[4], Hossein Askari Rad[5], Razieh Avan[4], Asadollah Mohseni Kiasari[6], Pouneh Ebrahimi[7]

[1] *Pharmaceutical Research Center, Faculty of Pharmacy, Mazandaran University of Medical Sciences, Sari, Iran.*
[2] *Student Research Committee, Faculty of Pharmacy, Mazandaran University of Medical Sciences, Sari, Iran.*
[3] *Immunogenetics Research Center, Faculty of Medicine, Mazandaran University of Medical Sciences, Sari, Iran.*
[4] *Student Research Committee, Department of Clinical Pharmacy, Mazandaran University of Medical Sciences, Sari, Iran.*
[5] *Faculty of Pharmacy, Mazandaran University of Medical Sciences, Sari, Iran.*
[6] *Faculty of Medicine, Mazandaran University of Medical Sciences, Sari, Iran.*
[7] *Department of Chemistry, Faculty of Basic Sciences, Golestan University, Gorgan, Iran.*

Keywords:
- Propranolol
- Pharmacokinetics
- Pharmacodynamic
- Iranian Population
- Polymorphism

Abstract

Purpose: Propranolol is the most widely used treatment for cardiovascular diseases. Dosage range in our patients is usually less than the amount mentioned in references. The aim of the present study was to clarify whether pharmacokinetic differences are able to justify the need for the fewer doses in our patients or not.

Methods: Twenty healthy volunteers (10 male) at heart center of Mazandaran University of Medical Sciences were studied. Samples of blood were collected before a single oral dose (40 mg) of Propranolol. Blood samples were taken up to 9 hours after dose. Total plasma concentration of Propranolol was measured by HPLC. Population Pharmacokinetic analysis was performed using population pharmacokinetics modeling software P-Pharm.

Results: The mean value for oral plasma clearance (CL/F) was 126.59 ml/hr. The corresponding values for apparent volume of distribution (V/F), t1/2 beta, maximum blood concentration (C max), and time to reach the maximum blood concentration (T max) were 334.12 Lit, 1.98 hr, 40.25 ng/ml, and 1.68 hr, respectively. The observed mean values of V/F of propranolol in the present study were comparable with those reported in the literature. However, the mean values of CL/F of propranolol in current study was significantly higher than those reported in other population (P-value<0.001).

Conclusion: This study has confirmed that the pharmacokinetic differences are not able to justify over-responsiveness of Iranian population to propranolol. Pharmacodynamic differences in responding to beta blocker drugs by Renin secretion or having a different sensibility to beta receptors might play a role in making our population have a different response to propranolol.

Introduction

Propranolol is a nonspecific beta-blocker that was presented as the first beta blocker in 1960.[1] It is used in various cases, and mainly to treat high blood pressure,[2] cardiac arrhythmias,[3,4] thyrotoxicosis,[5] migraine headaches,[6] and psychiatric diseases.[7] In recent studies, the beneficial effects of the drug to inhibit angiogenesis,[8] treatment of different types of cancer,[9-12] and hemangioma in children[13] has been established. The dosage range of propranolol is very broad and the maintenance dose and maximum dose listed in reference books are much higher than the usual dose in our patients. For example, the recommended dose of propranolol at the beginning of the treatment of hypertension is mentioned to be 80 milligrams per day and the gradual increase to the maintenance dose of 80-320 mg per day.[14] Many complications such as hypotension, bradycardia, depression, fatigue, sexual disorders and weight gain have been reported after taking beta blockers so the drug at the proper dose is necessary.[15,16] Despite the widespread use of propranolol, the suitable dosage range is not clear in Iranian population. It is believed that our patients are not able to tolerate high dosage of propranolol that is mentioned in the references. It seems that the intensification of pharmacodynamic effects of the drug, especially bradycardia or hypotension prevents prescribing a standard dose of the medication. The mean pharmacokinetic parameters of propranolol in healthy volunteers in previous studies, (clearance equal to 0.96 ±0.3 Lit/kg/hr, the volume of distribution equal to 4.3 ±0.6 Lit/kg, half-life equal to 3.4 ±0.4 (hour) and oral bioavailability equal to 26±10%), has been declared.[17,18] Given the uncertainty of pharmacokinetic parameters of

***Corresponding author:** Ebrahim Salehifar, Email: Esalehifar@mazums.ac.ir propranolol in our population, this study was conducted to determine pharmacokinetic parameters of propranolol in a sample of healthy volunteers of Iranian population.

Materials and Methods

This study was conducted on 20 healthy volunteers (10 men) at the Fatemeh Zahra educational hospital of Mazandaran University of Medical Sciences. Each subject gave his or her written informed consent to participation in the study, which was approved by the Research Ethics Committee of Mazandaran University of Medical Sciences (approval number 2.3.84-458).

Those who agreed to participate underwent a short clinical examination and gave details of their age, sex, weight, and their medical history was collected. Electrocardiography was performed on all the participants. Only healthy adults, non-smokers and non-consumers of any inhibitor drugs (e.g., cimetidine, ketoconazole, erythromycin, clarithromycin) or metabolism inducer (e.g., rifampin, phenytoin, carbamazepine and clarithromycin) in the past two weeks were recruited. Exclusion criteria included: pregnancy, bradycardia (heart rate less than 55 beats per minute), low blood pressure (systolic pressure below 110 mmHg or mean arterial pressure below 70 mmHg) and disapproval of health of various organs in physical examination. After an overnight fasting, a sample of 5 ml blood (analyzed to confirm abstinence) was collected. The subjects received a single oral dose of 40 mg tablet of propranolol (Tolid daroo) with 250 ml water. They were fasted over 2 h post-dose and peripheral venous blood samples (5 ml) were taken at 0.5, 1, 2, 3, 6, 8, and 9 hours post dose. After centrifugation for 5-min (1000 g), the plasma samples were stored at -20 °C until analysis. Urinary pH of the volunteers was measured at the 0 and 4 hours. The plasma concentration of propranolol was treated according to the method of Hermansson J et al.[19] 500 ml of thawed sample was mixed with 250 µl of zinc sulfate (0.07 molar) and 250 µl of sodium Hydroxide (1 molar). The mixture was vortex-mixed for 2 min. After centrifugation for 15 min at 3000 rpm the upper layer was transferred to a 1 ml tube and centrifuged for the second time at 1100 rpm for 5 minutes to obtain a clear solution and a 100 µl aliquot for 3 consecutive times, injected onto the HPLC. The chromatographic separation of propranolol was performed on a C8 analytical column (5 µm particle size, L × I.D. 15 cm × 4.6 mm) using an isocratic mobile phase of water- acetonitrile-methanol (65:25:5, v/v), 0.3% triethylamine. The pH of mobile phase was adjusted to 3.5 by means of phosphoric acid 85% and degassed by Knaver degaser, and delivered at a flow-rate of 0.5ml /min. The detector used was a UV, set at 233 nm wavelength.

Pharmacokinetics analysis

Pharmacokinetics analysis was carried out using population pharmacokinetics modeling software P-Pharm (P-Pharm., version 1.5. InnaPhase, Ceretil, France). Various population pharmacokinetic models were fitted to the data. Selection of the best model was based on the lowest value of the Akaike Information Criteria (AIC), visual inspection of residuals for systematic error and the predicted versus actual concentration plots. Initial estimates of the pharmacokinetics parameters were derived from values reported in the literature. Non parametric methods were used to calculate AUC and drug elimination constant (K_e). Statistical analysis was performed using SPSS for Windows (ver.16, SPSS Inc., Chicago, USA). For comparing non-paired clinical data, an independent samples t-test was used. In all cases $p < 0.05$ was taken as statistically significant.

Results and Discussion

The demographic characteristics of volunteers in present study are summarized in Table 1. There were no significant differences in the characteristics of patients between males and females (independent sample t-test), except for weight, and height ($p = \geq 0.046$). The weight and height were significantly higher in males than in females ($p<0.001$).

Table 1. Characteristics of the participants who completed the study.

-	Male (N=10)	Female (N=10)	P-value
Age (year)	27.3 ± 5.8	27.5 ± 7.2	0.95
Height (cm)	174.9 ± 4.5	161 ± 3.9	<0.001
Weight (kg)	73.4 ± 5	59.9 ± 7.6	<0.001
BMI*	24 ± 1.1	23.2 ± 3.3	0.46

*BMI: Body Mass Index = Weight $_{(kg)}$ / [Height $_{(m)}$] ^{2}

A two-compartment pharmacokinetic model with first-order input, first-order distributional rate constants and first-order elimination provided a significantly better fit to the concentration-time profiles compared than other models. A heteroscedastic error model (1/y^2) was more appropriate for all the analytes. A lognormal distribution best described the inter-subject variability in all population pharmacokinetic parameters. The population–derived Bayesian predicted vs observed total plasma concentrations and population mean and individual bayesian model fit to propranolol concentrations are shown in Figure 1, and Figure 2, respectively.

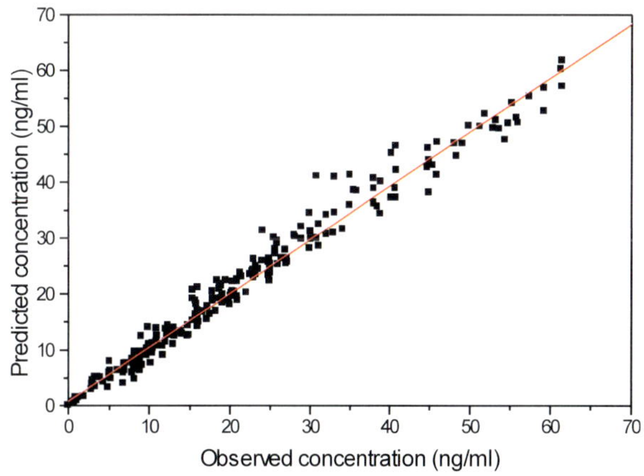

Figure 1. Population–derived Bayesian predicted vs observed total plasma concentrations after fitting of plasma concentration of propranolol calculated from the best fitted model

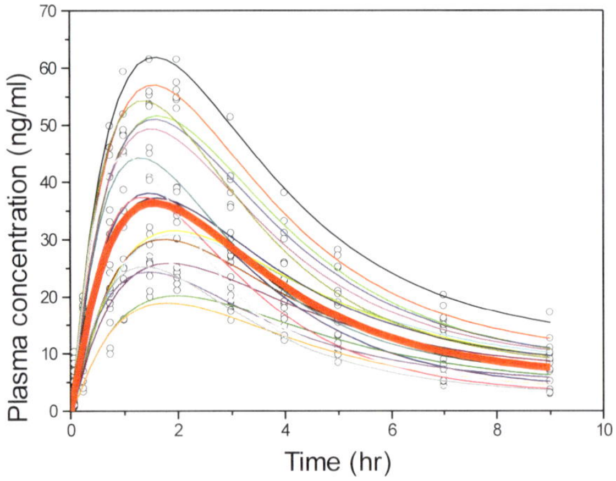

Figure 2. Population (bold line) and individual bayesian model fit to propranolol concentrations

Mean disposition and absorption pharmacokinetic parameter values for propranolol obtained from the best PK model and nonparametric analysis and the pharmacodynamics parameters are listed in Table 2 , and Table 3, respectively.

With the exception of the Ka, there were no significant differences in any PK parameters of propranolol between males and females ($p \leq 0.1$). The Ka was significantly higher in females than in males ($p=0.009$).

Mean pharmacodynamic parameters including heart rate and blood pressure of the volunteers are listed in Table 3.

Table 2. Dose, pharmacokinetic parameters and urine pH of the participated volunteers

Variable	Male (N=10)			Female (N=10)			P-value
	Mean±SD	Max	Min	Mean±SD	Max	Min	
Dose (mg/kg)	0.55 ± 0.04	0.61	0.49	0.68 ±0.09	0.8	0.58	0.001
Cp_{max} (ng/ml)	35.9 ± 12.1	56	22.1	44.6 ±14.5	61.4	21	0.17
T_{max} (min)	105 ±16.6	120	90	96 ± 24	120	60	0.33
Vd (Lit)	360.9 ±114.8	609.4	221.7	307.4 ± 144.9	633.7	198.9	0.37
Vd (Lit/Kg)	4.95 ± 1.6	8.24	2.95	5.28 ±2.84	11.74	2.88	0.76
Cl (Lit/hr)	128.4 ±51.6	232.1	80	124.7 ±47.7	210.3	65.6	0.87
Cl (Lit /Kg/hr)	1.77 ± 0.79	3.36	1.03	2.17 ±1.02	4.12	0.95	0.34
Ka (hr^{-1})	0.5 ± 0.03	0.56	0.45	0.56 ± 0.06	0.66	0.47	0.009
T½α (hr)	0.77 ± 0.13	0.95	0.58	0.70 ± 0.14	0.9	0.44	0.28
T½β (hr)	19.7 ± 5.7	32.5	13.3	17.4 ± 6.4	33	12.21	0.4
T½ (hr)	2.1 ± 0.84	3.6	1.1	1.83 ± 0.75	3.1	0.67	0.41
$AUC_{0\text{-}2}$ (ng×hr/ml)	32.7 ± 11.4	51.8	16.3	43.8 ± 16.4	63.51	16.14	0.1
AUC 0-10 (ng×hr/ml)	169.2 ± 52.8	257.1	107.4	194.5 ±72.1	313.9	97.2	0.38
$AUC_{0\text{-}\infty}$ (ng×hr/ml)	169.6 ± 52.8	257.4	107.9	194.8 ± 72	314.1	97.8	0.38
pH at time zero urine	5.9± 0.74	7	5	5.7 ±0.82	7	5	0.57
pH at time 4hr urine	6.4 ± 0.52	7	6	6.1 ± 0.57	7	5	0.23

AUC: area under the curve; Cp: concentration; CL: clearance; Vd: volume of distribution

Table 3. Heart rate and blood pressure of the volunteers after taking a single dose of 40 mg propranolol

Variable (time; min)	Male (N=10)			P-value€ (within group)	Female (N=10)			P-value€ (within group)	P-value¥ (Between two groups)
	Mean±SD	Max	Min		Mean±SD	Max	Min		
SBP (0)	115±13.5	130	90		111 ±16.6	130	90	0.56	
SBP (180)	112±12.3	130	90	P = 0.024 (for SBP)	107 ± 14.2	120	90	0.41	P < 0.001 (for SBP)
SBP (360)	112 ± 6.3	120	100		105±15.01	130	90	0.19	
SBP (540)	104 ± 8.4	110	90		99 ± 13.7	120	80	0.34	
DBP (0)	82 ± 9.2	90	60		79 ± 9.95	90	60	0.49	
DBP (180)	82 ± 9.2	90	60	P = 0.27 (for DBP)	79 ± 9.95	90	60	0.49	P = 0.55 (for DBP)
DBP (360)	84 ± 11.7	100	60		81 ± 7.4	90	70	0.5	
DBP (540)	80 ± 8.2	90	60		80 ± 9.4	90	60	1	
HR (0)	65.4 ± 1.9	68	62		63.7 ± 2.9	67	60	0.15	
HR (45)	64.6 ± 2.6	68	60	P = 0.059 (for HR)	63.2 ± 1.8	66	60	0.19	P = 0.51 (for HR)
HR (180)	64.3 ± 3.3	68	60		63.4 ± 2.5	68	60	0.56	
HR (540)	63.5 ± 1.4	65	62		62 ± 2.3	66	60	0.14	

DBP: diastolic blood pressure; HR: heart rate; SBP: systolic blood pressure; €: P-value of repeated measure test within each sex; ¥: P-value of independent samples t-test

Changes in systolic blood pressure, following the administration of propranolol in the measured times in both genders, was significant and in changes of heart rate in male volunteers, there was marginally significant (the trend toward significance) (P=0.059). In hemodynamic variables and their changes in different times, there was no significant difference between male and female volunteers. In Table 4 pharmacokinetic parameters resulted from our study was compared with the average reported in the references.[17,18]

Table 4. Comparison of pharmacokinetic parameters resulted from the current study with the average reported in the references

-	This study	Other sources	Mean of differences	95% confidence interval	P-Value
Cl (Lit/kg/hr)	1.97± 0.91	0.096±0.3	+1.01	0.59 to 1.44	<0.001
Vd (Lit/kg)	5.11± 2.3	4.3± 0.6	+0.82	0.24 to 1.87-	0.123
$t_{1/2}$ (hr)	1.98± 0.8	3.4± 0.4	-1.41	-1.79 to -1.05	<0.001

CL: clearance; Vd: volume of distribution

The obtained clearance in our study is more than the average reported in the references and half-life is less than the average reported in the references (P<0.001). The volume of distribution was not significantly different with the amounts reported in the references.

Based on the above mentioned results, propranolol clearance was more than the average reported in the references, while its half-life was less and there was no significant difference in the volume of distribution of the drug. Propranolol is metabolized to 14 metabolites, through 3 major pathways including Glucuronidation, side chain oxidation and ring-oxidation.[20] Regarding the previous studies, cytochrome P450 2D6, is the main enzyme responsible for propranolol, that 50 to 90 percent of -4 hydroxylation of the drug is performed by this enzyme. Previous studies have shown that oral clearance of propranolol is higher in black people due to the higher activity of hepatic metabolic pathways.[21,22] However in the study about the effects of 2D6 genotypes on the side effects and effectiveness of Metoprolol in the treatment of hypertension,[9] despite the influence of these factors on pharmacokinetic of the drug, it was not associated with side effects of beta blocker or its effectiveness.[23] In another study on the racial differences in pharmacokinetic propranolol, it was found that CYP1A2 metabolism pathway plays a role in 4-hydroxylation of propranolol, as well as CYP2D6, and the formation of metabolites resulting from these metabolic pathways, is considerably higher in African- American race than in Asian race. These racial differences in drug metabolism are related to the effectiveness or toxicity of the drug[24] and pharmacokinetic parameters of propranolol. Although in our study, the minimum concentration (Cp_{max}) in women was %24.2 more than men (44.6ng/ml against 35.1ng/ml). But these differences were not statistically significant. In the study of Xie and Chen in china, Cp_{max} in women and their AUC were respectively %99 and %74 more than men, the results were statistically significant. Moreover, half-life of the drug in women was longer than in men.[25] In another study on the difference of propranolol metabolic clearance in both genders it has been observed that after administration of 80 mg of the oral drug, there has been no significant difference in volume of distribution and half-life of the drug. Nevertheless, plasma level of the drug after oral administration was higher in women than in men. These results correspond to the results from our study. In addition, Walle et al found that oral clearance of propranolol in women was considerably less than in men.[26] In our study, the average half-life of Propranolol in women was not statistically different with men, though numerically half-life was lower in women (1.83 hr against 2.1 hr). Considering the equation t1/2=0.693*Vd/Cl, the two factors of clearance and volume of distribution can affect half-life. The more volume of distribution and the less clearance results in a longer half-life of a drug. Comparing volume of distribution and clearance in two genders imply no significant statistical difference between two genders. Yet numerically, volume of distribution and clearance of the drug is higher in women than in men. Changes of Vd can't justify shorter half-life in women. On the other hand, comparison of clearance in two genders (2.17 L/kg/hr against 1.77 L/kg/hr) signifies that the speed of drug metabolism is more in women than in men and can justify a shorter half-life in women. In other words, in women the increase of clearance is more than the increase of Vd. Eventually, the half-life of the drug has been decreased to some extent. The area under the curve or the bioavailability after oral administration had been inversely associated with intrinsic clearance of liver. The Changes in intrinsic clearance leads to changes in the amount of the drug withdrawal in the first-pass effect in the liver, but has little impact on clearance and half-life of the drug.[27] Therefore due to the lack of significant difference in the area under the curve, the liver metabolism capacity determining the intrinsic clearance of propranolol was not significantly different in two genders. As expected, systolic blood pressure of volunteers has decreased over time and after receiving propranolol. This decrease was significant in both genders unlike systolic blood pressure, changes in diastolic blood pressure over time was not significant. In this study, there were inclinations to an decrease in heart rate after single dose of the drug; similar results were obtained in study of Pharmacodynamic and pharmacokinetic of a single dose of 40 mg sublingual and oral propranolol in patients with high blood pressure.[28]

Comparing two genders no difference was observed in Pharmacodynamic parameters including heart rate, systolic and diastolic blood pressure. These results are compatible with pharmacokinetic parameters (volume of distribution, clearance and half-life) that were not significantly different between two genders.

In our study, the average clearance was 126.59 ml/h and the maximum and minimum clearance was 232.11 and 65.63, respectively. Several interpersonal changes are expected due to the effects of gender, race and age on the stable plasma concentration of the drugs metabolized by liver such as propranolol.[27,29] In some studies it has been shown that oral clearance of propranolol is higher in African-Americans rather than the white people.[21,30,31] In the study of Sowinski et al, the clearance in black and white people were 5036±4175 ml/min and 2854±879 ml/min respectively.[21] Similar results were obtained by L-Isomer of propranolol.[30] Unlike the study of Sowinski et, the average oral clearance was the same in black and white people in a study conducted in the United States (clearance range between 42.1 ml/min/kg and 54.5 ml/min/kg).[31] The average clearance in our study (1.97 L/hr/kg equal to 32.8 ml/min/kg) was less than the mentioned studies. In Wilson and colleagues study clearance of propranolol was 1040±120 ml/kg/hr (17.3 ml/min/kg) that is in the range of the average clearance mentioned in references 0.96 L/kg/hr (equal to 16 ml/min/kg).[32] Clearance in our study was more than the average clearance mentioned in the references (Table 4). The average volume of distribution had been 334.12 Lit (0.11±2.3 L/kg). Maximum and minimum volume of distribution was 633.73 Lit and 98.93 Lit, respectively. The volume of distribution obtained from our study had no significant difference with the average mentioned in the references. In the study conducted in Poland, the volume of distribution of propranolol was 5±1.2 L/kg, which was within the range of volume of distribution obtained in our study.[33] In another study conducted in Malaysia by Zain-Hamid R and colleagues, volume of distribution following a single 20 mg dose of propranolol was 543.89±292.91 L which was more than the results from our study.[34] Although in our study pharmacokinetic parameters of propranolol were examined as a single dose, but it has shown that the value of distribution with repeated doses decreases due to saturated tissue attachment of the drug.[34] Half-life of propranolol in our study was 1.98±0.8 hour, which was less than the average mentioned in the references.[17,18] In the study Castleden and George in England, half-life of the drug following the administration of a single oral dose of 40 mg in healthy volunteers was reported 217±13 minutes (equal to 3.61±0.22 hours).[35] In another study in the same country, half-life of the drug was reported 4.7±0.9.[36] Although there is a limitation in terms of the low number of participants in our study, the increased clearance and volume of distribution of subjects in our study suggest that the decrease of half-life was a consequence of a more increase in clearance rather than an increase in volume of distribution. In poor metabolizer people, following the administration of certain doses of the drug, there was more increase in the concentration of the drug, longer elimination half-life and an increase in the inhibition of beta. Therefore, administration of standard doses of beta blocker might cause the outbreak of dose-dependent side effects.[37] One of propranolol metabolites is 4-Hydroxypropranolol resulted from drug oxidation in the route of P450 cytochrome. This metabolite in people with low metabolic capacity is less than that in extensive metabolizer people. Yet, in the study of Lennard and colleagues, it was demonstrated that the average plasma concentrations were similar after a single oral dose of 80 mg in two groups of people with low and normal metabolic capacity. This indicates that oxidation phenotype is not the main determinant of drug levels and dose-dependent side effect s.[38] It seems that pharmacokinetic differences in our patients can't justify their being over- responsive to beta blockers. Unexpectedly clearance of the drug studied volunteers was higher and their half-life was lower than the average mentioned in the references. Regarding the identifying of polymorphism in beta blockers,[39] the differences in beta receptor expression in our population might justify pharmacodynamics differences. Several studies have been conducted on the polymorphism of beta- adrenergic receptors and its effects on changes in responding to the beta blocker treatment in different population. Also in the study of Parvez et al., it is indicated that people suffering from atrial fibrillation with common polymorphism of adrenergic beta-1 receptors, as Arg389Gly, give a better response to the treatments and need different doses of beta blocker and calcium blocker drugs.[40] As long as hemodynamic responses to propranolol is different in various races and countries due to genetic differences, there has been conducted several studies in various populations. As an example it has been observed that people with genotype homozygote C/C188 take more benefits from treatment of liver cirrhosis with propranolol rather than patients with C/T188 genotype heterozygote.[41] In another study it was observed that patients with cirrhosis and portal vein hypertension had different responses to propranolol, calculated by reduction of variceal pressure. That is, patients with Gly16-Glu/Gln27 genotype homozygote had shown more decrease in variceal pressure rather than Arg16-Gln27 homozygote people. Also, patients with heterozygote genotype had an intermediate response between within two homozygote genotypes.[42] There are as well such studies about other beta blocker drugs. For instance, it is observed that in people with ADRB1 Arg389Gly polymorphism, there is a dose-response relation between plasma Renin activity and Metoprolol concentrations in healthy male Caucasian people. It seems that in these people (Gly/Gly), plasma Renin activity is inhibited in lower Metoprolol concentrations and they need lower doses to inhibit neurohormonal hyperactivity.[43] In another study, it was observed that Arg 389Gly polymorphism has an important effect on the decrease in heart rate caused by carvedilol in patients with heart failure along with atrial fibrillation, but such effect is not true about Bisoprolol.[44] Results have shown that homozygote mutant genotype ADRB1 1165G>C is associated with the increase in effectiveness of Metoprolol in treating hypertension, that suggest the selection of anti-hypertension according to genotype of patients.[45] Furthermore, in Korean patients suffering from heart failure, it was observed that people with ADRB1 Gly389X genotype, have shown a better response to Bisoprolol compared to Arg389Arg genotype. These results show that treatment with beta-blocker goes to treatment of each person separately, on the basis of genotype.[46] Another study indicates a 10 times difference in the effects of Esmolol on exercise-induced tachycardia in people with ADRB1 389 genotype.[47] Furthermore, according to previous studies, in people with ADRb1-389 Arg/Arg genotype, a higher dose of beta blocker is needed to achieve a treatment response rather than in people with Gly genotype carriers.[48]

According to the results of the above-mentioned studies, the Pharmacodynamic difference of Propranolol in the present study may be associated with polymorphism of beta-adrenergic receptors in the population under study and its effect on the increase in responsiveness to this drug. It is worth to conduct future studies about polymorphism of beta receptors in order to investigate Pharmacodynamic differences in our population.

Conclusion

According to the results of this study, it seems that pharmacokinetic differences are not able to explain over-responsiveness of our patients to propranolol. Pharmacodynamic differences in responding to beta blocker drugs by Renin secretion or having a different sensibility to beta receptors might play a role in making our population have a different response to propranolol.

Acknowledgments

This study was an approved research project sponsored by Deputy of Research and Technology, Mazandaran University of Medical Sciences, to which the authors express their appreciation and thanks. We also declare our acknowledgment to the personnel of Fatemeh Zahra Hospital Laboratory as well as to all of the volunteers participated in this study.

Ethical Issues

The approval number of the study was 2.3.84-458. The ethical standards were met according to Fifth revision of Declaration of Helsinki.

Conflict of Interest

The authors report no conflicts of interest.

References

1. Emilien G, Maloteaux JM. Current therapeutic uses and potential of beta-adrenoceptor agonists and antagonists. *Eur J Clin Pharmacol* 1998;53(6):389-404.
2. Zacharias FJ, Cowen KJ, Prestt J, Vickers J, Wall BG. Propranolol in hypertension: a study of long-term therapy, 1964-1970. *Am Heart J* 1972;83(6):755-61.
3. Friedman LM, Byington RP, Capone RJ, Furberg CD, Goldstein S, Lichstein E. Effect of propranolol in patients with myocardial infarction and ventricular arrhythmia. *J Am Coll Cardiol* 1986;7(1):1-8.
4. A randomized trial of propranolol in patients with acute myocardial infarction. I. Mortality results. *JAMA* 1982;247(12):1707-14.
5. Zonszein J, Santangelo RP, Mackin JF, Lee TC, Coffey RJ, Canary JJ. Propranolol therapy in thyrotoxicosis. A review of 84 patients undergoing surgery. *Am J Med* 1979;66(3):411-6.
6. Weber RB, Reinmuth OM. The treatment of migraine with propranolol. *Neurology* 1972;22(4):366-9.
7. Hayes PE, Schulz SC. Beta-blockers in anxiety disorders. *J Affect Disord* 1987;13(2):119-30.
8. Lamy S, Lachambre MP, Lord-Dufour S, Beliveau R. Propranolol suppresses angiogenesis in vitro: Inhibition of proliferation, migration, and differentiation of endothelial cells. *Vascul Pharmacol* 2010;53(5-6):200-8. doi: 10.1016/j.vph.2010.08.002
9. Al-Wadei HA, Al-Wadei MH, Schuller HM. Prevention of pancreatic cancer by the beta-blocker propranolol. *Anticancer Drugs* 2009;20(6):477-82. doi: 10.1097/CAD.0b013e32832bd1e3
10. Kozanoglu I, Yandim MK, Cincin ZB, Ozdogu H, Cakmakoglu B, Baran Y. New indication for therapeutic potential of an old well-known drug (propranolol) for multiple myeloma. *J Cancer Res Clin Oncol* 2013;139(2):327-35. doi: 10.1007/s00432-012-1331-y
11. Liao X, Che X, Zhao W, Zhang D, Bi T, Wang G. The beta-adrenoceptor antagonist, propranolol, induces human gastric cancer cell apoptosis and cell cycle arrest via inhibiting nuclear factor kappab signaling. *Oncol Rep* 2010;24(6):1669-76.
12. Powe DG, Entschladen F. Targeted therapies: Using beta-blockers to inhibit breast cancer progression. *Nat Rev Clin Oncol* 2011;8(9):511-2. doi: 10.1038/nrclinonc.2011.123
13. Hasan M, Rahman M, Hoque S, Zahid Hossain AK, Khondker L. Propranolol for hemangiomas. *Pediatr Surg Int* 2013;29(3):257-62. doi: 10.1007/s00383-012-3220-5
14. Weber MA, Schiffrin EL, White WB, Mann S, Lindholm LH, Kenerson JG, et al. Clinical practice guidelines for the management of hypertension in the community: A statement by the american society of hypertension and the international society of hypertension. *J Clin Hypertens (Greenwich)* 2014;16(1):14-26. doi: 10.1111/jch.12237
15. Ko DT, Hebert PR, Coffey CS, Sedrakyan A, Curtis JP, Krumholz HM. Beta-blocker therapy and symptoms of depression, fatigue, and sexual dysfunction. *JAMA* 2002;288(3):351-7.
16. Leslie WS, Hankey CR, Lean ME. Weight gain as an adverse effect of some commonly prescribed drugs: A

systematic review. *QJM* 2007;100(7):395-404. doi: 10.1093/qjmed/hcm044
17. Colangelo PM, Blouin RA, Steinmetz JE, McNamara PJ, DeMaria AN, Wedlund PJ. Age and propranolol stereoselective disposition in humans. *Clin Pharmacol Ther* 1992;51(5):489-94.
18. Brown JH, Taylor P, Hardman J, Limbird L, Molinoff P, Ruddon R. Goodman and Gilman's the pharmacological basis of therapeutics. New york, USA: Mc Graw Hill; 2001.
19. Hermansson J, Grahn A, Hermansson I. Direct injection of large volumes of plasma/serum on a new biocompatible extraction column for the determination of atenolol, propranolol and ibuprofen. Mechanisms for the improvement of chromatographic performance. *J Chromatogr A* 1998;797(1-2):251-63.
20. Walle T, Walle UK, Olanoff LS. Quantitative account of propranolol metabolism in urine of normal man. *Drug Metab Dispos* 1985;13(2):204-9.
21. Sowinski KM, Lima JJ, Burlew BS, Massie JD, Johnson JA. Racial differences in propranolol enantiomer kinetics following simultaneous i.V. And oral administration. *Br J Clin Pharmacol* 1996;42(3):339-46.
22. Yoshimoto K, Echizen H, Chiba K, Tani M, Ishizaki T. Identification of human cyp isoforms involved in the metabolism of propranolol enantiomers--n-desisopropylation is mediated mainly by cyp1a2. *Br J Clin Pharmacol* 1995;39(4):421-31.
23. Zineh I, Beitelshees AL, Gaedigk A, Walker JR, Pauly DF, Eberst K, et al. Pharmacokinetics and cyp2d6 genotypes do not predict metoprolol adverse events or efficacy in hypertension. *Clin Pharmacol Ther* 2004;76(6):536-44. doi: 10.1016/j.clpt.2004.08.020
24. Johnson JA, Herring VL, Wolfe MS, Relling MV. Cyp1a2 and cyp2d6 4-hydroxylate propranolol and both reactions exhibit racial differences. *J Pharmacol Exp Ther* 2000;294(3):1099-105.
25. Xie HG, Chen X. Sex differences in pharmacokinetics of oral propranolol in healthy chinese volunteers. *Zhongguo Yao Li Xue Bao* 1995;16(5):468-70.
26. Walle T, Walle UK, Cowart TD, Conradi EC. Pathway-selective sex differences in the metabolic clearance of propranolol in human subjects. *Clin Pharmacol Ther* 1989;46(3):257-63.
27. Walle T, Walle UK, Olanoff LS, Conradi EC. Partial metabolic clearances as determinants of the oral bioavailability of propranolol. *Br J Clin Pharmacol* 1986;22(3):317-23.
28. Mansur AP, Avakian SD, Paula RS, Donzella H, Santos SR, Ramires JA. Pharmacokinetics and pharmacodynamics of propranolol in hypertensive patients after sublingual administration: Systemic availability. *Braz J Med Biol Res* 1998;31(5):691-6.
29. Shand DG. Pharmacokinetic properties of the beta-adrenergic receptor blocking drugs. *Drugs* 1974;7(1):39-47.
30. Johnson JA, Burlew BS. Racial differences in propranolol pharmacokinetics. *Clin Pharmacol Ther* 1992;51(5):495-500.
31. Sharoky M, Perkal M, Turner R, Lesko LJ. Steady state relative bioavailability and pharmacokinetics of oral propranolol in black and white north americans. *Biopharm Drug Dispos* 1988;9(5):447-56.
32. Wilson TW, Firor WB, Johnson GE, Holmes GI, Tsianco MC, Huber PB, et al. Timolol and propranolol: Bioavailability, plasma concentrations, and beta blockade. *Clin Pharmacol Ther* 1982;32(6):676-85.
33. Wojcicki J, Jaroszynska M, Drozdzik M, Pawlik A, Gawronska-Szklarz B, Sterna R. Comparative pharmacokinetics and pharmacodynamics of propranolol and atenolol in normolipaemic and hyperlipidaemic obese subjects. *Biopharm Drug Dispos* 2003;24(5):211-8. doi: 10.1002/bdd.357
34. Zain-Hamid R, Ismail Z, Mahendra Raj S, Shuaib IL, Mohsin SS. The pharmacokinetics of single dose vs steady-state doses of propranolol in cirrhotic malay patients. *Malays J Med Sci* 2002;9(1):16-20.
35. Castleden CM, George CF. The effect of ageing on the hepatic clearance of propranolol. *Br J Clin Pharmacol* 1979;7(1):49-54.
36. Murdoch DL, Thomson GD, Thompson GG, Murray GD, Brodie MJ, McInnes GT. Evaluation of potential pharmacodynamic and pharmacokinetic interactions between verapamil and propranolol in normal subjects. *Br J Clin Pharmacol* 1991;31(3):323-32.
37. Pirmohamed M, Park BK. Cytochrome p450 enzyme polymorphisms and adverse drug reactions. *Toxicology* 2003;192(1):23-32.
38. Lennard MS, Jackson PR, Freestone S, Tucker GT, Ramsay LE, Woods HF. The relationship between debrisoquine oxidation phenotype and the pharmacokinetics and pharmacodynamics of propranolol. *Br J Clin Pharmacol* 1984;17(6):679-85.
39. Vrydag W, Alewijnse AE, Michel MC. Do gene polymorphisms alone or in combination affect the function of human beta3-adrenoceptors? *Br J Pharmacol* 2009;156(1):127-34. doi: 10.1111/j.1476-5381.2008.00014.x
40. Parvez B, Chopra N, Rowan S, Vaglio JC, Muhammad R, Roden DM, et al. A common beta1-adrenergic receptor polymorphism predicts favorable response to rate-control therapy in atrial fibrillation. *J Am Coll Cardiol* 2012;59(1):49-56. doi: 10.1016/j.jacc.2011.08.061
41. Zhang F, Duan X, Zhang M, Li Z, He Q, Wang Y, et al. Influence of cyp2d6 and β2-adrenergic receptor gene polymorphisms on the hemodynamic response to propranolol in chinese han patients with cirrhosis. *J Gastroenterol Hepatol* 2016;31(4):829-834. doi: 10.1111/jgh.13198
42. Kong DR, Wang JG, Sun B, Wang MQ, Chen C, Yu FF, et al. Beta-2 adrenergic receptor gene polymorphism and response to propranolol in cirrhosis. *World J Gastroenterol* 2015;21(23):7191-6. doi: 10.3748/wjg.v21.i23.7191

43. Petersen M, Andersen JT, Jimenez-Solem E, Broedbaek K, Hjelvang BR, Henriksen T, et al. Effect of the arg389gly beta(1)-adrenoceptor polymorphism on plasma renin activity and heart rate, and the genotype-dependent response to metoprolol treatment. *Clin Exp Pharmacol Physiol* 2012;39(9):779-85. doi: 10.1111/j.1440-1681.2012.05736.x
44. Rau T, Dungen HD, Edelmann F, Waagstein F, Lainscak M, Dimkovic S, et al. Impact of the beta1-adrenoceptor arg389gly polymorphism on heart-rate responses to bisoprolol and carvedilol in heart-failure patients. *Clin Pharmacol Ther* 2012;92(1):21-8. doi: 10.1038/clpt.2012.18
45. Wu D, Li G, Deng M, Song W, Huang X, Guo X, et al. Associations between adrb1 and cyp2d6 gene polymorphisms and the response to beta-blocker therapy in hypertension. *J Int Med Res* 2015;43(3):424-34. doi: 10.1177/0300060514563151
46. Lee HY, Chung WJ, Jeon HK, Seo HS, Choi DJ, Jeon ES, et al. Impact of the beta-1 adrenergic receptor polymorphism on tolerability and efficacy of bisoprolol therapy in korean heart failure patients: Association between beta adrenergic receptor polymorphism and bisoprolol therapy in heart failure (abba) study. *Korean J Intern Med* 2016;31(2):277-87. doi: 10.3904/kjim.2015.04
47. Muszkat M, Hoofien A, Orlanski-Meyer E, Makhoul H, Porat E, Davidson EM, et al. The common arg389gly adrb1 polymorphism affects heart rate response to the ultra-short-acting beta(1) adrenergic receptor antagonist esmolol in healthy individuals. *Pharmacogenet Genomics* 2013;23(1):25-8. doi: 10.1097/FPC.0b013e32835afde6
48. Fiuzat M, Neely ML, Starr AZ, Kraus WE, Felker GM, Donahue M, et al. Association between adrenergic receptor genotypes and beta-blocker dose in heart failure patients: Analysis from the hf-action DNA substudy. *Eur J Heart Fail* 2013;15(3):258-66. doi: 10.1093/eurjhf/hfs175

Hybrid Scaffolds of Hyaluronic Acid and Collagen Loaded with Prednisolone: an Interesting System for Osteoarthritis

Farhad Mohammadi[1], Soliman Mohammadi Samani[1,2], Nader Tanideh[3], Fatemeh Ahmadi[1,2]*

[1] *Department of Pharmaceutics, School of Pharmacy, Shiraz University of Medical Sciences, Shiraz, Iran.*
[2] *Research Center for Nanotechnology in Drug Delivery, School of Pharmacy, Shiraz University of Medical Sciences, Shiraz, Iran.*
[3] *Department of Pharmacology, Stem Cell and Transgenic Research Center, Shiraz University of Medical Sciences, Shiraz, Iran.*

Keywords:
· Scaffold
· Hyaluronic acid
· Collagen
· Implantable disk
· Thermo-sensitive gel
· Cartilage regeneration

Abstract

Purpose: Cartilage regeneration by using polymeric scaffolds is a new option for treatment of osteoarthritis. A good scaffold for tissue engineering should copy the characteristics of natural extracellular matrix. The purpose of this study was to make a dosage form with proper reliability and stability for cartilage repair.

Methods: Hybrid scaffolds containing different ratios of hyaluronic acid (HA) and collagen were prepared and loaded with prednisolone as anti-inflammatory agent. Two different dosage forms (lyophilized implantable disk and thermo-sensitive gels) were examined. A scaffold of cross-linked HA was used as control. Different characterization tests were considered including differential scanning calorimetry (DSC), scanning electron microscopy, mechanical evaluations, and drug release.

Results: The physical and chemical performance of hybrid-scaffolds was better than HA scaffold. Increasing the concentration of HA and collagen improved the physical and chemical characteristics. Regarding the mechanical properties of the hybrid scaffold, the pore size was 20-200μm, compressive modulus was 54.77±0.31 kPa, more than 1200% water uptake was observed after 4 days, gelation temperature was 32±0.16°C, gelation time was 2.4±0.1 min, and drug release was controlled for 5 days by Higuchi release kinetic model.

Conclusion: It seems that this porous hybrid scaffold could be a suitable choice in cartilage regeneration as well as a controlled-release system for delivery of prednisolone in osteoarthritis.

Introduction

Defects and injuries of the cartilages are significant causes of dysfunction and disability of knee and other organs. Cartilage diseases such as different types of arthritis affect nearly three quarters of the people during the lifetime.[1] Among the various strategies of treating cartilage defects, tissue engineering has grown rapidly thanks to the application of natural, synthetic or hybrid polymers. They are used in scaffolding as space filling agents, delivery vehicles for proteins or drugs, and 3D structures that establish cells and present the stimuli required for tissue regeneration.[2]

The scaffold material and its characteristics differ according to the type and final application of the tissue.[3] Some natural materials used as scaffolds are collagen, fibrin, gelatin, agarose, alginate, chitosan and hyaluronic acid (HA). Studies evaluated various synthetic polymers namely poly(acrylic acid) (PAA), poly(propylene fumarate-co-ethylene glycol) (P (PF-co-EG)), poly(ethylene oxide) (PEO), poly(vinyl alcohol) (PVA), poly(lactic-co-glycolic acid) (PLGA), poly(lactic acid) (PLA) and hybrid materials of synthetic and natural polymers.[4,5]

The scaffold structure should be porous which provides the required mechanical stability for adequate cell substitution and facilitates the transfer of oxygen and nutrients. The inflammatory responses and hypersensitivity reactions with scaffolds of natural polymers are not much important due to their biodegradable and biocompatible nature.[6]

Cartilage repair is one of the extensively studied fields in tissue engineering. Simulating the extracellular matrix is a suitable approach for regeneration of cartilage tissue. HA is one of the main constituents of extracellular matrix found in the connective tissue. Collagen is a biocompatible and biodegradable material that helps the adhesion and regeneration of cells.[7] HA is considered as the main constituent in constructing the preliminary framework. Meanwhile, collagen plays the role of interpenetrated protein fiber in the network to improve the mechanical characteristics of the scaffold and to remain for a longer time in the body and then release the drug in a controlled manner. Lu et al. reported that a combination of these materials was more helpful for

***Corresponding author:** Fatemeh Ahmadi, Email: ahmadi_f@sums.ac.ir

cartilage regeneration and provided an appropriate environment for tissue repair.[8]
Corticosteroids reduce the inflammation and pain, especially in moderate to severe cases of osteoarthritis, and improve the joints function for a limited time (about four weeks). Therefore, they can be used as an adjuvant treatment for cartilage repair. To our knowledge there was no report on loading anti-inflammatory drugs in polymeric scaffolds for cartilage tissue regeneration. Thus, the present research used HA and collagen to make a combined polymeric scaffold for cartilage tissue regeneration. The aim was to fabricate a porous and mechanically-stable scaffold loaded with prednisolone as an anti-inflammatory agent. The scaffolds of HA as well as combination of HA and collagen were designed and loaded with drug; and the rheological properties, swelling, degradation and release profiles were studied.

Materials and Methods

Preparation of HA and HA/collagen scaffolds

To prepare the HA-based scaffold, 2 ml of distilled water was adjusted to pH 3.5 by dropwise adding of the necessary amounts of acetic acid (Merck; Germany). Two mg prednisolone (Iran Hormone Co., Iran) was added to the solution, and homogenized by using an IKA T10basic, Ultra-Turrax homogenizer (IKA-Werke, Germany) to dissolve. Then, HA (Sigma-Aldrich, Czech Republic) was added to the mixture and the solution was stirred at 1500 rpm for 1 h at 4°C to make an aqueous solution containing 0.1% prednisolone and 1% HA. Poly ethylene glycol diglycidyl ether (Sigma-Aldrich, Czech Republic) as crosslinking agent was added to the aqueous solution to provide a 0.25% solution. The mixture was stirred for 30 min, and then, left to react in a reactor (Labtech, DAIHAN LABTECH) at 35°C for 1 h.
To make disk-shaped HA scaffold, the reacted solution was poured into each well of a 96-well plate (Falcon, USA), frozen at -80°C, and then freeze-dried (CHRIST, Alpha 2-4 LDPlus, Germany). Similar procedure was used to fabricate the combined scaffolds; i.e., 0.1, 0.2 and 0.4% of collagen (Type I, Rat tail, Millipore, Germany) was added to the HA aqueous solution. The obtained mixture was stirred at 1500 rpm for 1 h at 4°C. The same amount of PEGDGE was added to each of the prepared combined aqueous solutions, mixed homogenously, and then permitted to react in the incubator at 35°C for 1 h.
Each reacted mixture was poured in each well of a 96-well plate, frozen at -80°C, and freeze dried. In order to prepare an injectable dosage form, each formulation was added to an aqueous solution containing 18% of poloxamer 407(Sigma-Aldrich; Germany) at 25°C and stirred to provide a thermo-sensitive gel. Finally, the gels were sterilized by filtration through 0.22-μ filter. Table 1 shows the concentration of HA and collagen in different formulations prepared.

Table 1. Composition of formulations and results of physical tests

Formulations	HA (mg/ml)	Collagen (mg/ml)	Compressive modulus (kPa)	Gelation temperature (°C)	Gelation time (min)
F_1	10	-	41.26 ± 0.35	33 ± 0.18	3.5 ± 0.07
F_2	5	1	39.86 ± 0.20*	37 ± 0.21*	4.5 ± 0.04*
F_3	10	1	46.37 ± 0.56*	34 ± 0.09*	3.8 ± 0.01*
F_4	10	2	48.43 ± 0.18*	35 ± 0.12*	4 ± 0.08*
F_5	10	4	50.94 ± 0.36*	37 ± 0.33*	5.2 ± 0.11*
F_6	20	1	54.77 ± 0.31*	32 ± 0.16*	2.4 ± 0.1*

Formulations F_2 to F_6 showed significant difference in comparison to F_1. (*p-value<0.05)

Differential scanning calorimetry

In order to determine whether HA cross-linked and made the network, differential scanning calorimetry (DSC) was done. Thermal analysis was carried out by using DSC 302 (BAHR Thermoanalyse GmbH, Germany). 10 mg HA, 20 μl PEGDGE and 20 mg cross-linked HA were hermetically sealed within the DSC pans and heated in the range of 25-300°C at a rate of 10°C/min under 60 cc/min of nitrogen gas flow; Al_2O_3 was used as the reference material. All samples were tested in triplicates.[9]

Surface morphology of implantable disks

To observe the surface morphology of the prepared disks, scaffolds were scanned by a scanning electron microscope (SEM, S-800, HITACHI, Tokyo, Japan). Prior to scanning, each sample was coated with a thin layer of gold within an ion sputter. Observation was done by 200 x magnification at an alternating voltage of 5 KV. The pore size of the lyophilized disks was measured from SEM images using Digimizer software, version 4.1.1.0 (MedCalc Software).[10]

Compression test of implantable disks

Cylindrical lyophilized hydrogels (10×3 mm diameter×height) were prepared for compression tests. Lyophilized disks were swelled in distilled water for 2 h and then compressed at constant force rate of 0.1N/minute up to a maximum of 2 N at room temperature by CT3 Texture Analyzer (Brookfield, USA). The test was done three times for each formulation on different samples. The specific software of instrument was used to calculate the compressive modulus from stress-strain curve.[10]

Swelling measurement of implantable disks

The lyophilized disks were weighed and immersed in distilled water at 25°C. At predetermined times, one of the disks was removed, wiped with filter paper to remove the excess water, and weighed again. The water uptake of lyophilized hydrogels was calculated by Equation 1:

Equation 1: $\%\ \text{Water uptake} = W_t\text{-}W_0/W_0 \times 100$

Herein, W_0 was the weight of the lyophilized sample and W_t was the weight of the swollen sample.[10,11]

In vitro degradation test of implantable disks

The lyophilized cylindrical hydrogels prepared with different concentrations of HA and collagen, were placed in a 50-ml glass beaker containing 20 ml phosphate buffered saline (PBS). The samples were shaken in a shaker incubator at 50 rpm at 37.5°C. On 1, 4, 7, 14, 28 days after starting the test, each scaffold was removed and rinsed with distilled water, freeze-dried, and then weighed. Percentage of the remaining lyophilized hydrogels was calculated based on Equation 2.

Equation 2: $\%\ \text{Degradation (t)} = Wd_{(0)} - Wd_{(t)}/Wd_{(0)} \times 100$

In this equation, $W_d(0)$ was the weight of the lyophilized sample and $W_d(t)$ was the weight of the sample removed at the predetermined time.[12]

Measurement of gelation temperature for thermo-sensitive gels

A glass beaker containing 50 ml of the thermo-sensitive gel was connected to a water circulator bath. A temperature sensor was connected to a digital thermometer probe and immersed in the gel. The heating rate was 1°C/min and stirring rate was set to 80 rpm. Gelation temperature was defined as the temperature showed on the thermometer when the magnetic bar stopped rotating due to gel formation.[13]

Measurement of gelation time for thermo-sensitive gels

To evaluate the gelation time of thermo-sensitive gel formulations by the inverted tube test, 900 µl of PBS, equilibrated at 37°C, was poured into a 2-ml microcentrifuge tube (QC LAB, Southampton, UK). 100 µl of the gel solution was poured into the tube and incubated at 37°C. At 2, 5, 10, 15, and 20 minute intervals, the tubes were inverted to verify possible flowability of the gel. The time at which the gel did not flow was considered as the gelation time.[13]

Drug release measurement

The release tests were performed by the membrane-less model since this method allows direct contact between dosage forms (gels and implantable disks) and release medium; thus, the erosion of dosage forms can be studied.[14] The dosage forms were placed in 25 ml beakers, and 20 ml PBS solution containing 0.1% sodium lauryl sulfate (SLS) equilibrated at 37°C was poured precisely. The beakers were put in the shaker incubator (Jal Tajhiz, JSH20LUR, Iran) at 37±0.05°C. The samples were withdrawn at predetermined time points; 0.5, 2, 6, 12, 18 hours and 1, 2, 3, 4, 5 days, and the release medium was completely replaced with fresh medium kept at 37 °C. The concentration of prednisolone in each sample was quantified by high-performance liquid chromatography (HPLC) (CECIL, CE 4200) in 243 nm. The results were shown as percentage of prednisolone released against time. A similar study was performed for prednisolone powder dissolved in release media to prove that the sink condition was provided. All experiments were done in triplicate.

Statistical analyses

Quantitative results were expressed as mean±SD. The statistical differences were analyzed by ANOVA test, and p-values < 0.05 were considered significant.

Results and Discussion

Cartilage diseases and defects like osteoarthritis or rheumatoid arthritis are the most important causes of knee and low back pain. Cartilage degenerative diseases usually need surgeries or other invasive procedures. The use of tissue engineering and biomaterials improve the outcome of therapeutic procedures. Use of biomaterials as scaffolds allows the stem cells or growth factors to attach to the scaffold surface or be load into it.[15] Although previous studies evaluated the effect of prednisolone on treatment of osteoarthritis, this material was never loaded into the combined polymeric formulations. The present study developed a porous and mechanically-stable combined scaffold loaded with prednisolone as an anti-inflammatory agent in two usable dosage forms.

DSC study

Distinct difference was observed between DSC thermograms of HA and cross-linked HA. Figure 1 shows the thermograms of HA, PEGDGE and cross-linked HA. In the HA thermogram, a wide endothermic peak was seen about 100°C which was related to the loss of moisture after the early drying process. About 250°C, a sharp exothermic peak was seen which could possibly be related to the degradation of HA.

In the thermogram of cross-linked HA, sharp exothermic peaks were also observed at higher temperatures due to the increase in chemical stability of the polymer after crosslinking. Seemingly, the first peak revealed conversion into a less-ordered phase, and the second showed thermal degradation. In the thermogram of PEGDGE, an exothermic peak with the onset about 200°C might be associated with flashing of PEGDGE. Similar results were reported by Collins and Birkinshaw.[16,17] Comparison of the thermograms (a) and (c) in Figure 1 revealed that HA was cross-linked under the reaction condition.

Surface morphology of implantable disks

Figure 2 shows the morphology of implantable disks with different concentrations of HA and collagen. SEM images exhibited homogeneous distribution and interconnected porous structure of the implantable disks. Pore size of the implantable disks ranged 20-200 μm. The pore sizes between 100-500 μm can improve the cell proliferation, but the smaller sizes make the implantable disks more compact and more stable.[18] The existence of pores in scaffolds is one of the perquisites for a scaffold used in tissue engineering, since the pores help passage of necessary nutrients during the growth of tissues and cells.[19] In the current study, the pore size decreased by increasing the concentration of HA and collagen, because the concentration of HA as main network backbone fibers and collagen as interpenetrated fibers increased simultaneously. The results are parallel with those of the previous studies on HA scaffolds.[20] Surface area of the porous framework is a significant feature in the proliferation and differentiation of cells. Increasing the concentration of HA and collagen decreased the pore size, which caused increment in the surface area of the implantable disks. However, the strength and stability of implantable disks are important only for a few weeks because a controlled release dosage form is required. Therefore, a balance between these two characteristics should be addressed.

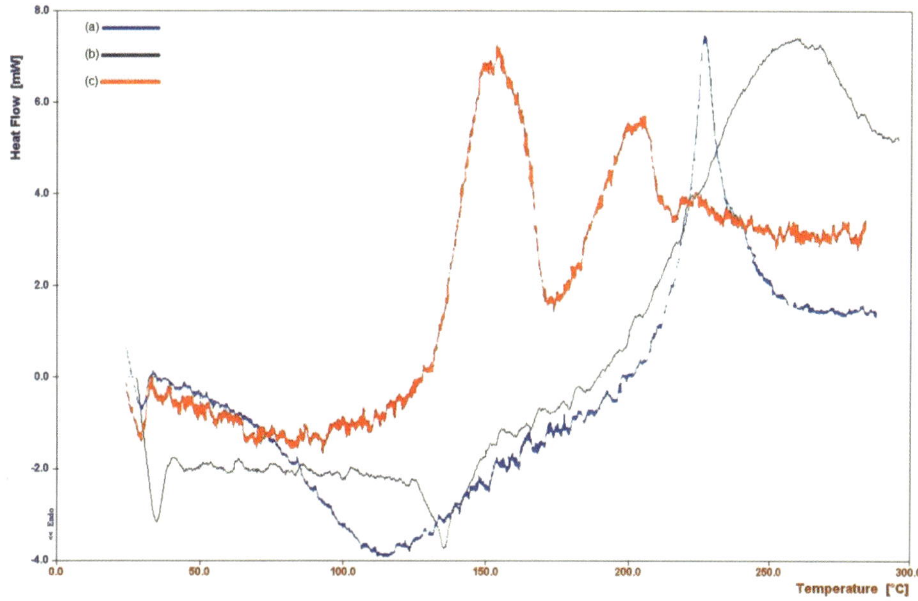

Figure 1. DSC thermograms of (a) HA, (b) PEGDGE, (c) crosslinked HA

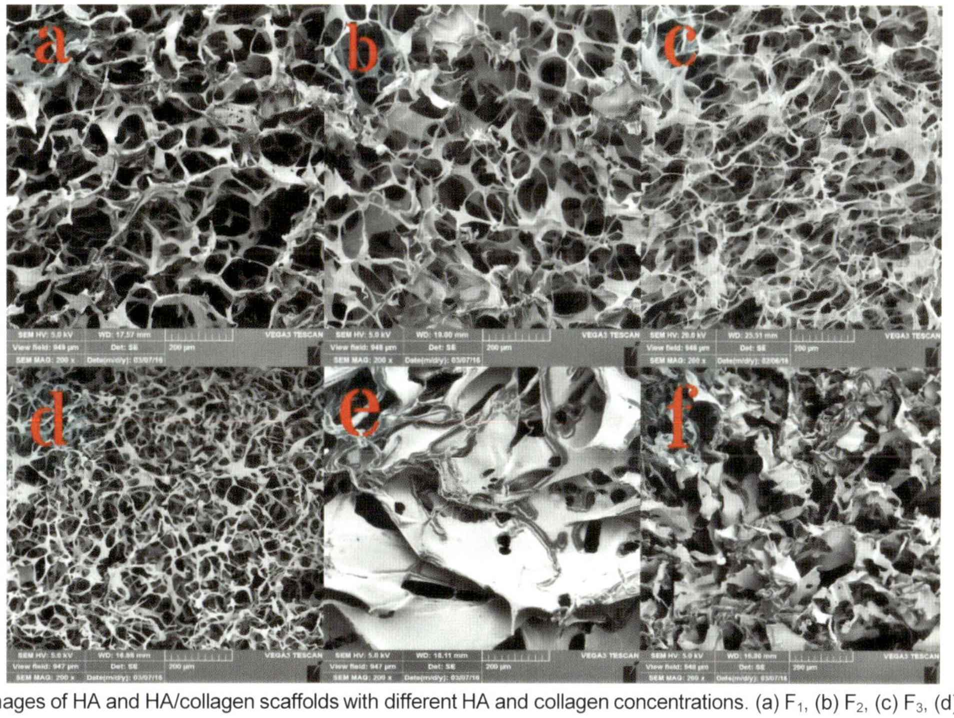

Figure 2. SEM images of HA and HA/collagen scaffolds with different HA and collagen concentrations. (a) F_1, (b) F_2, (c) F_3, (d) F_4, (e) F_5, (f) F_6.

Compression test of implantable disks

Table 1 presents the compressive modulus of implantable disks calculated by mechanical measurements. The nominal stress (σ_{nom}) and strain (ε) were determined by Equation 3.

Equation 3: $\sigma nom = F/A_0$

Equation 4: $\varepsilon = 1 - \lambda$

Equation 5: $\sigma nom = G\,(\lambda - \lambda^{-2})$

In these equations, F is the force required to compress the disks, A_0 is the cross-sectional area of the disks and λ is the deformation ratio (deformed length/initial length). Compressive modulus (G) factor were computed as a ratio of the stress and (λ- λ^{-2}) in the linear region of the curves at 20% strain. For example, Figure 3 shows the stress-strain curve of formulation 6. Addition of collagen to the formulation made it stronger than the disk fabricated with HA per se. increasing the concentration of HA and collagen increased the compressive modulus, which consequently provided higher strength against compressive strain. Nonetheless, increasing the HA concentration is more effective on the strength of formulations than increasing the collagen concentration. Zhang et al.,[10] Kim et al.,[12] Chen et al.[21] and Vikingsson et al.[22] reported similar results.

Cartilage as a tissue that is affected by different stresses like compressive, strain and tension, should be strong enough to resist these stresses. The negative charges of HA and collagen attract water molecules. This hydration effect increased the compressive strength of the tissue. Moreover, collagen is a kind of fibrous protein with negative charge in which three polypeptide chains form a stable helical structure. Thus, increase in the concentrations of HA and collagen improves the mechanical properties.[12]

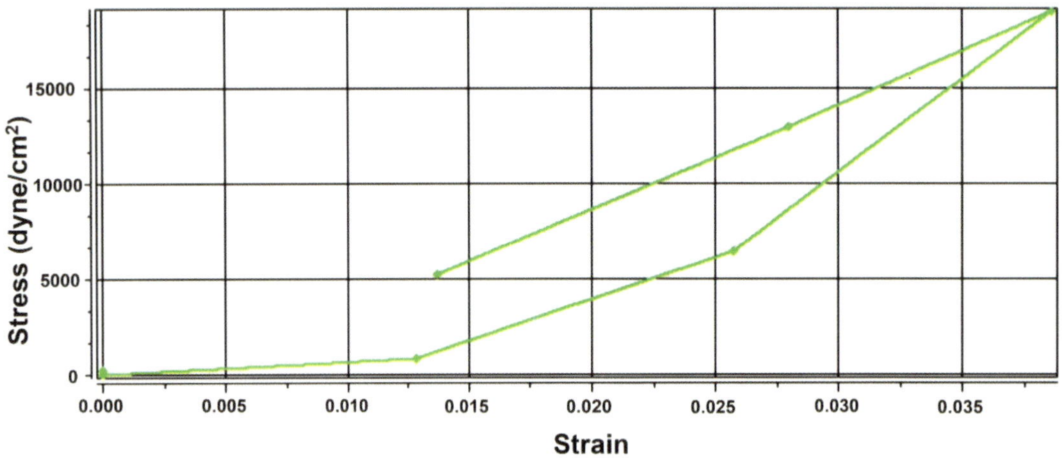

Figure 3. Stress-strain curve of F_6 formulation

Swelling measurement of implantable disks

The swelling profiles of implantable disks are shown in Figure 4. Accordingly, the percentage of water uptake was directly related to the concentration of HA and collagen. The effect of HA was higher and increasing the HA concentration caused higher percentage of swelling. Both HA and collagen are charged molecules and hydrophilic materials which attract water molecules; so, raising the concentration of HA and collagen increases the amount of water uptake. It seems that the polysaccharide structure of HA totally presents higher number of charges than the three polypeptide chains of collagen. The percentage of swelling affects the diffusion of signaling molecules and nutrients in scaffolds; hence, the higher concentration of HA and collagen would be preferred.[23]

In vitro degradation test of implantable disks

Figure 5 shows the degradation of implantable disks of formulations 1 to 6 in PBS at 37°C. Accordingly, increase in the concentration of HA and collagen decreased the amount and rate of degradation. It could be supposed that increase in the concentration of HA and collagen caused the polymer chains to be more ordered and massive, and consequently enhanced the durability of the structure, as proved in SEM images.[24] The effect of HA and collagen concentration in this test was almost similar; meanwhile, collagen was marginally more effective in stability of implantable disks.

Gelation temperature of thermo-sensitive gels

Results of measuring the gelation temperature of the gel formulations are presented in Table 1. All formulations would be converted into gel in the body after injection. It was detected that, increasing the HA concentration resulted in reduced gelation temperature; and inversely, increasing the collagen concentration resulted in increased gelation temperature.

Gelation time of thermo-sensitive gels

Table 1 shows the results of gelation time test. This test was done at 37°C and the results showed that all formulations converted to gel at the body temperature in less than five minutes. By increasing the HA concentration, the gelation time decreased; whereas, increasing the collagen concentration resulted in increased gelation time.

As the temperature increases, dehydration of hydrophobic polyoxypropylene blocks causes poloxamer molecules aggregate and change into micelles; which is the initial step in the gelation process. These spherical micelles have a dehydrated polyoxypropylene core with an outer layer of hydrated swollen polyoxyethylene chains. This micellization occurs when the samples are adequately concentrated. Organized packing of micelles causes gelation. Collagen might be able to interact with micelles, make bonds, and cause delay in the gelation process. Actually, after injection, a short gelation time would be useful in order to decrease the risk of dilution with physiological fluids and local depletion at the injection site.[25]

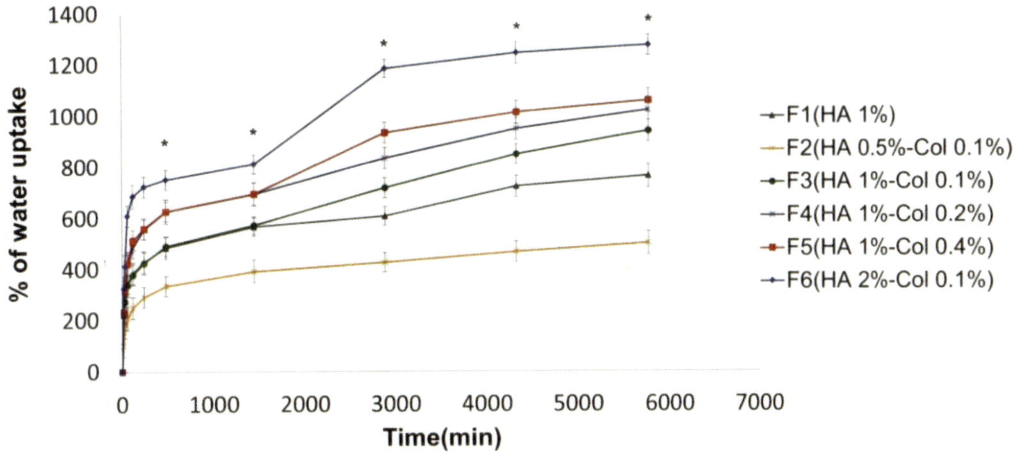

Figure 4. Swelling profile of implantable disk formulations F_1-F_6. Formulations F_2 to F_6 showed significant difference at determined times compared with F_1. (*p-value <0.05)

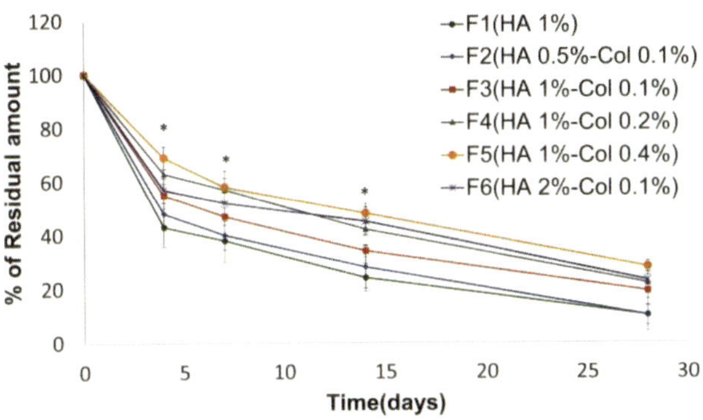

Figure 5. Degradation profile of implantable disk formulations F_1-F_6. Formulations F_2 to F_6 showed significant difference at determined times in comparison to F_1. (*p-value <0.05)

Drug release measurement

Intrinsic solubility of prednisolone in water is 1:1300; but, use of sodium lauryl sulfate (SLS) increased this ratio up to 1:100 and provided the sink condition.[26] Prednisolone powder was dissolved in the dissolution medium, and the samples were withdrawn and quantified at predetermined time points. It was done to show that the prednisolone release in sustained manner was not related to the limited dissolution rate of prednisolone (Figure 6).

Having separately tested the gels and implantable disks (Figure 6), it was found that at least 60% of the prednisolone was dissolved in the first point of the dissolution profile. It can be concluded that at least within the first 24 h, the prednisolone release from dosage forms was not related to low solubility of prednisolone.[27]

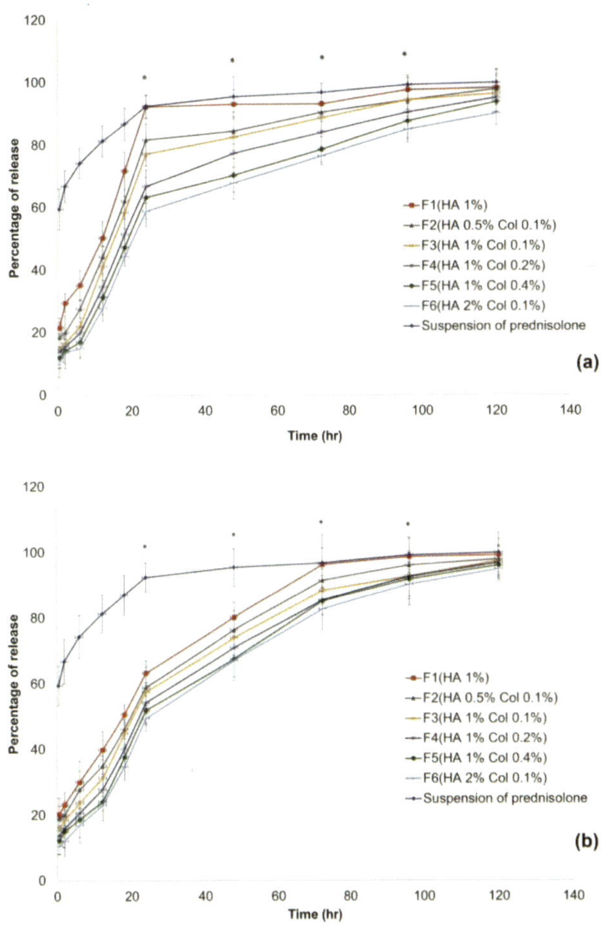

Figure 6. (a) Release profiles of implantable disk formulations F_1-F_6. (b) Release profiles of gel formulations F_1-F_6. Formulations F_2 to F_6 showed significant difference at determined times compared with F_1. (*p-value <0.05)

Figure 6 depicts some general trends like the fact that all the formulations were able to sustain the release of drug for more than 100 h. The release of the drug from these formulations was completed within 120 h. Increasing the concentration of HA and collagen resulted in significant decrease of prednisolone release. Although the effect of HA and collagen concentration on the release kinetic was the same, HA concentration provided more pronounced effects. This might be related to the structure of the scaffolds whose main backbone is HA, while prednisolone was just entrapped in this network. Release of drug from gel formulations was slower than implantable disk formulations, because poloxamer creates an additional barrier around the gel formulations and causes slower water penetration and consequently more long-lasting release behavior could be seen.

Korsmeyer-Peppas release model is often used to analyze the release mechanism of polymeric pharmaceutical dosage forms. This model is of great help particularly when the release mechanism is not known or when more than one type of release phenomena is involved. Kinetic of release for all formulations was better fit to Higuchi release kinetic based on the regression coefficients square calculated in Table 2. Based on the release data and fitting experimental results of M_t and M_∞ in the time range, diffusion exponent (n) for the two dosage forms was calculated (Equation 6) to be 0-0.5 ($0<n<0.5$).

It seems that the release mechanism for all scaffolds were the Fickian diffusion. This mechanism describes the condition in which the rate of diffusion is slower than the rate of chain relaxation.[13] Based on the degradation and swelling profiles of implantable disks in the first five days, about 50% of each disk was remained and swelled by more than 200% during the studied period. It could be concluded that these hybrid polymeric dosage forms are matrix systems that the drug transport and release through them is mainly provided by diffusion mechanism.[28-30]

Equation 6: $M_t/M_\infty = kt^n$

Herein, n is diffusional exponent, k is kinetic parameter, M_t and M_∞ are the absolute cumulative amounts of prednisolone released at time t and infinite time using the Korsmeyer-Peppas model.[31]

Statistical Analysis

According to the results of different tests and one-way ANOVA, the formulation F_6 of implantable disks and thermo-sensitive gels was significantly different from other formulations and was chosen to be examined in the ongoing *in vivo* study.

Table 2. Results of fitting release data of implantable disk and gel formulations to different kinetic models.

Formulations	R^2_{0i}	R^2_{0g}	R^2_{1i}	R^2_{1g}	R^2_{Hi}	R^2_{Hg}	R^2_{pi}	R^2_{pg}	k_{pi}	k_{pg}	n_{pi}	n_{pg}
F1	0.9575	0.9781	0.977	0.9852	0.9831	0.9887	0.897	0.8919	0.24	0.21	0.3519	0.283
F2	0.971	0.9713	0.9834	0.9875	0.9841	0.9831	0.8601	0.8568	0.18	0.19	0.3848	0.2808
F3	0.9682	0.9656	0.9835	0.9742	0.991	0.9831	0.8447	0.8473	0.15	0.16	0.4271	0.3127
F4	0.9553	0.9781	0.9871	0.9857	0.9899	0.9871	0.8324	0.8523	0.14	0.14	0.4011	0.3326
F5	0.9792	0.9603	0.9835	0.9715	0.9864	0.9894	0.8265	0.8304	0.12	0.13	0.4172	0.3393
F6	0.962	0.9593	0.9805	0.9752	0.9901	0.9922	0.8177	0.8519	0.11	0.11	0.4226	0.3763

R^2_{0i} = Regression coefficient square of zero order model for implantable disks; R^2_{0g} = Regression coefficient square of zero order model for gels; R^2_{1i} = Regression coefficient square of first order model for implantable disks; R^2_{1g} = Regression coefficient square of first order model for gels; R^2_{Hi} = Regression coefficient square of Higuchi model for implantable disks; R^2_{Hg} = Regression coefficient square of Higuchi model for gels; R^2_{pi} = Regression coefficient square of exponential model for implantable disks; R^2_{pg} = Regression coefficient square of exponential model for gels; k_{pi} = kinetic parameter of exponential model for implantable disks; k_{pg} = kinetic parameter of exponential model for gels; n_{pi} = diffusion exponent of exponential model for implantable disks; n_{pg} = diffusion exponent of exponential model for gels.

Conclusion

Based on the findings of this study, it can be concluded that hybrid formulations are superior to formulations containing HA per se. All of the formulated scaffolds were porous and had interconnected pores, suggesting that the scaffolds are useful for the growth of cells and tissues. Furthermore, increasing the concentration of HA and collagen improves the mechanical properties.

Regarding the release test, gel formulations showed more sustained release profile. However, both systems showed Higuchi release kinetic at least for the first 24 h. It can be claimed that hybrid scaffolds (implantable lyophilized disk and injectable gel) can be easily applied as useful dosage forms for cartilage tissue regeneration.

Acknowledgments

This paper was part of a thesis written by Farhad Mohammadi for the partial fulfillment of PhD degree. It was financially supported by Shiraz University of Medical Sciences (Grant# 94-7585).

Ethical Issues

Not applicable.

Conflict of Interest

The authors declare no conflict of interests.

References

1. Hunziker EB. Articular cartilage repair: Basic science and clinical progress. A review of the current status

and prospects. *Osteoarthritis Cartilage* 2002;10(6):432-63. doi: 10.1053/joca.2002.0801

2. Sharma C, Gautam S, Dinda AK, Mishra NC. Cartilage tissue engineering: Current scenario and challenges. *Adv Mater Lett* 2011;2(2):90-9.
3. Buckwalter JA, Mankin HJ. Articular cartilage repair and transplantation. *Arthritis Rheum* 1998;41(8):1331-42.
4. Gohel MC, Parikh RK, Nagori SA, Jena DG. Fabrication of modified release tablet formulation of metoprolol succinate using hydroxypropyl methylcellulose and xanthan gum. *AAPS PharmSciTech* 2009;10(1):62-8. doi: 10.1208/s12249-008-9174-1
5. Perera G, Barthelmes J, Bernkop-Schnurch A. Novel pectin-4-aminothiophenole conjugate microparticles for colon-specific drug delivery. *J Control Release* 2010;145(3):240-6. doi: 10.1016/j.jconrel.2010.04.024
6. Kreuz PC, Steinwachs MR, Erggelet C, Krause SJ, Konrad G, Uhl M, et al. Results after microfracture of full-thickness chondral defects in different compartments in the knee. *Osteoarthritis Cartilage* 2006;14(11):1119-25. doi: 10.1016/j.joca.2006.05.003
7. Hunziker EB. The elusive path to cartilage regeneration. *Adv Mater* 2009;21(32-33):3419-24. doi: 10.1002/adma.20080195
8. Lu Q, Ganesan K, Simionescu DT, Vyavahare NR. Novel porous aortic elastin and collagen scaffolds for tissue engineering. *Biomaterials* 2004;25(22):5227-37. doi: 10.1016/j.biomaterials.2003.12.019
9. Collins MN, Birkinshaw C. Comparison of the effectiveness of four different crosslinking agents with hyaluronic acid hydrogel films for tissue-culture applications. *J Appl Polym Sci* 2007;104(5):3183-91. doi: 10.1002/app.25993
10. Zhang L, Li K, Xiao W, Zheng L, Xiao Y, Fan H, et al. Preparation of collagen–chondroitin sulfate–hyaluronic acid hybrid hydrogel scaffolds and cell compatibility in vitro. *Carbohydr Polym* 2011;84(1):118-25. doi: 10.1016/j.carbpol.2010.11.009
11. Park H, Guo X, Temenoff JS, Tabata Y, Caplan AI, Kasper FK, et al. Effect of swelling ratio of injectable hydrogel composites on chondrogenic differentiation of encapsulated rabbit marrow mesenchymal stem cells in vitro. *Biomacromolecules* 2009;10(3):541-6. doi: 10.1021/bm801197m
12. Kim HJ, Kim KK, Park IK, Choi BS, Kim JH, Kim MS. Hybrid scaffolds composed of hyaluronic acid and collagen for cartilage regeneration. *Tissue Eng Regen Med* 2012;9(2):57-62. doi: 10.1007/s13770-012-0007-7
13. Bermudez JM, Grau R. Thermosensitive poloxamer-based injectables as controlled drug release platforms for veterinary use: Development and in-vitro evaluation. *Int Res J Pharm Pharmacol* 2011;1(6):109-18.
14. Holland TA, Tabata Y, Mikos AG. Dual growth factor delivery from degradable oligo(poly(ethylene glycol) fumarate) hydrogel scaffolds for cartilage tissue engineering. *J Control Release* 2005;101(1-3):111-25. doi: 10.1016/j.jconrel.2004.07.004
15. Calderon L, Collin E, Velasco-Bayon D, Murphy M, O'Halloran D, Pandit A. Type II collagen-hyaluronan hydrogel--a step towards a scaffold for intervertebral disc tissue engineering. *Eur Cell Mater* 2010;20:134-48.
16. Collins MN, Birkinshaw C. Physical properties of crosslinked hyaluronic acid hydrogels. *J Mater Sci Mater Med* 2008;19(11):3335-43. doi: 10.1007/s10856-008-3476-4
17. Strom A, Larsson A, Okay O. Preparation and physical properties of hyaluronic acid-based cryogels. *J Appl Polym Sci* 2015;132(29):1-11. doi: 10.1002/app.42194
18. Touyama R, Inoue K, Takeda Y, Yatsuzuka M, Ikumoto T, Moritome N, et al. Studies on the blue pigments produced from genipin and methylamine. Ii. On the formation mechanisms of brownish-red intermediates leading to the blue pigment formation. *Chem Pharm Bull* 1994;42(8):1571-8. doi: 10.1248/cpb.42.1571
19. Touyama R, Takeda Y, Inoue K, Kawamura I, Yatsuzuka M, Ikumoto T, et al. Studies on the blue pigments produced from genipin and methylamine. I. Structures of the brownish-red pigments, intermediates leading to the blue pigments. *Chem Pharm Bull* 1994;42(3):668-73. doi: 10.1248/cpb.42.668
20. Vikingsson L, Gomez-Tejedor JA, Gallego Ferrer G, Gomez Ribelles JL. An experimental fatigue study of a porous scaffold for the regeneration of articular cartilage. *J Biomech* 2015;48(7):1310-7. doi: 10.1016/j.jbiomech.2015.02.013
21. Chen J, Zhou R, Li L, Li B, Zhang X, Su J. Mechanical, rheological and release behaviors of a poloxamer 407/ poloxamer 188/carbopol 940 thermosensitive composite hydrogel. *Molecules* 2013;18(10):12415-25. doi: 10.3390/molecules181012415
22. Vikingsson L, Claessens B, Gomez-Tejedor JA, Gallego Ferrer G, Gomez Ribelles JL. Relationship between micro-porosity, water permeability and mechanical behavior in scaffolds for cartilage engineering. *J Mech Behav Biomed Mater* 2015;48:60-9. doi: 10.1016/j.jmbbm.2015.03.021
23. Spiller KL, Maher SA, Lowman AM. Hydrogels for the repair of articular cartilage defects. *Tissue Eng Part B Rev* 2011;17(4):281-99. doi: 10.1089/ten.TEB.2011.0077
24. Gupta D, Tator CH, Shoichet MS. Fast-gelling injectable blend of hyaluronan and methylcellulose for intrathecal, localized delivery to the injured spinal cord. *Biomaterials* 2006;27(11):2370-9. doi: 10.1016/j.biomaterials.2005.11.015
25. Drury JL, Mooney DJ. Hydrogels for tissue engineering: Scaffold design variables and applications. *Biomaterials* 2003;24(24):4337-51. doi: 10.1016/S0142-9612(03)00340-5

26. Moffat AC, Osselton MD, Widdop B, Galichet LY. Clarke's analysis of drugs and poisons. 3rd ed. USA: Pharmaceutical Press; 2005.
27. Kurakula M, Mohd AB, Samhuidrom, A PR, Diwan PV. Estimation of prednisolone in proliposomal formulation using RP HPLC method. *Int J Res Pharm Biomed Sci* 2011;2(4):1663-9.
28. Ahmadi F, Giti R, Mohammadi-Samani S, Mohammadi F. Biodegradable scaffolds for cartilage tissue engineering. *GMJ* 2017;6(2):70-80. doi: 10.22086/GMJ.V6I2.696
29. Fu Y, Kao WJ. Drug release kinetics and transport mechanisms of non-degradable and degradable polymeric delivery systems. *Expert Opin Drug Deliv* 2010;7(4):429-44. doi: 10.1517/17425241003602259
30. Ranjha NM, Ayub G, Naseem S, Ansari MT. Preparation and characterization of hybrid ph-sensitive hydrogels of chitosan-co-acrylic acid for controlled release of verapamil. *J Mater Sci Mater Med* 2010;21(10):2805-16. doi: 10.1007/s10856-010-4134-1
31. Liechty WB, Kryscio DR, Slaughter BV, Peppas NA. Polymers for drug delivery systems. *Annu Rev Chem Biomol Eng* 2010;1:149-73. doi: 10.1146/annurev-chembioeng-073009-100847

Comparative Study of Different Combinational Mucoadhesive Formulations of Sumatriptan-Metoclopramide

Mitra Jelvehgari[1,2], Hadi Valizadeh[1,2]*, Sanam Ziapour[3,4], Mahdieh Rahmani[4], Seyed Hassan Montazam[5], Saieede Soltani[1]

[1] *Drug Applied Research Center, Tabriz University of Medical Sciences, Tabriz, Iran.*
[2] *Faculty of Pharmacy, Tabriz University of Medical Sciences, Tabriz, Iran.*
[3] *Biotechnology Research center, Tabriz University of Medical Sciences, Tabriz, Iran.*
[4] *Student Research Committee, Tabriz University of Medical Sciences, Tabriz, Iran.*
[5] *Department of Microbiology, Bonab Branch, Islamic Azad University, Bonab, Iran.*

Keywords:
- Mucoadhesive
- Buccal
- Transmucosal
- Sumatriptan
- Metoclopramide

Abstract
Purpose: Sumatriptan succinate (Sum) is a Serotonin 5- HT1 receptor agonist, used in the treatment of migraine. It is absorbed rapidly but incompletely when taken orally and underwent first - pass metabolism, resulting in a low bioavailability of about 15%. The aim was to design mucoadhesive buccal discs and sublingual films of Sum and metoclopramide (Met) combined to improve their bioavailability.
Methods: In the current study, the microparticles and films were prepared by emulsion solvent diffusion (ESD) and solvent casting methods, respectively. Buccal-mucoadhesive microparticles and films with different drug to polymer ratios were prepared and characterized by encapsulation efficiency, particle size, DSC (Differential Scanning Calorimetric), folding endurance, mucoadhesive property and drug release studies.
Results: The best drug/s to polymer ratios in films and microparticles were 1:2.7:8 (SM_2) and 1:4:6 (SM_4), respectively. The film of SM_2 showed 11.01 mg weight, 123 µm thickness and 300 folding endurance. The production yield was 107.33% for SM_4 microparticles, 323.59 µm for mean particle size and 94.53% for loading efficiency (for Sum) and 104.18% (for Met). The DSC showed no stable characteristic of Sum and Met in the drug loaded films/discs and revealed amorphous form and transition of hydrate to anhydrous form for Met. The films exhibited very good mucoadhesive properties and shorter retention time (15-30 s) in comparison with the discs (130 min). The results showed that the discs prepared had slower release than the films ($p<0.05$).
Conclusion: Films and discs of Sum-Met combinations were successfully prepared with improved release and mucoadhesive properties.

Introduction

Migraine is recognized as a common neurovascular disorder which displays recurrent episodes of immobilizing headache and autonomic nervous system dysfunction. Neurological aura symptoms are also observed in some patients.[1,2] Nonspecific treatments such as antiemetics are prescribed in treating any kind of pain, and specific therapies such as triptans are exclusively effective in treating migraine and related disorders.[3,4] Triptans are frequently prescribed in the treatment of acute migraine attacks as they are potent in providing wide efficacy and tolerability.[1,5]
Sumatriptan succinate (Sum) as a 5-HT1receptor agonist is employed in the removal of symptoms of migraine headaches. However, due to severe nausea or vomiting during the migraine attacks and low oral bioavailability (15%) because of high first-pass metabolism, the oral treatment proves unsatisfactory.[6,7]
This medication is commercially available as oral tablet, nasal spray and subcutaneous injection.[8]
The antiemetic properties of metoclopramide (Met) apparently are a result of antagonism of its central and peripheral dopamine receptors. Met is ordinarily prescribed for the treatment of nausea and vomiting. This drug is highly water soluble and is swiftly absorbed after oral administration. It has a short biological half-life (4.5 h) and is commonly administered in a dose of 10 to 15 mg four times per day in order to maintain effective concentrations throughout the day. In long -term therapy, fluctuation in the plasma concentration, with high concentration

***Corresponding author:** Hadi Valizadeh, Email: valizadeh@tbzmed.ac.ir peaks are common for drugs with rapid absorption and elimination.

Hydroxypropyl methylcellulose is an odorless and tasteless, white to slightly off-white, fibrous or granular, free-flowing powder that is a synthetic modification of the natural polymer, cellulose. The reason for its widespread acceptance include (1) solubility characteristics of the polymer in gastrointestinal fluid, and in organic and aqueous solvent systems, (2) noninterference with tablet disintegration and drug availability, (3) flexibility, chip resistance and absence of taste and odor, (4) stability in the presence of heat, light, air or reasonable levels of moisture, (5) ability to incorporate color and other additives into the film without difficulty.

Thin-film and disc-buccal drug delivery benefit a dissolving film or oral drug to be administered via absorption in the mouth (buccally or sublingually) and/or in small intestines (enterically). Film is prepared using hydrophilic polymers that rapidly dissolve upon the tongue or buccal cavity, and delivers the drug to the systemic circulation through dissolution when a contact is made with liquid. Thin dissolvable films of drugs delivered sublingually are potent to trigger the beginning of action, lower the dosing, and increase the efficacy and safety profile of the medication.[9]

Therefore the objectives of this work are; to develop a new drug delivery system for Sum which could be administered through the buccal (discs prepared from microspheres)/sublingual (film) route, to particularly target the mucous region in order to result in a rapid relief by fast onset of action; to increase bioavailability; and to avoid the second dose administration. Its sublingual film and buccal disc applications may be better alternatives that also reduce the side effects associated with oral and parental therapy.[7]

Oral transmucosal absorption generally occurs rapidly because of the rich vascular supply to the mucosa and the lack of a stratum corneum epidermidis. This minuscule barrier to drug transport results in a rapid rise in blood concentration level. Oral transmucosal administration has the advantage in avoiding the enterohepatic circulation and instaneous destruction by gastric acid or partial first-pass effects of hepatic metabolism.[10]

Sublingual and buccal medications are prepared either in the form of small, quick dissolving tablets, or in sprays, lozenges and liquid suspensions. The administration of these medications is through placing the medication in the mouth, either under the tongue (sublingual), or between the gum and the cheek (buccal). This form of medication administration is very adequate as it bypasses the digestive system and is absorbed in the blood flow in minutes. Should administered properly, sublingual and buccal therapies act within 1 to 5 min of administration.[11]

Hence the present study aimed to prepare and evaluate sublingual film/buccal discs of sumatriptan combined with methoclopramide and using bioadhesive polymer, in order to improve the therapeutic efficacy of these drugs and reduce their dose dependent side effects and frequency of administration in treating migraine.

Materials and methods

Materials

Sumatriptan succinate (Sum), metoclopramide hydrochloride (Met), HPMC (E-15), ethanol, dichloromethane, potassium dihydrogen phosphate, sodium hydroxide, sodium chloride, potassium chloride, sodium sulfate, ammonium acetate, urea, lactic acid, liquid paraffin, span 80 and propylene glycol were obtained from Merck (Darmstadt, Germany). All solvents and reagents were of analytical grade.

Experimental methods

Preparation of Sum and Met combined film

Sublingual films of Sum and Met combined were prepared by solvent casting technique using a film forming mucoadhesive polymer. HPMC was accurately weighed (200 mg) and dissolved in 2.5 ml of ethanol. The beaker containing polymer and ethanol was kept aside for 5 min for the polymer to swell. Next, 2.5 ml of dichloromethane was added to the above polymer solution and the dispersion was stirred. Then, one drop of propylene glycol (0.030 g) was added to the polymer solution. Sum drug was accurately weighed with a different drug-to-polymer ratio (50, 66.7 and 100 mg) and then dissolved in 2 ml of water in beaker. In second step, Met drug was weighed with a constant amount (25 mg) and added to the Sum solution beaker. The drugs' solution was then added to the polymer solution and mixed thoroughly with a magnetic stirrer. The solution was utterly poured into the glass Petri dish placed over a flat surface. Then an inverted funnel was placed over the dish to prevent sudden evaporation. The mould containing the polymeric solution of drug was kept for 12 h at room temperature to dry. After drying, the films were observed and checked for possible imperfections upon their removal from the moulds. They were covered with wax paper and kept in desiccators until the evaluation tests were conducted. These new films were examined in order to identify and select the film showing the best characteristics (Table 1).

Preparation of Sum and Met combination microparticles

Microparticles of Sum and Met were prepared using HPMC polymer with different drugs-to-polymer ratios (1:4:6, 1:4:10 and 1:4:14 w/w). Briefly, HPMC (300, 500 and 700 mg) was dissolved in 2.5 ml of ethanol and 2.5 ml of dichloromethane by stirring at 500 rpm with magnetic stirrer. Drugs were then added to polymeric solution and stirred until complete dissolution. Then the resultant drug-polymer suspension was injected using a 5 ml syringe into 100 ml of light liquid paraffin with 3 g of span 80 and propylene glycol (0.030 g) while stirring to form an O1/O2 emulsion. Stirring was continued for 2 h and then 25 ml of petroleum ether was added at 600 rpm until complete solvent evaporation and microspheres' formation. After another 2 h, the hardened microparticles were collected by filtration and washed with three portions of 30 ml petroleum ether and air dried at room temperature for 24 h. Microspheres were allowed to be dried at room temperature (Table 1).

Table 1. Sumatriptan succinate combined with methoclopramide hydrochloride films/discs with different drug to polymer ratios prepared by solvent casting and (O1/O2) emulsion solvent diffusion method, respectively

Formulation code	Drug to polymer ratio	Metoclopramide hydrochloride (mg)	Sumatriptan succinate (mg)	HPMC (mg)	water (ml)	dichloromethane (ml)	ethanol (ml)	Liquid paraffine (ml)	Petrulum ether (ml)	Span 80 (g)	Propylen glycol (g)
SM1	1:2:8	25	50	200	2	2.5	2.5	-	-		0.03
SM_2	1:2.7:8	25	66.7	200	2	2.5	2.5	-	-		0.03
SM_3	1:4:8	25	100	200	2	2.5	2.5	-	-		0.03
SM_4	1:4:6	50	200	300	-	2.5	2.5	100	25	3	0.03
SM_5	1:4:10	50	200	500	-	2.5	2.5	100	25	3	0.03
SM_6	1:4:14	50	200	700	-	2.5	2.5	100	25	3	0.03

Characterization of buccoadhesive microparticles' studies

Determination of loading efficiency and production yield

The loading efficiency was calculated using the following formula:

$$\text{Loading efficiency (\%)} = (\text{actual drug content in microparticles/theoretical drug content}) \times 100 \qquad \text{Eq. (A-1)}$$

The production yield of the microparticles was determined by dividing the final weight of the polymeric particles to the initial weight of the raw materials. Each determination was performed in triplicate.

Frequency distribution analysis

Samples of microparticles were analyzed for frequency distribution with calibrated optical microscope, fitted with a stage and an ocular micrometer. Small quantities of microsphere were spread on a clean glass slide and the average particle size of 60, frequency distribution and mean particle size were determined in each batch using scion image and sigma plot software packages.

Disc production and physicochemical characterization

Each disc contained 100 mg of Sum and Met microspheres (with different drug-to-polymer ratios of 1:4:6, 1:4:10, 1:4:14). The discs were round and flat with an average diameter of 6 ± 0.1 mm compressed with a constant compression force (2 tones). Hardness of the discs was determined for six discs using Erweka hardness tester (Erweka, Germany). Friability of the prepared discs was assessed using friability tester (Erweka, Germany).

Characterization of buccoadhesive film studies

Appearance of the films was appraised by observing the color, elegance, stickiness and texture.

Weight uniformity of films

Six films of size $1\times1cm^2$ of every formulation were individually weighed in a digital balance (Sartorius, Germany) and the weight variation was calculated.

Thickness uniformity of the films

Thickness of films was measured using digital vernier calipers at five different points (one center and four corners) of the film and the average was calculated (Mitutoyo, Japan).[12]

Folding endurance

The folding endurance of each film was decided by counting the number of times the film (size $1x1\ cm^2$) could be folded repeatedly (folded or broken up to 300 times), which was supposed reasonable to reveal good film properties.[13]

Moisture content loss and moisture absorption

The films were accurately weighed and kept in desiccators containing: a) anhydrous calcium chloride and b) 100ml of saturated solution of aluminum chloride, which maintained 76% and 86% humidity (RH). After 3 days, the films were taken out and weighed. The moisture content (%) was determined by calculating the moisture loss (%) using the following formula:[13]

$$\text{Moisture content (\%)} = \text{Initial weight} - \text{final weight} / \text{Initial weight} \times 100 \qquad \text{Eq. (A-2)}$$

The moisture absorption was also calculated using the following formula:[13]

$$\text{Moisture absorption (\%)} = \text{Final weight} - \text{initial weight} / \text{Initial weight} \times 100 \qquad \text{Eq. (A-3)}$$

Drug content and content uniformity

The films (five samples of each film) were analyzed for the content uniformity by dissolving $1\times1cm^2$ films in 10 ml phosphate buffer, pH 6.8, with simultaneous shaking for several hours. The absorbance of the solution (Sum and Met) was measured by UV spectrophotometer at 227.4 (Sum) and 272.4 (Met) nm. All experiments were performed in triplicate.

Characterization of buccoadhesive film/microparticles' studies

Differential Scanning Colorimetry (DSC)

The physical state of drug in the microspheres was analyzed by Differential Scanning Calorimeter (Shimadzu, Japan). The thermograms were obtained at a scanning rate of 10 °C/min conducted over a temperature range of 25-300 °C.

Determination of surface pH

The surface pH of formulations was determined using a combined glass electrode in order to investigate their possible side effects *in vivo.* An acidic or alkaline formulation causes the irritation of mucosal membrane and hence this is an important parameter in developing a mucoadhesive dosage form. The discs/films were first allowed to swell by keeping them in contact with 5 ml phosphate buffer and pH 6.8 for 4 h in 50 ml beakers. pH was then noted by bringing the electrode near the surface of the formulation and allowing equilibration for 1 min. Surface pH was measured at predetermined time intervals (0, 60, 90, 120, and 240 min). The experiments were carried out in triplicate.

Disc swelling studies

Bioadhesive preparations can swell in the presence of saliva. The swelling rate of buccoadhesive discs was evaluated by placing the accurately weighed discs (W_1) in 50 ml phosphate buffer solution (pH 6.8) at 37 °C. Swelling was measured at predetermined time intervals (15, 30, 60, 90 and 120 min). Then the discs were removed from the beaker after carefully removing the excess surface water using the filter paper. The swollen disc was weighed again (W_2) and the swelling index were calculated accordingly:

$$\text{Swelling index} = (W_2 - W_1)/ W_1 \times 100 \qquad \text{Eq. (B-1)}$$

Initial diameter of the film (1x1 cm^2) was determined when placed in a phosphate buffer solution and incubated at 37±1°C was (D_1). Then swollen film diameter was re-measured (D_2) at regular intervals (up to 1 h) and the swelling index was calculated using the following formula:[14,15]

$$\text{Swelling index} = D_2 - D_1/D_1 \qquad \text{Eq. (B-2)}$$

Ex vivo mucoadhesion time

Sheep were used in this study. The animals were fed and watered ad libitum. They were kept in the Animal House at a controlled ambient temperature of 25±2 °C with 50±10% relative humidity and a 12-h light/ 12-h dark cycle. The present study was conducted according to the Guide for the Care and Use of Laboratory Animals of Tabriz University of Medical Sciences, Tabriz-Iran (National Institutes of Health Publication No 85-23, revised 1985). The selected film/discs were subjected to *ex vivo* mucoadhesion test. The disintegration medium contained 900 ml phosphate buffer, pH 6.8, maintained at 37 °C. A segment of sheep buccal mucosa, 3 cm long, was glued to the surface of a glass slab and vertically attached to the disintegration apparatus (Erweka, Germany).[16] The mucoadhesive films/discs were hydrated from one surface and then brought into contact with the mucosal membrane. The glass slab was so vertically fixed to the apparatus that allowed it to move up and down; thus, the film was completely immersed in the buffer solution at the lowest point and was out at the highest point. The time demanded for complete erosion or detachment of the films from the mucosal surface was recorded. The experiment was performed in triplicate.

Bioadhesion strength

The tensile strength required to detach the bioadhesive films/discs from the mucosal surface was applied as a measure of the bioadhesive performance. The apparatus was locally assembled. The device mainly composed of a two-arm balance (Figure 1).

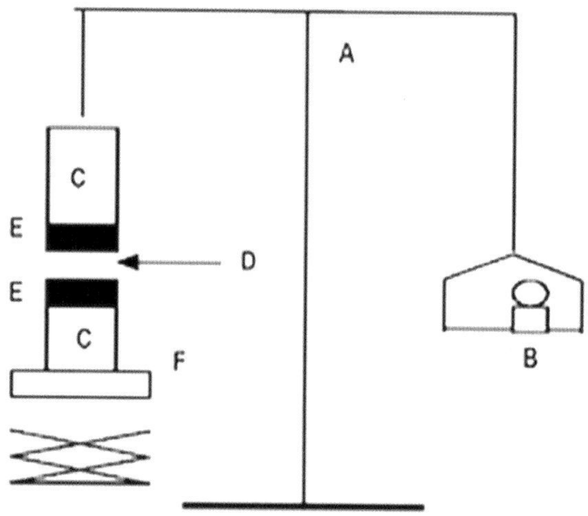

Figure 1. Bioadhesive force measuring device: (A) modified balance; (B, E) glass vial; (C) discs; (D) tissue; (F) Weights; (G) height-adjustable pan.

The mucoadhesive forces of films were measured by means of the mucoadhesive force-measuring device,[16] using the tissue cut from sheep buccal mucosa. The pieces of mucosa were stored frozen in phosphate buffer, pH 7.4, and thawed to room temperature before use. At the time of testing, a section of mucosa was secured to the upper glass vial (C) using a cyanoacrylate adhesive (E). The diameter of each exposed mucosal membrane was 1.5 cm. The vials were equilibrated and maintained at 37 °C for 10 min. Next, one vial with a section of tissue (E) was connected to the balance (A) and the other vial was fixed on a height-adjustable pan (F). To expose the tissue on this vial, a constant amount of films (D) was applied. The height of vial was so adjusted that the films/discs could adhere to the mucosal tissues of both vials. Immediately, a constant force of 0.5 N was applied for 2 min to ensure the intimate contact between the tissues and the samples. The vial was then moved upwards at a constant speed and connected to the balance. Weights were added at a regular rate to the pan on the other side of the modified balance of the used device until the two vials were separated. During measurement, 150 μl of phosphate buffer at pH 6.8 was evenly spread onto the surface of the test membrane. The bioadhesive force, noticed as the detachment stress in g/cm^2, was determined from the minimal weights that detached the tissues from the surface of each formulation using the following equation:[16]

$$\text{Detachment Stress}\left(g/cm^2\right) = \frac{m}{A} \qquad \text{Eq. (B-3)}$$

Where *m* is the weight added to the balance in grams and *A* is the area of tissue exposed. Measurements were repeated three times for each of the films. All the above three experiments were conducted in triplicate.

Permeation studies

The *in vitro* permeation study of the Sum and Met combined films/discs through the buccal mucosal of sheep was performed using Franz diffusion cell at 37 ± 0.2 °C. Freshly obtained buccal mucosa was mounted between the donor and receptor compartments so that the smooth surface of the mucosa faced the donor compartment. The films/discs were placed on the mucosa and the compartments were clamped together. The donor compartment was filled with 3 ml simulated saliva, pH 6.8 (sodium chloride 4.50 g, sodium sulfate 0.30 g, potassium chloride 0.30 g, urea 0.20 g, ammonium acetate 0.40 g, lactic acid 3 g, and distilled water up to 1,000 mL, adjusting pH of the solution to 6.8 by 1 M NaOH solution). The receptor compartment was filled with 22-25 ml phosphate buffer, pH 7.4, and stirred with a magnetic bead at 700 rpm.[17]

Three milliliters of sample were withdrawn at predetermined time intervals and analyzed for drugs at 228 (Sum) and 272.4 (Met) nm.

In vitro release studies

In vitro release studies were carried out using an incubator shaker at 37 ±0.5 °C, at a stirring speed of 50 rpm. Films/discs were fixed on glass slides and placed at the bottom of beaker. The studies were performed for all formulations (Sum and Met combination) in triplicate, using 50 ml (37 °C, 50 rpm) of isotonic phosphate buffer (pH 6.8) as the dissolution medium. An aliquot of 3 ml sample was withdrawn at regular intervals and replaced immediately with an equal volume of fresh phosphate buffer (pH 6.8). Samples were then analyzed at 226.6 (Sum) and 272 (Met) nm with UV spectrophotometer.

Histopathological evaluation of mucosa

Histopathological evaluation of tissue incubated in phosphate buffer, pH 6.8, was compared with that treated with sublingual mucoadhesive films/discs delivered from mucoadhesion time test. The tissue was fixed with 10% formalin, routinely processed, and embedded in paraffin. The sections were cut and stained with hematoxylin and eosin on glass slides. A pathologist, blinded to the study, worked on detecting any damage to the tissue and assessed the sections on the light microscope.[17]

Results and Discussion

Mucoadhesive drug delivery system is a high potential means that is applied in delivering drugs to the body through targeting the stratified squamous epithelium which is supported by a connective tissue lamina propria in buccal mucosal membrane.[18] Drug penetration into the membrane first leaves behind a net of capillaries and arteries in lamina propria and then reaches the systemic circulation through the internal jugular vein.[19] This drug delivery system benefits from bioadhesion property of determined water soluble polymers which become adhesive on hydration and hence could be used in targeting buccal mucosa (lining of the cheek) to the systemic circulation.[20] The mucoadhesive drug delivery system suggests apparently some advantages. For example, the system enhances drug bioavailability as a result of avoidance of first-pass metabolism; if it encounters toxicity, effortlessly terminates the therapy and removes the dosage form from the buccal cavity; this system requires less frequency of administration and therefore shows a better patient compliance; it significantly reduces the costs and dose-related local or systemic side effects by targeting the disease sites or tissues; and in steady-state levels, it shows a reduction in fluctuation.[21] Thus, adhesive mucosal dosage forms have been prepared in the form of adhesive tablets (discs), adhesive gels, and adhesive patches (films) for oral delivery.[22] In transmucosal delivery, the demanded quantity of mucoadhesive polymer was supplied with required volume of solvent system and vortexed to allow the polymer to swell. The required quantity of drug was also dissolved in a small volume of solvent system and added to the polymer solution and mixed well.

In the present study, we prepared the sublingual films and mucoadhesive microspheres containing Sum and Met combinations by solvent casting technique and evaporation/extraction technique, respectively. The drug delivery system was formulated as a matrix. The physicochemical and mucoadhesive characteristics of all the formulations are shown in Table 2.

All the formulations were smooth, flexible, colorless (transparent), non-sticky and elegant in appearance, except for SM_3 film (dark color) (Figure 2).

The cut films were 1x1 cm^2 in size. The weight and thickness of SM films were in the range of 9.5-14.02 mg and 110.3-243 μm, respectively (Table 2). The SM_1 and SM_2 films resisted the breakage upon folding them for more than 300 times at the same place (Table 2).

The content of films was in the range of 1.03-1.80 mg/cm^2 (Sum) and 0.59-0.57 mg/cm^2 (Met), respectively. Though there was a small change in the loss of drug (Sum and Met) among the formulations, more uniformity was observed for films (96.63-100%,SM film, Sum combined with Met); 99.78-100%, SM' film, Met combined with Sum) as shown in Table 2.

Table 2. Effect of drug to polymer ratio on physicochemical characteristics and mucoadhesivity of sumatriptan combined with methoclopramide films/discs

Variables	Formulation code					
	SM_1	SM_2	SM_3	SM_4	SM_5	SM_6
Met :Sum: HPMC ratio	1:2:8	1:2.7:8	1:4:8	1:4:6	1:4:10	1:4:14
Weight variation (mg ± SD)	9.50 ± 2.50	11.01 ± 0.80	14.02 ± 1.20	99.85 ± 2.50	100.01 ± 2.80	99.02 ± 1.20
thickness (µm± SD)	110.30 ± 0.03	123 ± 0.007	243 ± 0.05	-	-	-
Folding endurance (n±SD)	>300±7	>300±10	89 ± 12	-	-	-
Drug content (%±SD)	**Sum:** 1.03 ± 0.33	1.15 ± 0.60	0.23 ± 0.02	15 ± 0.06	16.70 ± 0.23	19.90 ± 0.1
	Met: 0.59 ± 0.50	0.60 ± 0.80	0.57 ± 0.74	3.80 ± 0.06	4.30 ± 0.06	5.48 ± 0.06
Loading Efficiency (%±SD)	**Sum:** -	-	-	94.53±3.58	62.64±1.58	41.25±1.32
	Met: -	-	-	104.18±2.33	64.56±3.75	41.80±1.06
Content uniformity (%±SD)	**Sum:** 100 ± 0.02	98.59 ± 0.02	96.63 ±0.02	100 ± 0.12	97.49 ± 0.32	95.33 ± 0.22
	Met: 100 ± 0.01	99.9 ± 0.01	95.78 ± 0.06	100 ± 0.03	98.9 ± 0.01	94.59 ± 0.26
Production Yield (%±SD)	99.10 ± 9.1	100 ± 6.60	99.40 ± 2.30	107.33±3.78	88±9.16	69.66±6.65
Particle size (%±SD)	-	-	-	323.59±16.98	316.22±17.78	549.54±19.50
Absorbed moisture (% ± SD)	0.79 ± 0.44	1.06 ± 0.95	4.52 ± 1.79	-	-	-
Moisture loss (% ± SD)	0.79 ± 0.04	0.73 ± 0.08	2.85 ± 0.66	-	-	-
Surface pH (±SD)	6.6 ± 0.2	6.8 ± 0.1	6.9 ± 0.1	6.8 ± 0.00	6.8 ± 0.04	6.8 ± 0.02
Swelling index (%±SD)	19.85 ± 0.02	20 ± 0.01	14.18 ± 0.02	15.67 ± 0.82	16.20 ± 0.17	17.47 ± 0.41
Mucoadhesive strength (g/cm^2±SD)	134.81 ± 13.1	127.61 ± 8.4	120.50 ± 6.6	0.8 ± 0.16	1.11± 0.16	1.38 ± 0.09
Residence time (min±SD)	0.42 ± 0.002	0.33 ± 0.014	0.5 ± 0.004	61± 12.77	78 ± 19.67	130 ± 8.86

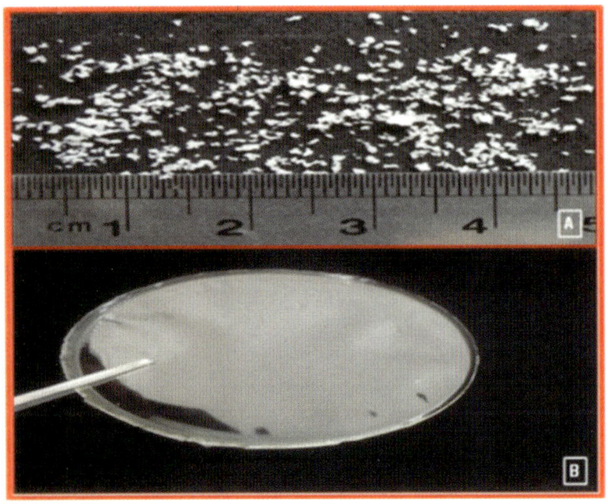

Figure 2. Optical microscopic photograph of mucoadhesive of sumatriptane combined with metoclopramide 2A: microparticle; 2B: film.

The optical image showed that the microspheres obtained from all the formulations had almost spherical shape with smooth surface microspheres (Figure 2). Particle analysis of microspheres prepared is shown in Table 2. An increase in the ratio of polymers from 1:4:6 to 1:4:14 resulted in a significant effect on the mean particle size of microparticles. The data scrutinizing showed that all obtained microparticles adhered to a log-probability distribution. The mean particle size significantly varied according to the amounts of polymer used for the preparation of microspheres; this may be due to a difference in the viscosity of polymer solutions, as high viscosity of the polymer solution (SM_6; 1:4:14 ratio) requires a high shearing energy to break the droplets of emulsion. Microspheres containing 700 mg HPMC were larger in comparison to other microspheres because this polymeric solution had more viscosity.

It is worth mentioning that an increase in the concentration of polymer in the internal phase leads to the increase in the size of microspheres. This occurs as at a higher concentration, polymer solution represents more viscosity which in turn requires more energy to break the droplets of dispersed phase.

Rank order of percentage drug loading for various formulations was found to be as follows: $SM_4>SM_5>SM_6$.

Percentage drug loading efficiency of microspheres was found in the range of 54.73 to 72.24% (Table 2). Formulation SM_6 (1:4:14 ratio) containing 50 mg Met, 200 mg Sum and 700 mg HPMC showed a maximum percentage of drug loading efficiency about 71.26% (for Sum) and 72.24% (for Met) because these microspheres had larger size as compared to other formulations. Whereas formulation SM_4 (1:4:6 ratio) containing 300 mg HPMC showed the minimum percentage of drug loading efficiency around 54.73% (for Sum) and 60.28% (for Met), because these microspheres were small in size, which resulted in more loss of drug from surface during washing of microspheres.

The percentage of moisture absorption was shown to range from 0.79±0.44 to 4.52±1.79% for films and 15.67±0.82 to 17.47±0.41% for discs. The moisture loss measured as 1.62-1.41% (for films) is shown in Table 2.

The percentage swelling of different microparticles'/discs' formulations was shown at different time intervals. The results depicted that all microsphere formulations swelled slowly when immersed in 0.2 M phosphate buffer (pH 6.8). The percentage swelling of different microparticle formulations was found to be followed after 4 h of incubation. Percent swelling was observed to be 15.67±0.82% (SM_4), 16.20±0.17% (SM_5) and 17.47±0.41% (SM_6), respectively (Table 2). The effect of drug on the swelling features of polymer is primarily associated with the substituted groups of the polymer. The hydroxyl group in the molecules plays a remarkable role in the matrix integrity of the swollen hydrophilic cellulose matrices. The matrix integrity is determined by the amount and properties of the incorporated drug. For a mucoadhesive polymer to expand and create a proper macromolecular mesh of sufficient size, the hydration is required to occur. The hydration is also longed for mobility in the polymer chains in order to enrich the interpenetration process between polymer and mucin. Polymer swelling induces a mechanical entanglement and exposes the bioadhesive sites to hydrogen bonding and/or electrostatic interaction between the polymer and the mucous network.[23] However, the occurrence of optimum swelling and bioadhesion is accompanied by a critical degree of hydration of the mucoadhesive polymer.[13]

The variation in weight and thickness among the formulations may be observed as a result of difference in concentration of drugs (Sum and Met) used in the films (Table 2). The combination of Sum and Met Films did not show any cracks even after folding for more than 300 times. Hence it was supposed as the end point. The values were considered optimum as they revealed appropriate film properties. Numerous hydrophilic functional groups such as hydroxyl and carboxyl are present in mucoadhesive polymer (HPMC). These groups cause hydrogen to bond with the substrate (mucus), to swell in aqueous media, and thereby allow maximal exposure of potential anchor sites. Furthermore, swollen HPMC has the maximum distance between its chains. This distance results in an increased chain flexibility and efficient penetration of substrate. HPMC (with low molecular weights) either forms loose gels or dissolves quickly. Chain flexibility is a required factor in interpretation and entanglement of mucoadhesive HPMC polymer. When water-soluble polymer becomes cross-linked, the mobility of individual polymer chains reduces and in turn the effective length of the chain that is demanded for penetration into the mucous layer decreases. This reduction in turn results in the reduction of bioadhesive strength.[24,25]

The comparative percentage swelling for various formulations was in order of $SM_4> SM_5 > SM_6$. A high percentage swelling was observed in HPMC containing microspheres due to the presence of more hydroxyl group in the HPMC molecules. The weight of these formulations was increased to the extent of 30 to 110% from the initial value within 4 h (Table 2). Although the remarkable increase in surface area during swelling could develop drug release, the increase in diffusion path length of the drug may conversely postpone the release.

As the drug was uniformly dispersed in the matrix of polymer, a significantly good amount of drug was loaded in all the formulations. Hence, the loss of drug could be related to its aqueous insolubility. Sum and Met are water-soluble and does not begin settling down from medicated solutions when dispersed for removal of air bubbles. Thus, the solutions were casted as films containing utter amount of drugs.

Percentage moisture absorption was associated with the capacity of excipients in absorbing vapor-form water. The HPMC polymer used was hydrophilic. It is believed that initial moisture content acts as distinct factor in moisture absorption. Therefore the high moisture absorbing capacity was evinced in SM_3 (4.52%) and more moisture loss was observed in SM_1 (1.62%). The other films primarily had high moisture content as was confirmed by percentage moisture loss. There was an inverse association between these two parameters, that is, the higher the percentage moisture loss, the lower the moisture absorption and vice versa.[12]

All formulations were of pH 6.6-6.9 for film and 6.66-6.8 for discs, respectively and it may be concluded that the films were safe and non-irritating to the oral mucosa (Table 2).

The surface pH of all discs was within the range of salivary pH (5.13-5.96). No significant difference was found in the surface pH of different films and discs (Table 2).

The acidic or alkaline pH may cause irritation to the sublingual mucosa. It may also influence the drug release and the degree of polymer hydration. Therefore it was revealed that the surface pH of sublingual film/buccal discs may optimize the drug release as well as mucoadhesion. The surface pH of all formulations was determined within ±0.5 units of the buccal pH (6.6-6.9);

hence, it were anticipated no mucosal irritations and patient compliance was finally achieved.[26]

Pure Sum exhibited a sharp melting exothermic and endothermic peak around 173.27 °C and Met was melted at 184.59-208.75°C (Figure 3). The intensity of Sum drug fusion peak, however, for the film and disc formulations was disappeared.

Pure Met monohydrate has a very high melting point (184.59-208.75°C). The endothermic peak at around 95.80 °C occurs probably due to the transition of drug to the anhydrous form via loss of one mole of water. It is clearly observed from the thermogram of the films and discs (Figure 3) that the drugs (Sum and Met) peak has been disappeared. However in the thermogram of formulations, the endothermic peak corresponding to the drugs melting was absent, suggesting the amorphous state of the drugs (Sum and Met).

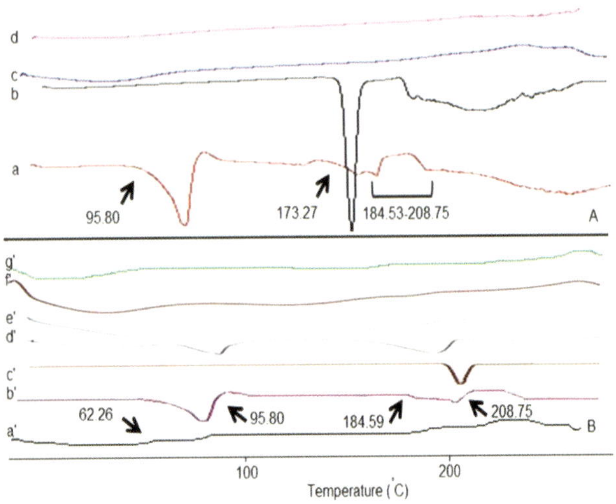

Figure 3. DSC thermogram of (A) film: sumatriptan (a); metoclopramide (b); HPMC (c); SM_2 (66.7 mg sumatriptan, 25 mg metoclopramide and 200 mg HPMC) (d); (B) disc: HPMC (a'); metoclopramide (b'); sumatriptan (c'); Physical mixture SM_4 (200 mg sumatriptan, 25 mg metoclopramide and 300 mg HPMC) (d'), SM_4 (e'); SM_5 (f'); SM_6 (g').

The DSC analysis of films/discs revealed a significant change in the melting point of Sum and Met drugs. This change illustrated a modification or interaction between the drug and polymer (Figure 3).

In vitro residence time determined the period of Sum adhering combined with Met films to the mucosa and it ranged from 25-30 s. All films showed low diameter swelling and the recorded swelling index for films was 14.18-20% after 4 h.

The *in vitro* residence time with mucosa for microparticles in phosphate buffer (pH 6.8) varied from 61 to 130 min (Table 2). Microparticles showed the highest mucoadesion in this study, and did not dissolve in 0.2 M phosphate buffer (pH 6.8) for about 4h. For SM_4 formulation, percentage of microparticles remaining was 61 min. SM_5 and SM_6 showed 78 and 130 min mucosa retentive time, respectively.

The results of *in vitro* bioadhesive strength study are shown in Table 2. The bioadhesion characteristics were affected by the concentration of bioadhesive polymer (HPMC). SM_1 films containing 1:2:8 ratios (Sum:Met:HPMC ratio) indicated the highest mucoadhesivity (134.81±13.1 g/cm^2). Conversely, SM_3 Formulations containing 1:4:8 ratios (Sum:Met:HPMC ratio) showed the lowest mucoadhesivity (120.5±6.6 g/cm^2).

The results of *in vitro* bioadhesive strength study for discs are also shown in Table 2. SM_6 Formulation containing 1:4:14 ratio (Met:Sum:HPMC) showed the highest mucoadhesivity (1.38±0.09 g/cm^2).

The integrity of Sum combined with Met films was lost early following their rapid uptake. Sum and Met drugs contain water-soluble molecules, which permit more water influx and result in quicker dissolution and erosion from mucosal surface. On the other hand, HPMC is a hydrophilic polymer and supposedly represents an affinity towards mucin comprising of 95% water. This property may be the reason for longer residence time (integrity of the films is lower). As it was also reported by several previous studies, the enhanced erosion rate was observed in some non-ionic polymers such as HPMC. The swelling behavior was assessed by measuring the diameter swelling. In the case of SM films supplied for sublingual (local) therapy uses, the contact area should have been as large as possible. This demand had to be balanced with patient compliance. Moreover, any excessive increase in the film diameter might have caused discomfort and/or dislodgment of the swollen film (lower than 20% swelling for Sum combined with Met films). In an *in vitro* mucoadhesion test performed by Nakanishi *et al.*,[27] the mucoadhesion force was dependant on the hydrogen bond made between the hydroxyl group in the polymer and mucus. It formed an ionic complex with hyaluronic acid that provided higher binding power. Bio-adhesive strength of formulation was increased due to a rise in the ratio of polymer. In the mucoadhesion process, this increase is required for swelling and expansion of the polymer chain as the interpenetration and entanglement of the polymer and the mucous networks supposedly are responsible for the adhesion.[28,29] Therefore, it seems that bioadhesives should swell and expand swiftly having contacted with water. For the hydrophilic polymer, hydration is responsible for the adhesion of polymer to the mucous membrane; as hydration makes these polymers sticky and hence they adhere to the mucous membrane. A high percentage of adhesion indicates that microspheres have excellent mucoadhesion to the mucosal tissue. HPMC interacts with the mucin and results in the adhesion of polymer to the mucin. The formulation films showed the highest mucoadhesivity, while the formulation discs indicated the lowest mucoadhesion strength due to the small size of microsphere which takes short time for solubilization. In this study, it was found no correlation between the bioadhesion force and the residence time of HPMC polymer. It seems that the high bioadhesive polymers do not necessarily inhabit any longer on the mucosal surface. Surface charge density and chain

flexibility are supposed to be preconditions for bioadhesion, whereas the residence time is basically dealt with the dissolution rate of the polymer.[30-32]
The release profiles for all films are showed in Figure 4. Films with high content uniformity or high drug entrapment showed a faster dissolution rate. Since more drugs are released from the films, it is supposed that more channels and pores are produced, contributing to the faster drug release rates. Comparison of various dissolution profiles is analyzed by several special measures including the dissolution $Rel_{0.5}$ (amount of drug release after 0.5h), $Rel_{0.75}$ (amount of drug release after 0.75h), Rel_8 (amount of drug release after 8h), efficiency (DE %) and the difference factor (F_1). The difference factor is used to determine whether the test product is different to the reference products (SM_1 formulation (1:2:8 ratio) is selected as reference formulation).

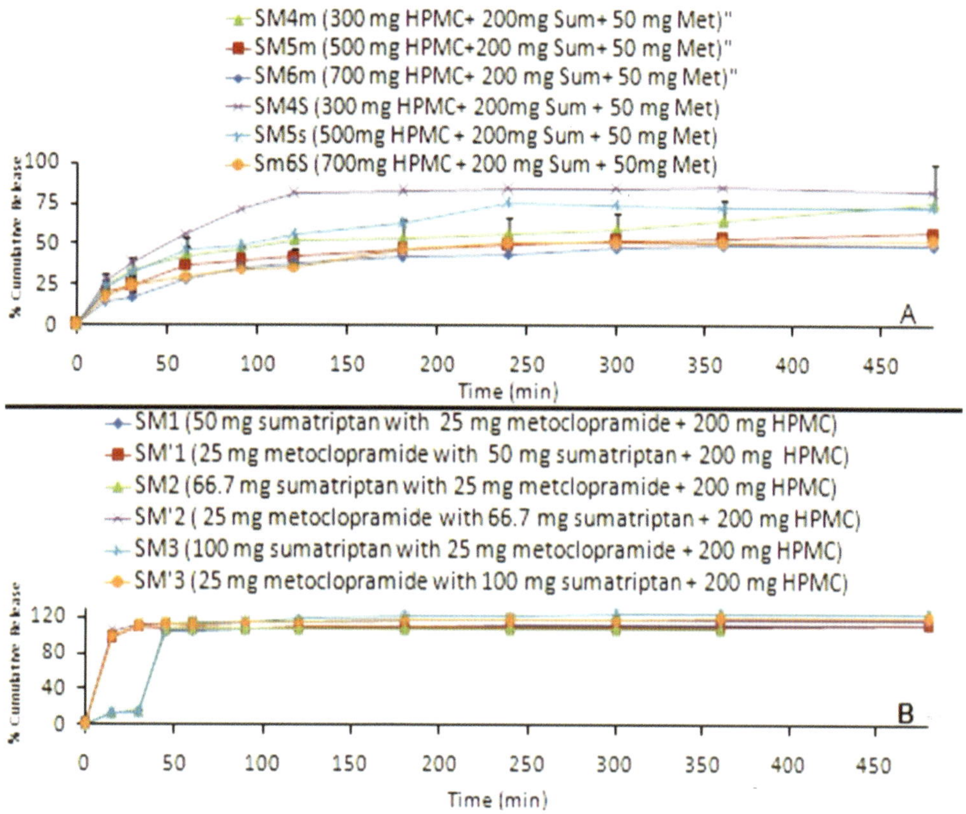

Figure 4. Cumulative percentage release of sumatriptan combined with metoclopramide from (A) films and (B) discs prepared with different drug to polymer ratios.

Accordingly, Figure 4 shows that the initial Sum drug releases ($Rel_{0.25}$) for the SM_1 to SM_3 formulations were low (12.60%, 12.42% and 12.67%, respectively) and $Rel_{0.5}$ was 103.10%, 105.82% and 112.57%, respectively. Moreover, Met drug release of SM' (SM) films shows that high burst effect for SM'_1 to SM'_3 formulations were high (96.10%, 102.83% and 99.43%, respectively) and $Rel_{0.5}$ was high, too (106.68%, 110.82% and 110.8%, respectively) (Figure 4B). The release of Met drug from SM films was faster than the release of Sum drug from SM films ($p<0.05$). During dissolution, HPMC containing films swelled forming a gel layer on the exposed mucous surfaces.
The release of drug from Sum combined with Met films with an increase in Sum concentration, and the interaction between the polymer and drug increased with the formation of a closer network, showed an increase in the diffusion of drug from the films (Figure 4A & 4B). The reason for the burst release ($Rel_{0.25}$) could be due to the presence of some pores and channels of polymer near to the surface of films. When water-soluble drugs (Sum and Met) did not show a tendency to migration or removal of air bubbles, thereby drug concentration is increased in the films and burst effect is induced.[12] The pores present in HPMC polymer act as channels for the entrance of liquid medium through the film surface and cause it to swell. Hydrogen bond between the hydroxyl groups of HPMC moiety and mucous surface decreases its porosity and permeability. Thus, if the ratio of drug to polymer be varied, the rate of release of drug could be controlled. Dissolution medium permeation into the films is facilitated due to the high swelling action of polymer which leads to more medium for the transport of the drug available. While the discs showed the least drug release, the drug release from microsphere was significantly affected by the size of microspheres. The increase in the polymer concentration led to an increase in the size of microspheres thus drug release from microspheres. Hence drug to polymer ratio was found to significantly decrease. SM_6 Formulation (1:4:14 ratio) showed the

fastest drug release among all the disc formulations as these microspheres are small in size.

logP values for Sum and Met were 0.67 and 2.76, exhibiting low permeability through buccal mucosa. Akin to other studies, the obtained results indicated that generally an increase in the ratio of drug to polymer resulted in a reduction in the release of Sum combined with Met from discs (Table 3 and Figure 4).[33]

Figure 4A draws a comparison of permeation of Sum combined with Met films and discs through sheep buccal mucosa for formulations containing different drug to polymer ratios. Slopes of the linear portion of release profiles were calculated. These slopes portrayed the rate of release or flux of Sum combined with Met from different formulations (Table 3). The highest fluxes and regression coefficient for films as SM_1 (reference formulation) formulations were 0.00182 mg/cm^2.min, 0.972 (Sum), and 0.00146 mg/cm^2.min, 0.940 (Met), respectively.

Table 3. Flux or amount of drug release per unit surface area after 4 h, permeability coefficient and regression coefficient for different formulation and comparison of various release characteristics of sumatriptan combined with methoclopramide from different film/disc formulations

Formulation code		$^{a}Rel_{0.5}$ (%±SD)	$^{b}Rel_{0.75}$ (%±SD)	$^{c}Rel_8$ (%±SD)	^{e}DE (%±SD)	$^{f}t_{50\%}$ (min±SD)	$^{g}f_1$	Flux [(mg/cm^2.min)/10^3]	Permeability coefficient [(cm/min)/10^3±SD]	r^2
SM_1	S_1	15.86±3.27	103.41±2.90	111.59±15.30	100.26±12.32	49.08±5.47	0	1.82±0.003	18.2±1.11	0.872
	M_1	109.87±3.71	106.67±3.04	110.75±4.71	93.85±10.24	138.16±14.52	0	1.46±0.002	50.34±7.45	0.940
SM_2	S_2	15.41±2.72	105.82±3.73	106.45±4.08	104.61±9.87	49.35±4.12	4.94	1.62±0.002	12.9±0.82	0.969
	M_2	116.63±1.72	110.82±1.54	117.80±5.06	106.37±12.14	143.71±14.78	14.80	1.23±0.001	38.44±5.63	0.959
SM_3	S_3	13.47±1.34	112.57±4.78	123.86±5.44	100.32±13.12	54.22±4.78	2.46	1.47±0.001	8.65±0.89	0.931
	M_3	108.54±7.03	110.80±1.59	118.23±4.42	116.60±14.39	71.23±6.25	23.94	1.02±0.0005	18.55±1.23	0.884
SM_4	S_1	37.99±3.30	56.74±6.32	83.28±1.19	92.77±13.32	54.01±4.96	13.30	1±0.0004	35.71±4.65	0.935
	M_1	37.30±7.11	42.24±12.33	75.49±25.38	66.94±5.64	106.28±6.25	32.28	0.8±0.0003	33.33±6.52	0.994
SM_5	S_2	32.7±4.06	46.02±4.48	72.62±0.80	55.32±5.98	52.82±3.69	46.48	0.8±0.0002	18.60±1.27	0.983
	M_2	23.74±6.57	37.17±11.87	58.21±1.65	56.43±4.25	176.75±25.14	43.66	0.72±0.0003	14.40±1.86	0.975
SM_6	S_3	24.01±3.77	29.91±2.02	51.62±0.56	48.36±6.21	54.29±3.69	52.74	0.65±0.0003	9.29±0.56	0.973
	M_3	17.30±3.46	27.83±3.92	49.44±0.27	40.72±2.17	113.63±21.10	61.38	0.45±0.0002	5.63±0.32	0.920

^{a} $Rel_{0.25}$ = amount of drug release after 15 min; ^{b} $Rel_{.75}$ = amount of drug release after 30 min; ^{c} Rel_8 = amount of drug release after 8h ;^{d}DE = dissolution efficiency; ^{e}t 50% = dissolution time for 50% fractions; ^{f} f_1 = Differential factor ($0<f_1<15$), SM_1(1:2:8 ratio) is selected as reference formulation.

Furthermore, Figure 4B draws a comparison of permeation of Sum and Met through buccal mucosa for formulations containing different drug to polymer ratios. Slopes of the linear portion of the release profiles were calculated. These slopes depicted the rate of release or flux of Sum and Met from different formulations (Table 3). The highest fluxes and regression coefficient for discs as SM_4 formulations were 0.001 mg/cm^2.min, 0.995 (Sum), and 0.0008 mg/cm^2.min, 0.994 (Met), respectively.

The pores present in HPMC polymer act as channels for the entrance of liquid medium through the microparticles wall and cause it to swell. The hydrogen bond between the hydroxyl groups of the carboxylic moiety and the carbonyl oxygen of ester group increases the degree of solidity of polymer and decreases its porosity and permeability. Thus, by varying the ratio of drug to polymer the release rate of Sum and Met could be controlled.

The microscopic observations indicated that none of the films and discs had a significant effect on the microscopic structure of mucosa. As shown in Figure 5, no cell necrosis was observed.

Cellular membrane was intact and no damage to the treated buccal mucosa was observed (was used in the bioadhesion strength test). Thus, the formulation containing microparticles appeared to be safe with respect to the buccal administration (Figure 5A, 5B & 5C).

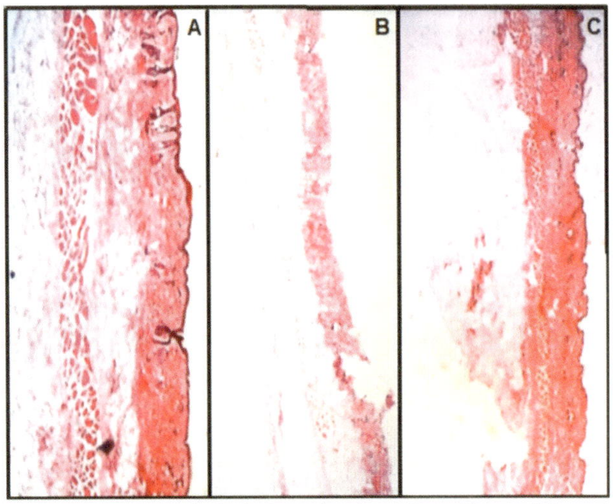

Figure 5. Histopathological evaluation of sections of buccal mucosal areas (A) un-treated (B) treated with film (C) treated with disc containing sumatriptan combined with methoclopramide (magnitude X).

Conclusion

In recent years, interest has been grown to develop a drug delivery system with the use of a mucoadhesive polymer (e.g., HPMC) that could attach to the related tissue or to the surface coating of the tissue to target various absorptive mucosa, buccally or sublingually. The mucoadhesive polymers could themselves exert some control over the rate and amount of drug release and thus contribute to the therapeutic efficacy of mucoadhesive drug delivery system. The buccal drug delivery system bypasses the liver and avoids the pre-systemic elimination in the gastrointestinal tract and increases bioavailability. The mucosa is relatively permeated with a rich blood supply. Two buccal and sublingual formulations of HPMC were prepared with HPMC polymer. Therefore, in the present study an attempt was made to study the mucoadhesive strength of different dosage forms by a straightforward *in vitro* method. Among the various Sum and Met combinations, the SM_3 formulation (100 mg Sum, 25 Met and 200 mg HPMC) was found to be the most suitable. The formulation SM_4 fulfilled the requirement of a proper buccal disc. The force of adhesion (g/cm^2) of different forms was found in the order of film > disc. The films showed the highest swelling as well as the highest mucoadhesive strength. It showed *in vitro* residence time up to 2.2 h. It followed *in vitro* drug release up to 112.57 % for 45 min and *in vitro* drug permeation up to 4 h. *In vitro* release studies of Sum and Met microparticles showed a significant difference in their release rate. The microparticles prepared showed a slow and controlled release over lengthened period of time when compared to the other mucoadhesive films. These results may suggest the potent application of films and microparticles as a suitable sustained release drug delivery system. These mucoadhesive films could be exploited in the effective and promising development of mucoadhesive drug delivery systems.

Acknowledgments

The financial support from Drug Applied Research Center and Research Council of Tabriz University of Medical Sciences is greatly acknowledged.

Ethical Issues

Not applicable.

Conflict of Interest

Authors certify that no actual or potential conflict of interests exists in relation to this article.

References

1. Lionetto L, Negro A, Casolla B, Simmaco M, Martelletti P. Sumatriptan succinate : Pharmacokinetics of different formulations in clinical practice. *Expert Opin Pharmacother* 2012;13(16):2369-80. doi: 10.1517/14656566.2012.730041
2. Cady R, Dodick DW. Diagnosis and treatment of migraine. *Mayo Clin Proc* 2002;77(3):255-61. doi: 10.4065/77.3.255
3. Matchar DB, Young WB, Rosenberg JH, Pietrzak MP, Silberstein SB, Lipton RB, et al. Evidence-based guidelines for migraine headache in the primary care setting: pharmacological management of acute attacks. *Neurology* 2000.
4. Diener HC, Kaube H, Limmroth V. A practical guide to the management and prevention of migraine. *Drugs* 1998;56(5):811-24. doi: 10.2165/00003495-199856050-00006
5. Silberstein SD. Practice parameter: Evidence-based guidelines for migraine headache (an evidence-based review): Report of the quality standards subcommittee of the american academy of neurology. *Neurology* 2000;55(6):754-62. doi: 10.1212/WNL.55.6.754
6. Silberstein SD, Lipton RB, Goadsby PJ. Headache in clinical practice. London: Martin Dunitz; 1998.
7. Shivanand K, Raju S, Nizamuddin S, Jayakar B. In vivo bioavailability studies of sumatriptan succinate buccal tablets. *Daru* 2011;19(3):224-30.
8. Desai HD, Shriley KL, Penzak SR, Strom JG, Hon YY, Spratlin V, et al. Pharmacokinetics in healthy volunteers of sumatriptan 25-mg oral tablet versus 25-mg extemporaneous suppository. *Int J Pharm Compd* 2003;7(6):481-4.
9. Perl MM, Rubin H, Schiraldi MT. Bioadhesive extruded film for intra-oral drug delivery and process. Google Patents 1987.
10. Notterman DA, Ward RM. Alternative routes of drug administration--advantages and disadvantages (subject review). *Pediatrics* 1997;100(1):143-52. doi: 10.1542/peds.100.1.143
11. Shojaei AH. Buccal mucosa as a route for systemic drug delivery: a review. *J Pharm Pharm Sci* 1998;1(1):15-30.
12. Nappinnai M, Chandanbala R, Balaijirajan R. Formulation and evaluation of nitrendipine buccal films. *Indian J Pharm Sci* 2008;70(5):631-5. doi: 10.4103/0250-474X.45402
13. Semalty M, Semalty A, Kumar G. Formulation and characterization of mucoadhesive buccal films of glipizide. *Indian J Pharm Sci* 2008;70(1):43-8. doi: 10.4103/0250-474X.40330
14. Bhupinder B. Sarita J. Formulation and evaluation of fast dissolving sublingual films of Rizatriptan Benzoate. *Int J Drug Dev Res* 2012;4(1):133-43.
15. Semalty A, Semalty M, Nautiyal U. Formulation and evaluation of mucoadhesive buccal films of enalapril maleate. *Indian J Pharm Sci* 2010;72(5):571-5. doi: 10.4103/0250-474X.78522
16. Wong CF, Yuen KH, Peh KK. An in-vitro method for buccal adhesion studies: importance of instrument variables. *Int J Pharm* 1999;180(1):47-57. doi: 10.1016/S0378-5173(98)00402-5
17. Shidhaye SS, Thakkar PV, Dand NM, Kadam VJ. Buccal drug delivery of pravastatin sodium. *AAPS*

PharmSciTech 2010;11(1):416-24. doi: 10.1208/s12249-010-9381-4

18. Hussein AA, Samein LH, Ghareeb MM, Salih OS. Effects of mucoadhesive polymers combination on the properties of lisinpril buccal tablets prepared by wet granulation method. *Int J Pharm Pharm Sci* 2013,5(4):340-3.
19. Chowdary KPR, Srinivas L. Mucoadhesive drug delivery systems: A review of current status. *Indian Drugs* 2000;37(9):400-6.
20. Sudhakar Y, Kuotsu K, Bandyopadhyay AK. Buccal bioadhesive drug delivery - A promising option for orally less efficient drugs. *J Control Release* 2006;114(1):15-40. doi: 10.1016/j.jconrel.2006.04.012
21. Takeuchi H, Yamamoto H, Kawashima Y. Mucoadhesive nanoparticulate systems for peptide drug delivery. *Adv Drug Deliv Rev* 2001;47(1):39-54. doi: 10.1016/S0169-409X(00)00120-4
22. Wong CF, Yuen KH, Peh KK. Formulation and evaluation of controlled release Eudragit buccal patches. *Int J pharm* 1999;178(1):11-22. doi: 10.1016/S0378-5173(98)00342-1
23. Roy S, Pal K, Anis A, Pramanik K, Prabhakar B. Polymers in mucoadhesive drug-delivery systems: a brief note. *Designed Monomers and Polymers* 2009;12(6):483-95. doi: 10.1163/138577209X12478283327236
24. Ludwig A. The use of mucoadhesive polymers in ocular drug delivery. *Adv Drug Deliv Rev* 2005;57(11):1595-639. doi: 10.1016/j.addr.2005.07.005
25. Wise DL. Handbook of pharmaceutical controlled release technology. CRC Press; 2000.
26. George M, Abraham TE. Polyionic hydrocolloids for the intestinal delivery of protein drugs: alginate and chitosan-a review. *J Control Release* 2006;114(1):1-14. doi: 10.1016/j.jconrel.2006.04.017
27. Nakanishi T, Kaiho F, Hayashi M. Improvement of drug release rate from carbopol 934p formulation. *Chem Pharm Bull (Tokyo)* 1998;46(1):171-3. doi: 10.1248/cpb.46.171
28. Andrews GP, Laverty TP, Jones DS. Mucoadhesive polymeric platforms for controlled drug delivery. *Eur J Pharm Biopharm* 2009;71(3):505-18. doi: 10.1016/j.ejpb.2008.09.028
29. Miyazaki Y, Ogihara K, Yakou S, Nagai T, Takayama K. In vitro and in vivo evaluation of mucoadhesive microspheres consisting of dextran derivatives and cellulose acetate butyrate. *Int J Pharm* 2003;258(1-2):21-9. doi: 10.1016/S0378-5173(03)00159-5
30. Nafee NA, Ismail FA, Boraie NA, Mortada LM. Mucoadhesive buccal patches of miconazole nitrate: in vitro/in vivo performance and effect of ageing. *Int J Pharm* 2003;264(1-2):1-14. doi: 10.1016/S0378-5173(03)00371-5
31. Nafee N, Schneider M, Schaefer UF, Lehr CM. Relevance of the colloidal stability of chitosan/PLGA nanoparticles on their cytotoxicity profile. *Int J Pharm* 2009;381(2):130-9. doi: 10.1016/j.ijpharm.2009.04.049
32. Jelvehgari M, Zakeri-Milani P, Khansari F. Mucoahhesive microspheres for gastroretentive delivery of metformine hydrochloride: In vitro evaluation. *Res Pharm Sci* 2012;7(5):S356.
33. Minami S, Suzuki H, Okamoto Y, Fujinaga T, Shigemasa Y. Chitin and chitosan activate complement via the alternative pathway. *Carbohydr Polym* 1998;36(2-3):151-5. doi: 10.1016/S0144-8617(98)00015-0

Sustained release Curcumin loaded Solid Lipid Nanoparticles

Parisa Jourghanian[1], Solmaz Ghaffari[2,3]*, Mehdi Ardjmand[4], Setareh Haghighat[5], Mahdieh Mohammadnejad[6]

[1] *Department of Chemical Engineering, Shahrood Branch, Islamic Azad University, Shahrood, Iran.*
[2] *Department of Medical Nanotechnology, Faculty of Advanced Sciences and Technology, Pharmaceutical Sciences Branch, Islamic Azad University, (IAUPS), Tehran, Iran.*
[3] *Young Researchers and Elite Club, Pharmaceutical Sciences Branch, Islamic Azad University, (IAUPS), Tehran, Iran.*
[4] *Department of Chemical Engineering, South Tehran Branch, Islamic Azad University, Tehran, Iran.*
[5] *Department of Microbiology, Faculty of Advanced Sciences and Technology, Pharmaceutical Sciences Branch, Islamic Azad University (IAUPS), Tehran, Iran.*
[6] *Quality Control Department, Tofigh Daru Research and Engineering Co. Tehran, Iran.*

Keywords:
- Curcumin
- Solid Lipid Nanoparticles
- Sustained release
- Freeze drying
- Particle size

Abstract

Purpose: curcumin is poorly water soluble drug with low bioavailability. Use of lipid systems in lipophilic substances increases solubility and bioavailability of poorly soluble drugs. The aim of this study was to prepare curcumin loaded Solid Lipid Nanoparticles (SLNs) with high loading efficiency, small particle size and prolonged release profile with enhanced antibacterial efficacy.

Methods: to synthesize stable SLNs, freeze- Drying was done using mannitol as cryoprotectant. Cholesterol was used as carrier because of good tolerability and biocompatibility. SLNs were prepared using high pressure homogenization method.

Results: optimized SLNs had 112 and 163 nm particle size before and after freeze drying, respectively. The prepared SLNs had 71% loading efficiency. 90% of loaded curcumin was released after 48 hours. Morphologic study for formulation was done by taking SEM pictures of curcumin SLNs. Results show the spherical shape of curcumin SLNs. DSC studies were performed to determine prolonged release mechanism. Antimicrobial studies were done to compare the antimicrobial efficacy of curcumin SLNs with free curcumin. DSC studies showed probability of formation of hydrogen bonds between cholesterol and curcumin which resulted in prolonged release of curcumin. Lipid structure of cholesterol could cause enhanced permeability in studied bacteria to increase antibacterial characteristics of curcumin.

Conclusion: the designed curcumin SLNs could be candidate for formulation of different dosage forms or cosmeceutical products.

Introduction

Recently phytotherapeutics were prepared in nano size to improve pharmacokinetic and pharmacodynamics characteristics.[1] Curcumin, a phenolic compound from the plant Curcuma Longa as a traditional spice have many pharmacological activities including: anti-diabetic, anti-inflammatory, anti-cancer, anti-oxidant, antibacterial, anti-HIV and anti-aging activity and hepato protective activity as well as cardiovascular benefits.[2] According to Jadhav et al (2014), curcumin as a multifunctional phytoceutical, has been patented numerously.[1] Studies demonstrated that curcumin acts on multiplemolecular targets to selectively kill tumour cells with low intrinsic toxicity.[1,3-5] This compound is widely used in China, India and Iran as a spice and traditional herb.[6] The unexpected discovery that curcumin is also a powerful iron chelator has given new insight into its multimodal mechanisms of action in gaining control of age-related iron accumulations in the brain, heart, and liver.[7] Curcumin is a poorly water-soluble drug with low oral bioavailability and sensitive to photodegradation. Application of lipids for bioavailability enhancement of poor soluble drugs is promising. Since most of the components involved in formulation of solid lipid nanoparticles are of natural origin, they are compatible with components of biological membrane, and generally less toxicological risk is experienced.[8]

Nanoparticles (NPs) are colloidal particles in which the active ingredients are dissolved, entrapped in and/or is adsorbed or attached on to the particle.[9] Some advantages of nanotechnology in phytoceuticals include: the probability of designing sustained release systems, enhanced physicochemical stability, enhanced permeability, improves tissue distribution and enhanced solubility and bioavailability.[1] Many novel drug delivery strategies such as liposomes, nano- or micro- emulsions, polymeric NPs and solid lipid NPs, polymer conjugates, polymeric micelles, nanocrystals,

***Corresponding author:** Solmaz Ghaffari, Email: ghaffari.s@iaups.ac.ir nanogels, self-assemblies and cyclodextrin inclusion complexes have been described to increase solubility, bioavailability and delivery of curcumin.[10]

Solid lipid nanoparticles (SLNs) as colloidal carrier systems combine the advantages of traditional systems but avoid some of their major disadvantages. These colloidal systems have many important advantages, such as biocompatibility, good tolerability, and ease of scale-up.[11,12] SLNs have been studied as a drug-delivery system for the controlling of drug release.[13] Although SLNs used as carrier to sustain the release of lipophilic drugs but there are studies using SLN(s) for the delivery of hydrophilic drugs and peptides too. SLNs have been reported as drug carriers to treat neoplasms and tumour targeting.[9] Many studies were done to increase stability, solubility and efficacy of curcumin using nanotechnology.[9,14] Some studies were carried out to evaluate benefit of SLNs as a carrier system for curcumin for treatment of arthritis.[15] The findings emphasize that SLNs could be novel approach to deliver curcumin into the inflamed joints and improve its biopharmaceutical performance.[15] Curcumin SLNs were designed for treatment of lung cancer by Wang et al 2013.[16] As curcumin has been used widely in Iran, in the present study, curcumin loaded SLNs were synthesized to prolong drug release and enhance antibacterial effects.

Materials and Methods

Materials

Tween 80, ethanol and acetone were purchased from Merck, Germany and were used as surfactant and oily phase solvents, respectively. Curcumin was prepared by Sami Lab, India. Dialysis membrane was purchased from Sigma, Germany. All ingredients which were used to prepare phosphate buffer solution were purchased from Merck, Germany.

Preparation of Curcumin SLNs

Curcumin loaded SLNs were prepared using high pressure homogenization. 0.1 g tween 80 and 600 mg curcumin were added to 10 ml of purified water at room temperature, 600 mg of cholesterol was dissolved in mixture of ethanol and acetone on 3-1 ratio at 75-80 °C, then the hot oily phase was added to aqueous phase under homogenization at 11000 rpm and the mixture was homogenized for 7 minutes. While the mixture cooled to room temperature, SLNs formed.[13]

Particle size analysis

The evaluation of particle size was done using Malvern zeta sizer (ZEN3600) and confirmed by scanning electron microscopy (SEM).

Measurement of drug loading efficiency

For determination of drug loading efficacy (LE%) of curcumin solid lipid nanoparticles, the samples were centrifuged at 26,000 rpm for 35 minutes at -4 °C using Sigma laboratories centrifuge (Germany). The drug concentration in the supernatant was analyzed using UV spectrophotometer (Shimadzu, Japan) at 424 nm and LE% was calculated using reverse method applying following equation.[17]

$$Drug\ Loading\ efficacy\ (LE\ \%) = \frac{Drug_{total} - Drug_{supernatant}}{Drug_{total}} \times 100$$

Drug release study

Release study was performed using dialysis sack method by DO405 dialysis tubing 23-15mm (Sigma, Germany). 5 ml of each formulation was placed in dialysis membrane and immersed in 50 ml phosphate buffer pH 7.4 containing 0.1% Tween 80. Two ml samples were withdrawn in predetermined time intervals and drug concentration was measured at 424 nm using UV spectrophotometer. To ensure that sustained release profile is not due to membrane, curcumin dispersion in the same concentration with curcumin SLNs was studied under the same condition for release.

Morphology Study

Morphology of the nanoparticles was characterized by scanning electron microscopy (SEM). The nanoparticles were mounted on aluminum stubs; sputter- coated with a thin layer of Au-Pd and examined using an SEM (SEM XL30, Philips, Netherlands).

Freeze drying

To increase stability and shelf life, curcumin SLNs were lyophilized successfully. Lyophilization was done by using 5 and 15% mannitol as cryoprotectan at freezing temperature equal to -20° C for 24 hours and then particles were lyophilized for 48 hours by freeze-dryer (Lyotrap/ Plus,UK) at -40° C and pressure equal to 0.4 bar.

DSC Analysis

DSC thermograms were obtained using (Mettler, Switzerland). Certain amount of dried nanoparticle powder was crimped in a standard aluminum pan and heated from 25 to 400 °C at a heating rate of 10 °C/min under constant heating.

Antimicrobial Efficiency

To compare the antimicrobial activity of curcumin loaded nanoparticles with free curcumin, ''well diffusion test'' was carried out using E. coli (ATCC 25922) as the Gram-negative pathogenic strain and S. aureus (ATCC 25923) as Gram positive strain. In this study SLNs without curcumin was studied as blank. The antibacterial effect of curcumin against many bacterial strains including E.coli, S. aureus, S. epidermidis was reported by Zorofchian et al 2014. In this study the antibacterial efficiency of curcumin loaded SLNs was compared with the same concentration of free curcumin.[18]

Results and Discussion

Particle size

Particle size studies demonstrated that particles were 112 nm with PdI (Polydispersity index) equal to 0.114 before freeze drying. The particle size of nanoparticles was 163 and 306 nm when 5% and 15% mannitol was used as cryoprotectant, respectively. Therefore 5% mannitol was chosen as optimum cryoprotectant for further experiments. Particle size studies establish good size distribution before and after freeze drying. Figure 1a and 1b show the result of particle size distribution before and after freeze drying, respectively.

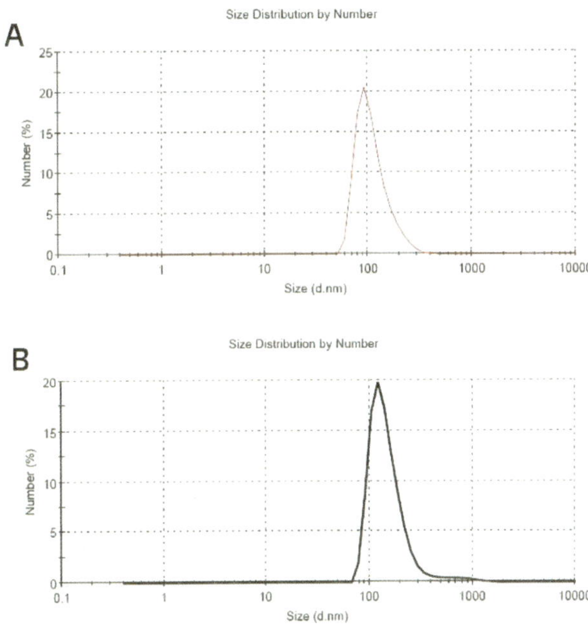

Figure 1. Particle size distribution of curcumin solid lipid nanoparticles before (A) and after (B) freeze drying.

Morphology study

SEM photograph of curcumin loaded SLNs was shown in Figure 2. According to SEM image, prepared SLNs showed spherical shape. The size distribution of particles was comparable to DLS.

Loading efficiency and drug release study

Using equation 1, loading efficiency was calculated as 70.4±1.2%. Figure 3, shows curcumin release profile. Release profile of curcumin from nanoparticles shows a prolonged manner. Results show that after 36 and 48 hours more than 85% and 92% of loaded curcumin released, respectively. More than 95% of curcumin released from free curcumin dispersion after less than one hour through dialysis membrane. Chen et al prepared prolonged release curcumin using liposomes as carrier, in their study after 48 hours less than 70% of loaded curcumin was released.[19] Other study was done to prepare unilamellar liposomes of curcumin analogue to increase hepatoprotective efficacy, in this study the active ingredients release was prolonged for 10 days.[20]

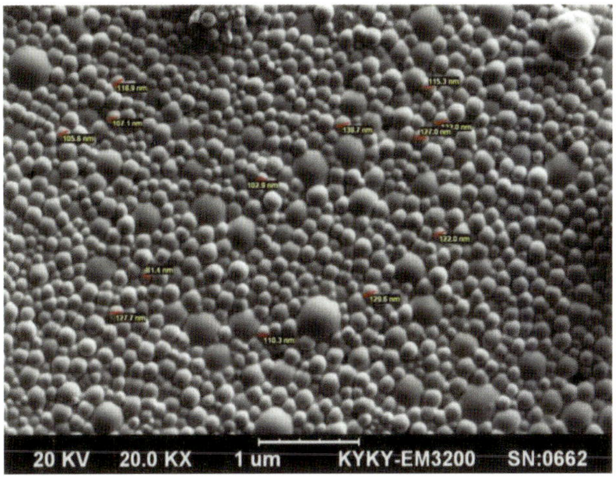

Figure 2. Scanning electron microscopy picture of curcumin solid lipid nanoparticles.

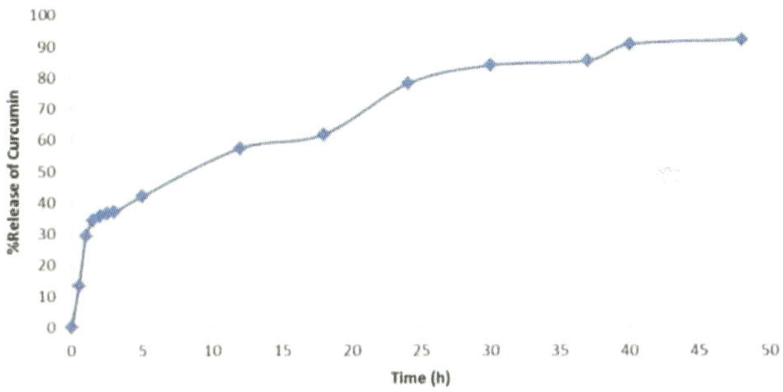

Figure 3. Curcumin release profile through SLNs.

DSC studies

Figure 4 shows DSC analysis results. DSC thermograms of pure cholesterol, curcumin and curcumin-loaded SLNs show that melting point of cholesterol has shifted from 80 °C to about 170 °C in the SLNs of curcumin. The melting temperature of curcumin is also seen at 185 °C in the thermogram of pure curcumin. Chemical structure of curcumin and cholesterol could support probability of hydrogen band formation between these two compounds which resulted in prolonged release from nanoparticles.

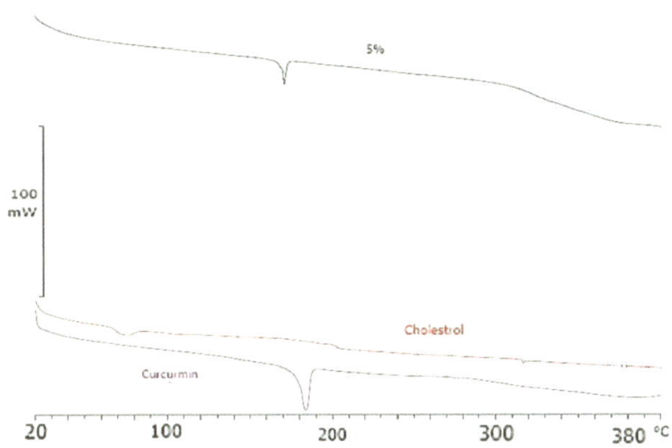

Figure 4. DSC thermograms of raw materials and freeze-dried curcumin SLNs.

Antimicrobial effect study

Figures 5a and 5b show increased antimicrobial effect of curcumin nanoparticles compared to free curcumin in same concentration on E.coli and S. aureus. In another study, the synergistic effect of curcumin and other antibacterial agents was observed.[21] Based on our findings, curcumin SLNs can be combined with other antibiotics in SLNs to reduce the MIC (Minimum Inhibitory Concentration) and MBC (Minimum Bactericidal Concentration) more. The reduction of MIC and MBC of some antibacterial agents loaded in SLNs was demonstrated before.[12,22]

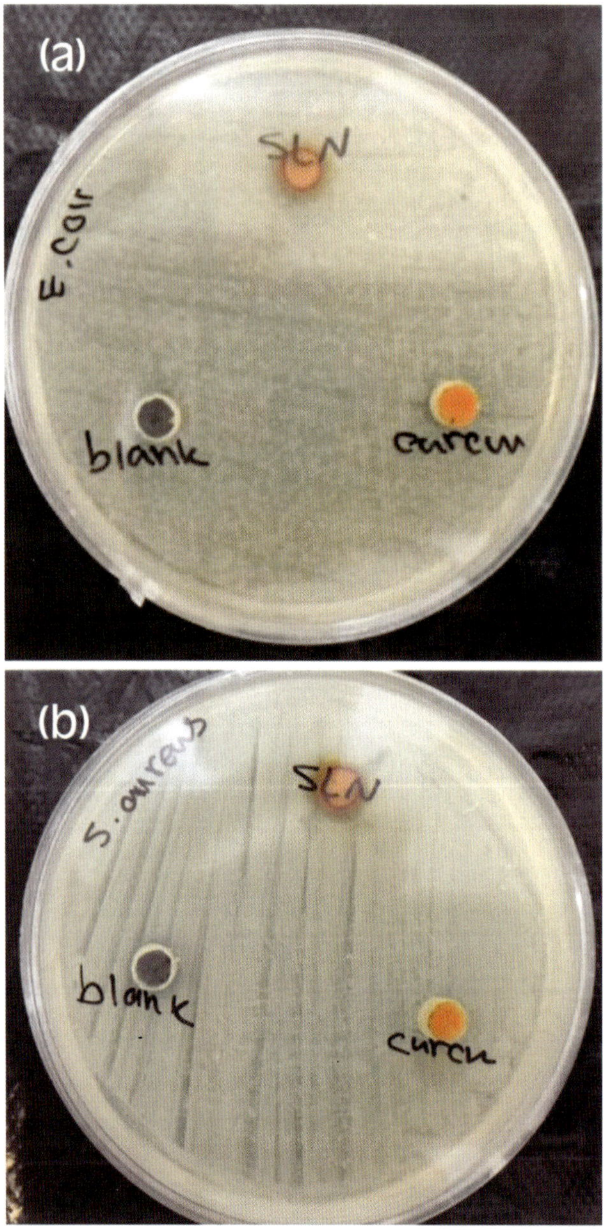

Figure 5. Photographs of the zone of inhibition produced by free curcumin and its SLNs against E.coli (a) and S. aureus (b).

Conclusion

Our results show that curcumin SLNs can be prepared and freeze dried with proper size, drug loading and release profile. Curcumin SLNs can be used in sustained release oral dosage forms to increase bioavailability, topical formulations for wound dressing, or anti-aging products. Since the particles are in proper size range, it is predictable that particles show enhanced permeability at site of action. Also the designed curcumin SLNs could be used to reach more MIC and MBC reduction in combination with other antibiotics for synergistic effects. According to Ronita et al study (2009) curcumin is effective against H. pylori,[23] so curcumin SLNs can be used with therapeutic protocols of H. pylori treatment.

Acknowledgments

Authors would like to thank Shahrood Branch and Pharmaceutical Sciences Branch, Islamic Azad University for financial and technical support and Tofigh Daru Co for technical support of this project. Authors are also grateful to Miss Hedieh Ghaffari for English editing of the manuscript and Dr. Tarane Gazori for scientific editing of the manuscript.

Ethical Issues

Not applicable.

Conflict of Interest

Authors declare no conflict of interest in this study.

References

1. Jadhav NR, Powar T, Shinde S, Nadaf S. Herbal nanoparticles: A patent review. *Asian J Pharm* 2014;8(1):58-69. doi: 10.4103/0973-8398.134101
2. Choudhary N, Singh SB. Potential therapeutic effect of curcumin - an update. *J Pharm Edu Res* 2012;3(2):64-7.
3. Ravindran J, Prasad S, Aggarwal BB. Curcumin and Cancer Cells: How Many Ways Can Curry Kill Tumor Cells Selectively? *AAPS J* 2009;11(3):495-510. doi: 10.1208/s12248-009-9128-x
4. Hasima N, Aggarwal BB. Targeting proteasomal pathways by dietary curcumin for cancer prevention and treatment. *Curr Med Chem* 2014;21(14):1583-94. doi: 10.2174/09298673113206660135
5. Mehta K, Pantazis P, McQueen T, Aggarwal BB. Antiproliferative effect of curcumin (diferuloylmethane) against human breast tumor cell lines. *Anticancer Drugs* 1997;8(5):470-81. doi: 10.1097/00001813-199706000-00010
6. Sun J, Bi C, Chan HM, Sun S, Zhang Q, Zheng Y. Curcumin-loaded solid lipid nanoparticles have prolonged in vitro antitumour activity, cellular uptake and improved in vivo bioavailability. *Colloids Surf B Biointerfaces* 2013;111:367-75. doi: 10.1016/j.colsurfb.2013.06.032
7. Jiao Y, Wilkinson Jt, Christine Pietsch E, Buss JL, Wang W, Planalp R, et al. Iron chelation in the biological activity of curcumin. *Free Radic Biol Med* 2006;40(7):1152-60. doi: 10.1016/j.freeradbiomed.2005.11.003
8. Romica C, Cristian D, Gabriela B, Stefan D. Improved solubilization of curcumin with a

microemulsification formulation. *The Annals of the University Dunarea de Jos of Galati Fascicle VI – Food Technology* 2011;35(2):46-55.
9. Nair R, Arun Kumar KS, Vishnu Priya K, Sevukarajan M. Recent Advances in Solid Lipid Nanoparticle Based Drug Delivery Systems. *J Biomed Sci and Res* 2011;3(2):368-84.
10. Li L, Braiteh FS, Kurzrock R. Liposome-encapsulated curcumin: In vitro and in vivo effects on proliferation, apoptosis, signaling, and angiogenesis. *Cancer* 2005;104(6):1322-31. doi: 10.1002/cncr.21300
11. Mehnert W, Mader K. Solid lipid nanoparticles: Production, characterization and applications. *Adv Drug Deliv Rev* 2001;47(2-3):165-96. doi: 10.1016/s0169-409x(01)00105-3
12. Ghaffari S, Varshosaz J, Saadat A, Atyabi F. Stability and antimicrobial effect of amikacin-loaded solid lipid nanoparticles. *Int J Nanomedicine* 2011;6:35-43. doi: 10.2147/IJN.S13671
13. Varshosaz J, Ghaffari S, Khoshayand MR, Atyabi F, Azarmi S, Kobarfard F. Development and optimization of solid lipid nanoparticles of amikacin by central composite design. *J Liposome Res* 2010;20(2):97-104. doi: 10.3109/08982100903103904
14. Krausz AE, Adler BL, Cabral V, Navati M, Doerner J, Charafeddine RA, et al. Curcumin-encapsulated nanoparticles as innovative antimicrobial and wound healing agent. *Nanomedicine* 2015;11(1):195-206. doi: 10.1016/j.nano.2014.09.004
15. Arora R, Kuhad A, Kaur IP, Chopra K. Curcumin loaded solid lipid nanoparticles ameliorate adjuvant-induced arthritis in rats. *Eur J Pain* 2015;19(7):940-52. doi: 10.1002/ejp.620
16. Wang P, Zhang L, Peng H, Li Y, Xiong J, Xu Z. The formulation and delivery of curcumin with solid lipid nanoparticles for the treatment of on non-small cell lung cancer both in vitro and in vivo. *Mater Sci Eng C Mater Biol Appl* 2013;33(8):4802-8. doi: 10.1016/j.msec.2013.07.047
17. Ghaffari S, Varshosaz J, Haririan I, Khoshayan MR, Azarmi S, Gazori T. Ciprofloxacin Loaded Alginate/Chitosan and Solid Lipid Nanoparticles, Preparation, and Characterization. *J Dispersion Sci Technol* 2012;33(5):685-9. doi: 10.1080/01932691.2011.579831
18. Moghadamtousi SZ, Kadir HA, Hassandarvish P, Tajik H, Abubakar S, Zandi K. A review on antibacterial, antiviral, and antifungal activity of curcumin. *BioMed Res Int* 2014;2014:186864. doi: 10.1155/2014/186864
19. Chen Y, Wu Q, Zhang Z, Yuan L, Liu X, Zhou L. Preparation of curcumin-loaded liposomes and evaluation of their skin permeation and pharmacodynamics. *Molecules* 2012;17(5):5972-87. doi: 10.3390/molecules17055972
20. Aukunuru J, Jonginapally S, Gaddam N, Burra M, Bonepally CR, Prabahakar K. Preparation, characterization and evaluation of hepatoprotective activity of an interavenous liposomal formulation of Bis-Demethoxy curcumin analogue (BDMCA). *Int J Drug Dev Res* 2009;1(1):37-46.
21. Mun SH, Joung DK, Kim YS, Kang OH, Kim SB, Seo YS, et al. Synergistic antibacterial effect of curcumin against methicillin-resistant staphylococcus aureus. *Phytomedicine* 2013;20(8-9):714-8. doi: 10.1016/j.phymed.2013.02.006
22. Alihoseyni F, Ghaffari S, Dabirsiaghi AR, Haghighat S. Preparation and evaluation of ampicillin solid lipid nanoparticles. *World J Pharm Sci* 2014;2(9):914-20.
23. De R, Kundu P, Swarnakar S, Ramamurthy T, Chowdhury A, Nair GB, et al. Antimicrobial activity of curcumin against helicobacter pylori isolates from india and during infections in mice. *Antimicrob Agents Chemother* 2009;53(4):1592-7. doi: 10.1128/AAC.01242-08

Investigating Effect of Rapamycin and Metformin on Angiogenesis in Hepatocellular Carcinoma Cell Line

Mandana Rastegar, Haji-Amin Marjani, Yaghoub Yazdani, Majid Shahbazi, Masoud Golalipour, Touraj Farazmandfar*

Medical Cellular and Molecular Research Center, Golestan University of Medical Sciences, Gorgan, Iran.

Keywords:
- Metformin
- Rapamycin
- Hepatocellular carcinoma

Abstract

Purpose: Human hepatocellular carcinoma is one of the most common causes of death in the world. Metformin and rapamycin may decrease the expression of VEGF protein and subsequently angiogenesis. The purpose of this study was to evaluate the effect of these two drugs on expression of VEGF protein and the cell proliferation in the hepatocellular carcinoma cell line (ATCC HB-8065).

Methods: HepG2 was cultured in RPMI-1640 medium at 37°C for 48h as a pre-culture and then treated by different concentrations of metformin (0, 5, 10 and 20 mM) and rapamycin (0, 5, 10 and 20 nM) at different times (12, 24 and 48 h). Cell viability was assessed by the MTT assay. Total RNA was extracted by the Trizol reagent and VEGF gene expression was analyzed by quantitative real-time PCR and was calculated by $2^{-\Delta Ct}$ method. The VEGF protein level was determined by Elisa assay. Finally, Apoptosis index was calculated by DAPI staining.

Results: Metformin and rapamycin significantly decrease cancer cells viability ($p<0.05$). Rapamycin but not metformin decreases VEGF gene expression in HepG2 cells. Metformin and rapamycin significantly induce cell apoptosis in hepatocellular carcinoma (HCC) cells.

Conclusion: Metformin and rapamycin have an anti-tumor effect on HCC. According to our data rapamycin might have an anti-angiogenesis effect via inhibition of VEGF expression. Our results provide an insight into future clinical strategies to improve chemotherapy outcomes in HCC.

Introduction

Hepatocellular carcinoma (HCC) is the most common primary malignant tumor of the liver and is the fourth leading cause of cancer-related death in the world.[1] HCC is seventh most common cancer in men and the ninth in women.[2] However, the increased prevalence of HCC in communities with a high risk, in men is higher than women.[3] HCC is an aggressive malignancy with poor prognosis. Current chemotherapeutic drugs are not effective to control tumor growth and drug resistance is a common problem in a successful therapy. Therefore, novel approaches in chemotherapy may be needed to improve the survival rate in patients with HCC.[4] The treatment with anti-angiogenic agents may be a promising approach to treat HCC. Angiogenesis is a complex process that is based on cooperation between various cells, such as pericytes, endothelial cells, fibroblasts and smooth muscle cells. These cells produce a variety of cytokines and growth factors that interact with other cells or with the extracellular matrix and affect migration, proliferation and angiogenesis.[5] Angiogenesis plays a key role in tumor growth, progression and metastasis. This uncontrolled growth is well established in many tumors such as ovarian,[6] lung,[7] colon,[8] prostate,[9] brain[10] and lymphoid[11] tumors. Inhibition of angiogenesis may be a valuable method for controlling cancer. Without angiogenesis, tumor growth potentially is limited due to lack of blood flow and proliferation factors. Metastatic potential of tumors develops through the increased angiogenesis. This process was performed by disrupting the balance between of pro-angiogenic and anti-angiogenic factors via increasing the presence of pro-angiogenic factors such as VEGF.[12] Some studies on angiogenesis inhibitors in animal models showed that angiogenesis inhibition can destroy many types of tumors.[13] Two strategies used in the development of anti-angiogenic agents include exogenous angiogenic inhibitors such as monoclonal antibody against VEGF, and endogenous inhibitors such as endostatin and angiostatin.[14]

Metformin is one of the oldest and most commonly used drugs in the treatment of type 2 diabetes that reduces blood sugar by decreasing insulin resistance, with no effect on insulin secretion.[15] Serious side effects of this drug are rare and mostly due to the simultaneous presence of other diseases in diabetic patients, and not by the drug itself.[16] Recently, several studies have shown

***Corresponding author:** Touraj Farazmandfar, Email: dr.farazmandfar@goums.ac.ir that metformin may reduce the risk of liver cancer.[17-19] Metformin interfere with glucose metabolism that leads to changes in the intracellular pathways. One of these changes is the increased expression of the enzyme 5' adenosine monophosphate-activated protein kinase (AMPK) in liver cells by which the mammalian target of rapamycin (mTOR) protein was inhibited.[20] It is known that increased expression of the protein mTOR leads to the increased expression of the transcription factor hypoxia-inducible factor 1-alpha (HIF1α) and this factor increases the intensity of vessel endothelial growth factor (VEGF).[21] Therefore, metformin indirectly increase VEGF. VEGF is a 45 kDa glycoprotein that increases angiogenesis and vascular endothelial cell proliferation. VEGF is one of the strongest and most important angiogenic factors in the body. VEGF is one of the most important angiogenesis factors that was overexpressed in many cancers.[22]

Rapamycin is known as an antibiotic and with a mechanism similar to metformin, inhibits mTOR and ultimately reduce VEGF expression. This drug is used as an immune suppressor to prevent organ rejection after liver transplantation.[23] Recently, several studies have shown that rapamycin in combination with other medicines reduced proliferation of HCC cells in vitro and animal models.[24,25]

Considering above evidences it can be concluded that drugs of metformin and rapamycin may indirectly reduce the expression of VEGF and subsequently decrease angiogenesis in cancerous tissues. Because the major effects of these drugs on liver cells, in this study, we evaluated the effect of these two drugs on VEGF expression and the cell proliferation in the liver carcinoma cell line.

Materials and Methods

Cell culture

The Human liver cancer cell line, HepG2 (ATCC HB-8065, Manassas, USA) was cultured in RPMI-1640 medium (Thermo Fisher Scientific, Massachusetts, USA), contained 10% fetal bovine serum (Invitrogen, Darmstadt, Germany) and 100 U/mL penicillin/streptomycin (Invitrogen, Darmstadt, Germany) in a CO2 incubator at 37°C for 48h as a pre-culture. The treatment program included concentrations of metformin (Sigma, Munich, Germany) (0, 5, 10 and 20mM) and rapamycin (Sigma, Munich, Germany) (0, 5, 10 and 20nM) at different times (12, 24 and 48 h).

MTT assay

Cell viability after drug treatment was investigated by a standard colorimetric assay using 3-(4 5-dimethylthiazol-2-yl)-2 5-diphenyltetrazolium bromide (MTT) reagent (Sigma, Munich, Germany. First, 5,000 cells were seeded in 100 μl medium in a 96-well plate (Thermo Fisher Scientific, Massachusetts, USA) and incubated at 37°C with 5 % CO2 for 24 hours before adding drugs to allow cell adhesion. Then the medium was removed and cells were washed with 50 μl Phosphate-buffered saline (PBS) that was then removed. Following cells were treated in triple tests with the different concentrations (0, 5, 10 and 20 mM of metformin and 0, 5, 10 and 20 nM of rapamycin) at different times (12, 24 and 48 h). 50 μl MTT solution (5 mg/ml in PBS) was added to each well and was incubated for 3 h at 37°C. The optical density was then measured at 570 nm using ELISA Plate Readers (BioTek, Winooski, USA).

Quantitative real-time PCR

Total RNA was extracted by the Trizol reagent (Thermo Fisher Scientific, Massachusetts, USA) according to manufacturer's protocol. First-strand complementary DNA (cDNA) was synthesized using SuperScript III First-Strand Synthesis System (Thermo Fisher Scientific, Massachusetts, USA) according to the manufacturer's instrument. The specific primers for VEGF were forward 5′-GGGCACTGCCTGGAAGATTCAG-3′ and reverse 5′-CTTCTCTTCGCCGGGACATCTG-3′, and for Glyceraldehyde 3-phosphate dehydrogenase (GAPDH) were forward 5′-GGTGGTCTCCTCTGACTTCAACA-3′ and reverse 5′-GTTGCTGTAGCCAAATTCGTTGT-3′, which were designed by GeneRunner software (version 5; Hastings, USA) and were reviewed in BLAST websites. Quantitative Real-time PCR was performed in triple tests in a detection System (Line-Gene K, BIOER, Hangzhou, China) by a real-time PCR kit (Thermo Fisher, Massachusetts, USA) as previously described.[26] PCR conditions started at one step initial denaturation (95°C for 3 min), followed by 40 cycles (95°C for 20 sec, 60°C for 20 sec, and 72°C for 20 sec). VEGF and GAPDH mRNA level were expressed as the cycle threshold (Ct) values. VEGF mRNA level normalized against GAPDH mRNA level and was calculated by $2^{-\Delta Ct}$ method.[27]

Elisa assay

To determine VEGF protein level, 5×10^3 HepG2 cells were seeded in a 96-well plate and were treated with the different concentrations at different times. VEGF concentrations were then measured by ELISA (Abcam, Cambridge, USA) for each well as previously described.[28]

Apoptosis index calculation

HepG2 Cells were fixed by Paraformaldehyde (Sigma, Munich, Germany) and stained by 4′,6′-diamidino-2-phenylindole dihydrochloride (DAPI) reagent (Sigma, Munich, Germany) according to the manufacturer's protocol. Cells were then investigated under a fluorescent microscope (Nikon, Shanghai, China) at a 100x magnification. Cells were counted in 10 randomized selected microscopic fields in which apoptotic cells were characterized by condensation, nuclear shrinkage and fragmentation. The apoptosis index (AI) percentage was calculated using the following formula: AI (%) = (apoptotic cells/total cells) × 100%.[4]

Statistical analysis

The experiment Data are expressed as the mean ± standard deviation. Data were analyzed using GraphPad software (version 6; San Diego, CA, United States). The difference between variables was performed by Student's t-test or one-way ANOVA test. A P value less than 0.05 was considered statistically significant.

Results and Discussion

Metformin and rapamycin decrease cancer cells viability

To evaluate the effects of metformin and rapamycin on HCC cells growth in vitro, cell viability of HepG2 Cells was assessed by MTT assay following treatment with metformin and rapamycin in various concentrations and at different times. MTT data showed that mean IC50 values from 3 independent experiments in times of 12, 24 and 48 h were 2.63 ± 0.52, 3.77 ± 0.69 and 3.74 ± 0.71 for metformin, and 3.83 ± 0.82, 3.54 ± 0.85 and 4.14 ± 0.91 for rapamycin. Results showed that both metformin and rapamycin inhibited the growth of HepG2 cells in a dose-dependent manner ($p < 0.05$) (Figure 1). It was also found that the lowest cell viability was seen in concentrations of metformin (10 mM) (Figure 1A) and rapamycin (10 nM) in 24 hours after treatment (Figure 1B). In addition, it was found that in combination with different concentrations of the two drugs, lowest survival cell viability was seen also in concentrations of metformin 10mM and rapamycin 10nM in 24 hours after treatment (Figure 1C).

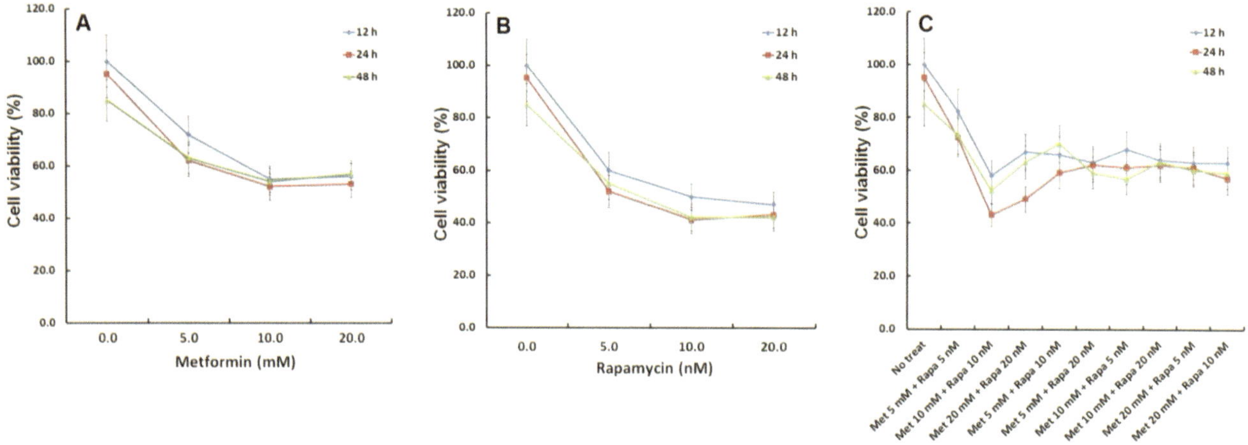

Figure 1. MTT assay for analyzing HepG2 cells viability after treatment with metformin and rapamycin. **(A)** Metformin has reduced hepatocarcinoma cells survival by about 50% in concentration 10 mM. **(B)** Rapamycin has reduced cells survival by about 60% in concentration 10mM. **(C)** The lowest survival is associated with cells treated by the combination of metformin 10mM and rapamycin 10 nM.

Rapamycin but not metformin decreases VEGF gene expression in HepG2 cells

To study the inhibitory effects of metformin and rapamycin on HepG2 cells growth, we examined the expression of *VEGF* gene, in cells treated with metformin (10 mM), rapamycin (10 nM) and the combination of two drugs after 24 hours. Our results in Figure 2 showed that metformin has no significant effect on *VEGF* gene expression in the treated HepG2 cells compared to the untreated cells. In contrast, rapamycin significantly reduces the *VEGF* gene expression in HepG2 cell line in comparison with untreated cells ($p = 0.012$). The combination of two drugs has also no significant effect on *VEGF* gene expression in HepG2 cells (Figure 2). Moreover, to confirm VEGF expression analysis, we determined VEGF protein level in HepG2 cells treated with two drugs and the results are shown in Figure 3. These results showed that metformin has no significant effect on *VEGF* gene expression in treated HepG2 cells. In contrast, Rapamycin significantly reduces the *VEGF* gene expression in HepG2 cells ($p = 0.013$). The combination of two drugs has also no significant effect on *VEGF* gene expression in treated HepG2 cells in comparison with untreated cells (Figure 3).

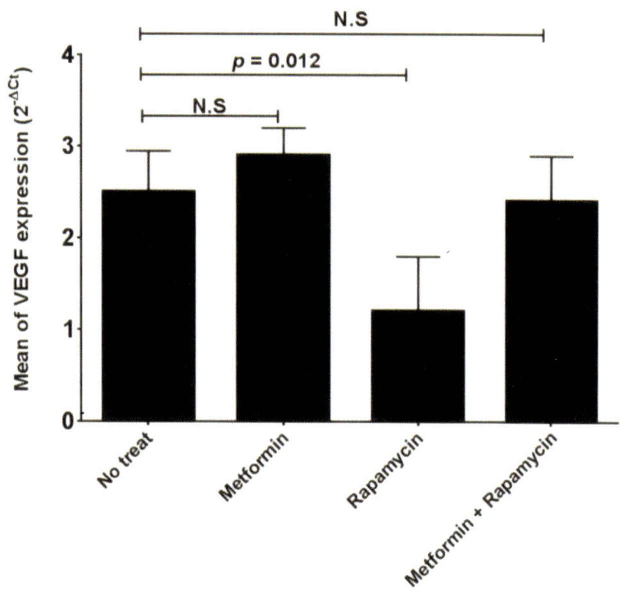

Figure 2. Quantitative real-time PCR for investigation of *VEGF* gene expression in HepG2 cells. Rapamycin but no metformin, significantly reduces the *VEGF* gene expression in the treated HepG2 cells in comparison with untreated cells. Metformin and rapamycin were used in concentrations of 10mM and 10nM respectively.

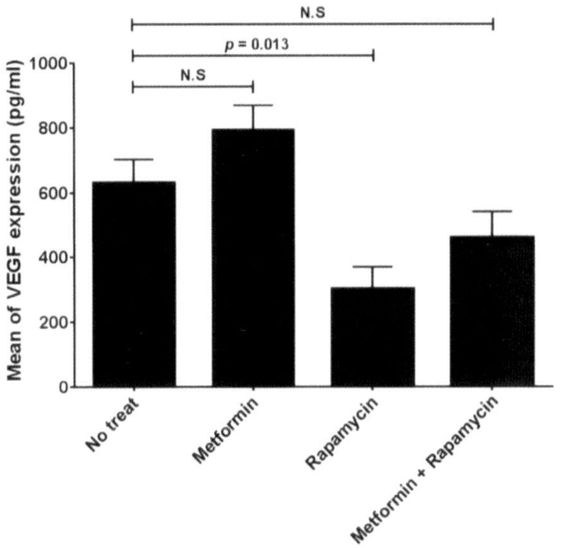

Figure 3. Elisa assay for determination of VEGF protein level in HepG2 cells. Rapamycin but no metformin significantly reduces the VEGF protein level in the treated HepG2 cells than untreated cells. Metformin and rapamycin were used in concentrations of 10mM and 10 nM respectively.

Metformin and rapamycin induce cell apoptosis

To investigate whether metformin and rapamycin induce cellular apoptosis, HepG2 cells were incubated with metformin (10mM), rapamycin (10nM) and the combination of two drugs at the same concentration. After 24 hours, nuclear morphology by DAPI staining was assessed (Figure 4). The results in Figure 5 showed that the apoptosis index in the treated cells with both drugs was significantly higher in comparison with untreated cells ($p < 0.001$).

Nowadays the use of VEGF pathway inhibitors in the angiogenesis is considered as a therapeutic strategy against cancer with a clinical validation.[12] In this study, we suggested that these agents should be used in combination with other therapeutic agents.[29] Therefore, further studies are needed to understand the effective combination therapies in reducing tumor angiogenesis and drug resistance. Despite significant advances in the control and treatment of malignant tumors, the search continues for new treatments and drugs. In this way, considering the molecular pathways involved in tumor growth and identify ways to control these pathways has attracted a more attention. The two drugs, which have been provided with specific molecular targets, are metformin and rapamycin. These two drugs indirectly inhibit expression of VEGF.[24] Therefore; it was assumed that these two drugs lead to reduced VEGF expression and subsequently to inhibit angiogenesis in tumors. Our results in this study showed that rapamycin but not metformin inhibits *VEGF* gene expression in HepG2 cells. Different effects of metformin treatment on gene expression can be due to several factors as mentioned in the Dallaglio et al. study in which they observed a paradoxical effect of metformin on endothelial and cancerous cells in the control of angiogenesis. They also concluded that effect of metformin on VEGF expression in each cell might be different.[30] These differences are probably due to the difference of cancerous cells in the resistance to a specific drug. The Miyoshi et al. in a study has shown that metformin inhibits angiogenesis in hepatocyte carcinoma cell line with no effect on VEGF expression.[31] The results of cell viability assay showed that metformin and rapamycin decrease cancer cells viability in HepG2 cells. This may be due to indirectly decrease of VEGF and subsequent activation of the phosphorylation of extracellular signal regulated kinase 1 (ERK1) and ERK2 as previously described.[32] In agreement with our study, the Wang et al. showed that rapamycin reduces VEGF expression. They found even a low dose of rapamycin is sufficient to prevent the progression of HCC tumors.[33] According to this study, it can be concluded that metformin can inhibit angiogenesis, but in the regulation of *VEGF* gene expression may demonstrate a dual effect. This dual effect probably depends on factors such as the type of cell, the duration of treatment, the drug concentration and other different signaling pathways. Confusion in this study may be due to the effect of combining the two drugs on VEGF expression. It seems that VEGF expression level in cells treated with the combination of two drugs is approximately equivalent to the average of expression level in cells treated with either drug separately. Although more comprehensive studies are needed to clarify it.

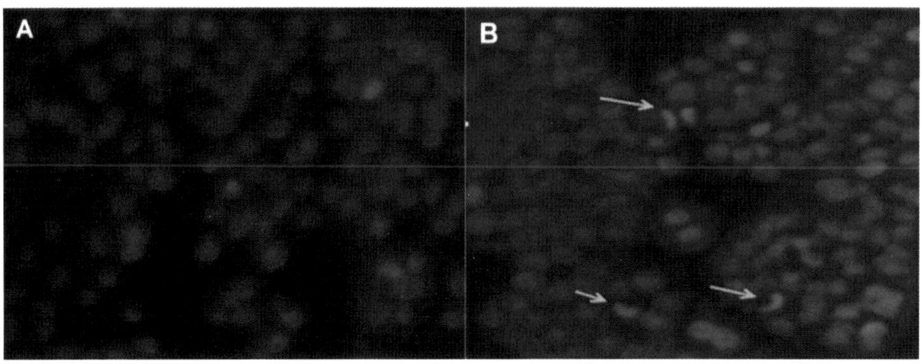

Figure 4. The nuclear morphological changes in HepG2 cells after treatment with metformin (10 mM) and rapamycin (10 nM). **(a)** The control cells showed intact nuclei with uniform shape and size. **(b)** Arrows indicate apoptotic bodies observed at 40X magnification under an inverted fluorescence microscope.

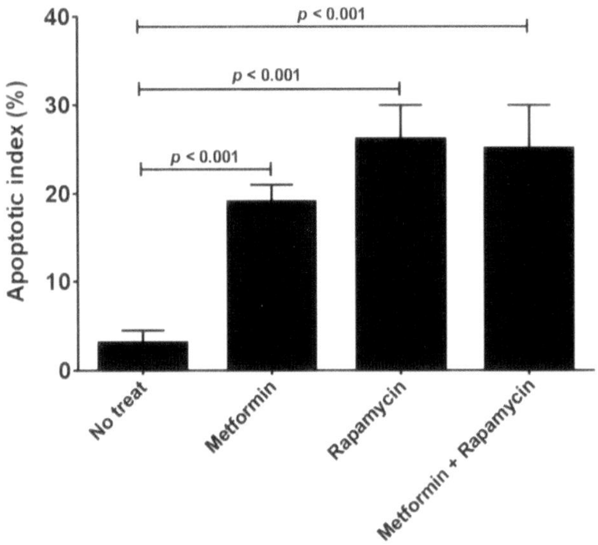

Figure 5. Apoptotic index analysis in the treated HepG2 cells with metformin (10 mM) and rapamycin (10 nM). Apoptosis index in the treated cells with both drugs (separately and in combination) was significantly high in comparison with untreated cells.

Conclusion

The differential effect of metformin and rapamycin on VEGF expression calls into question the use of mTOR inhibitors to target angiogenesis. Further analysis of the molecular pathways affected by both drugs may lead the authors to define new therapeutic strategies. This information may help to design a combination treatment to increase the efficacy of metformin and rapamycin in HCC.

Acknowledgments

This work was supported by the research department in Golestan University of Medical Sciences, Gorgan, Iran (Grant number 930705044).

Ethical Issues

Not applicable.

Conflict of Interest

The authors declare no conflict of interests.

References

1. Tsochatzis EA, Meyer T, Burroughs AK. Hepatocellular carcinoma. *N Engl J Med* 2012;366(1):92-3. doi: 10.1056/NEJMc1112501
2. Zhu RX, Seto WK, Lai CL, Yuen MF. Epidemiology of Hepatocellular Carcinoma in the Asia-Pacific Region. *Gut Liver* 2016;10(3):332-9. doi: 10.5009/gnl15257
3. Wang Z, Xiang Q, Li D, Li S. Correlation between gene expression and chromatin conformation of c-fos and N-ras in human liver and hepatoma. *Chin Med Sci J* 1991;6(1):6-8.
4. Qu Z, Zhang Y, Liao M, Chen Y, Zhao J, Pan Y. In vitro and in vivo antitumoral action of metformin on hepatocellular carcinoma. *Hepatol Res* 2012;42(9):922-33. doi: 10.1111/j.1872-034X.2012.01007.x
5. Taghizadeh S, Sankian M, Ajami A, Tehrani M, Hafezi N, Mohammadian R, et al. Expression Levels of Vascular Endothelial Growth Factors A and C in Patients with Peptic Ulcers and Gastric Cancer. *J Gastric Cancer* 2014;14(3):196-203. doi: 10.5230/jgc.2014.14.3.196
6. Shaw D, Clamp A, Jayson GC. Angiogenesis as a target for the treatment of ovarian cancer. *Curr Opin Oncol* 2013;25(5):558-65. doi: 10.1097/CCO.0b013e328363e0da
7. Hall RD, Le TM, Haggstrom DE, Gentzler RD. Angiogenesis inhibition as a therapeutic strategy in non-small cell lung cancer (NSCLC). *Transl Lung Cancer Res* 2015;4(5):515-23. doi: 10.3978/j.issn.2218-6751.2015.06.09
8. Sun W. Angiogenesis in metastatic colorectal cancer and the benefits of targeted therapy. *J Hematol Oncol* 2012;5:63. doi: 10.1186/1756-8722-5-63
9. Russo G, Mischi M, Scheepens W, De la Rosette JJ, Wijkstra H. Angiogenesis in prostate cancer: onset, progression and imaging. *BJU Int* 2012;110(11 Pt C):E794-808. doi: 10.1111/j.1464-410X.2012.11444.x
10. Jain RK, di Tomaso E, Duda DG, Loeffler JS, Sorensen AG, Batchelor TT. Angiogenesis in brain tumours. *Nat Rev Neurosci* 2007;8(8):610-22. doi: 10.1038/nrn2175
11. Ribatti D, Nico B, Ranieri G, Specchia G, Vacca A. The Role of Angiogenesis in Human Non-Hodgkin Lymphomas. *Neoplasia* 2013;15(3):231-8. doi: 10.1593/neo.121962
12. El-Kenawi AE, El-Remessy AB. Angiogenesis inhibitors in cancer therapy: mechanistic perspective on classification and treatment rationales. *Br J Pharmacol* 2013;170(4):712-29. doi: 10.1111/bph.12344
13. Bao S, Wu Q, Sathornsumetee S, Hao Y, Li Z, Hjelmeland AB, et al. Stem cell-like glioma cells promote tumor angiogenesis through vascular endothelial growth factor. *Cancer Res* 2006;66(16):7843-8. doi: 10.1158/0008-5472.CAN-06-1010
14. Watnick RS. The Role of the Tumor Microenvironment in Regulating Angiogenesis. *Cold Spring Harb Perspect Med* 2012;2(12):a006676. doi: 10.1101/cshperspect.a006676
15. DeFronzo RA, Goodman AM. Efficacy of metformin in patients with non-insulin-dependent diabetes mellitus. The Multicenter Metformin Study Group. *N Engl J Med* 1995;333(9):541-9. doi: 10.1056/NEJM199508313330902
16. Ben Sahra I, Le Marchand-Brustel Y, Tanti JF, Bost F. Metformin in cancer therapy: a new perspective for an old antidiabetic drug? *Mol Cancer Ther* 2010;9(5):1092-9. doi: 10.1158/1535-7163.MCT-09-1186

17. Donadon V, Balbi M, Mas MD, Casarin P, Zanette G. Metformin and reduced risk of hepatocellular carcinoma in diabetic patients with chronic liver disease. *Liver Int* 2010;30(5):750-8. doi: 10.1111/j.1478-3231.2010.02223.x
18. Chen TM, Lin CC, Huang PT, Wen CF. Metformin associated with lower mortality in diabetic patients with early stage hepatocellular carcinoma after radiofrequency ablation. *J Gastroenterol Hepatol* 2011;26(5):858-65. doi: 10.1111/j.1440-1746.2011.06664.x
19. Lee MS, Hsu CC, Wahlqvist ML, Tsai HN, Chang YH, Huang YC. Type 2 diabetes increases and metformin reduces total, colorectal, liver and pancreatic cancer incidences in Taiwanese: a representative population prospective cohort study of 800,000 individuals. *BMC Cancer* 2011;11:20. doi: 10.1186/1471-2407-11-20
20. Shackelford DB. Unravelling the connection between metabolism and tumorigenesis through studies of the liver kinase B1 tumour suppressor. *J Carcinog* 2013;12:16. doi: 10.4103/1477-3163.116323
21. Zhou J, Fan J, Wang Z, Wu ZQ, Qiu SJ, Huang XW, et al. Conversion to sirolimus immunosuppression in liver transplantation recipients with hepatocellular carcinoma: Report of an initial experience. *World J Gastroenterol* 2006;12(19):3114-8. doi: 10.3748/wjg.v12.i19.3114
22. Sahin F, Kannangai R, Adegbola O, Wang J, Su G, Torbenson M. mTOR and P70 S6 kinase expression in primary liver neoplasms. *Clin Cancer Res* 2004;10(24):8421-5. doi: 10.1158/1078-0432.CCR-04-0941
23. Semela D, Piguet AC, Kolev M, Schmitter K, Hlushchuk R, Djonov V, et al. Vascular remodeling and antitumoral effects of mTOR inhibition in a rat model of hepatocellular carcinoma. *J Hepatol* 2007;46(5):840-8. doi: 10.1016/j.jhep.2006.11.021
24. Forsythe JA, Jiang BH, Iyer NV, Agani F, Leung SW, Koos RD, et al. Activation of vascular endothelial growth factor gene transcription by hypoxia-inducible factor 1. *Mol Cell Biol* 1996;16(9):4604-13. doi: 10.1128/mcb.16.9.4604
25. Basu A, Contreras AG, Datta D, Flynn E, Zeng L, Cohen HT, et al. Overexpression of vascular endothelial growth factor and the development of post-transplantation cancer. *Cancer Res* 2008;68(14):5689-98. doi: 10.1158/0008-5472.CAN-07-6603
26. Daryani A, Sharif M, Dadimoghaddam Y, Souteh MB, Ahmadpour E, Khalilian A, et al. Determination of parasitic load in different tissues of murine toxoplasmosis after immunization by excretory-secretory antigens using Real time QPCR. *Exp Parasitol* 2014;143:55-9. doi: 10.1016/j.exppara.2014.05.008
27. Yazdani Y, Farazmandfar T, Azadeh H, Zekavatian Z. The prognostic effect of PTEN expression status in colorectal cancer development and evaluation of factors affecting it: miR-21 and promoter methylation. *J Biomed Sci* 2016;23:9. doi: 10.1186/s12929-016-0228-5
28. Farazmandfar T, Haghshenas MR, Shahbazi M. Inhibition of HIV-1 by a lentiviral vector with a novel tat-inducible expression system and a specific tropism to the target cells. *Hum Gene Ther* 2015;26(10):680-7. doi: 10.1089/hum.2015.031
29. Ebos JM, Lee CR, Cruz-Munoz W, Bjarnason GA, Christensen JG, Kerbel RS. Accelerated metastasis after short-term treatment with a potent inhibitor of tumor angiogenesis. *Cancer Cell* 2009;15(3):232-9. doi: 10.1016/j.ccr.2009.01.021
30. Dallaglio K, Bruno A, Cantelmo AR, Esposito AI, Ruggiero L, Orecchioni S, et al. Paradoxic effects of metformin on endothelial cells and angiogenesis. *Carcinogenesis* 2014;35(5):1055-66. doi: 10.1093/carcin/bgu001
31. Miyoshi H, Kato K, Iwama H, Maeda E, Sakamoto T, Fujita K, et al. Effect of the anti-diabetic drug metformin in hepatocellular carcinoma in vitro and in vivo. *Int J Oncol* 2013.
32. Gupta K, Kshirsagar S, Li W, Gui L, Ramakrishnan S, Gupta P, et al. VEGF prevents apoptosis of human microvascular endothelial cells via opposing effects on MAPK/ERK and SAPK/JNK signaling. *Exp Cell Res* 1999;247(2):495-504. doi: 10.1006/excr.1998.4359
33. Wang W, Jia WD, Xu GL, Wang ZH, Li JS, Ma JL, et al. Antitumoral activity of rapamycin mediated through inhibition of HIF-1alpha and VEGF in hepatocellular carcinoma. *Dig Dis Sci* 2009;54(10):2128-36. doi: 10.1007/s10620-008-0605-3

Interactions Between Sirolimus and Anti-Inflammatory Drugs: Competitive Binding for Human Serum Albumin

Arash Khodaei[1], Soheila Bolandnazar[1], Hadi Valizadeh[1], Leila Hasani[2], Parvin Zakeri-Milani[3]*

[1] *Drug Applied Research Center and Faculty of Pharmacy, Tabriz University of Medical Sciences, Tabriz, Iran.*
[2] *Department of Biological Sciences, Institute for Advanced Studies in Basic Sciences, Zanjan, Iran.*
[3] *Liver and Gastrointestinal Diseases Research Center and Faculty of Pharmacy, Tabriz University of Medical Sciences, Tabriz, Iran.*

Keywords:
· Sirolimus
· NSAIDs
· Protein binding
· Site I
· Site II
· Ultrafiltration

Abstract

Purpose: The aim of the present study was investigating the effects of three anti-inflammatory drugs, on Sirolimus protein biding. The binding site of Sirolimus on human serum albumin (HSA) was also determined.
Methods: Six different concentrations of Sirolimus were separately exposed to HSA at pH 7.4 and 37°C. Ultrafiltration method was used for separating free drug; then free drug concentrations were measured by HPLC. Finally, Sirolimus protein binding parameters was calculated using Scatchard plots. The same processes were conducted in the presence of NSAIDs at lower concentration of albumin and different pH conditions. To characterize the binding site of Sirolimus on albumin, the free concentration of warfarin sodium and Diazepam, site I and II specific probes, bound to albumin were measured upon the addition of increasing Sirolimus concentrations.
Results: Based on the obtained results presence of Diclofenac, Piroxicam and Naproxen, could significantly decrease the percentage of Sirolimus protein binding. The Binding reduction was the most in the presence of Piroxicam. Sirolimus-NSAIDs interactions were increased in higher pH values and also in lower albumin concentrations. Probe displacement study showed that Sirolimus may mainly bind to site I on albumin molecule.
Conclusion: More considerations in co-administration of NSAIDs and Sirolimus is recommended.

Introduction

Most of the drugs bind to tissue and plasma proteins in the body.[1] The protein binding of drugs is an important pharmacokinetic parameter affecting their biological activity, metabolism, distribution, and elimination.[2,3] The magnitude of the effect of a drug on the target organ is related to its free concentration. Human serum albumin (HSA) is the most abundant protein with a molecular weight of 65 – 69 KDa. Albumin is quantitatively the major binding protein for neutral and acidic drugs.[4,5] It can bind reversibly with different kind of ligands such as fatty acids, amino acids, steroids, metals for example calcium, copper and zinc, and numerous pharmaceuticals.[5,6] Drugs have two ligand-specific binding site namely, site- I and site-II to bind to human serum albumin.[5-7] The ligand selectivity is comparatively broader for these two sites, allowing a range of drug molecules to bind at these sites. This broad selectivity is considered to be a consequence of the significant allosteric effects in HSA and drug molecules can also interact nonspecifically with HAS.[5] HSA is responsible for maintaining the osmotic pressure of the blood and is a carrier of many molecules such as free fatty acids, bilirubin and various hormones (such as cortisone, aldosterone, thyroxin, etc.).[5,6] Since HSA has limited number of binding sites, it is expected that drugs or agents with high affinity to protein will displace others leading to higher plasma concentration and probable toxicity. This competitive displacement is more significant, when the binding occurs to the same sites on the protein. However competition ability of drugs depends on their binding affinities, relative concentration, and specificity of binding.[8-10]

Sirolimus (SRL, formerly Rapamycin: $C_{51}H_{79}NO_{13}$, CAS: 53123-88-9) is a lactone-lactam macrolide antibiotic that joined the immunosuppressant depot when it was approved by the Food and Drug Administration (FDA) for the prevention of kidney transplant rejection (Figure 1).[8,11] Sirolimus is metabolized by CYP3A4 in human liver.[12,13] The structure of this drug is related to tacrolimus but the mechanism of action of these drugs is different. It inhibits the second phase of T-cell activation.[14] In addition it binds to the FK (peptidyl-prolyl cis-trans isomerase) binding protein which modulates the activity of the mammalian Target of Rapamycin (mTOR). The mTOR inhibits Interleukin-2-mediated signal transduction, resulting in cell cycle stop in the G1-S phase and prevents cell cycle progression and

***Corresponding author:** Parvin Zakeri-Milani, Email: pzakeri@tbzmed.ac.ir

proliferation, hence blocks the response of T- and B-cell activation by cytokines. These properties of sirolimus allow it to be a possible chemotherapeutic agent against many types of solid tumor.[12,13,15]
In the present study the potential interactions between Sirolimus and NSAIDs at the level of protein binding displacement was investigated.

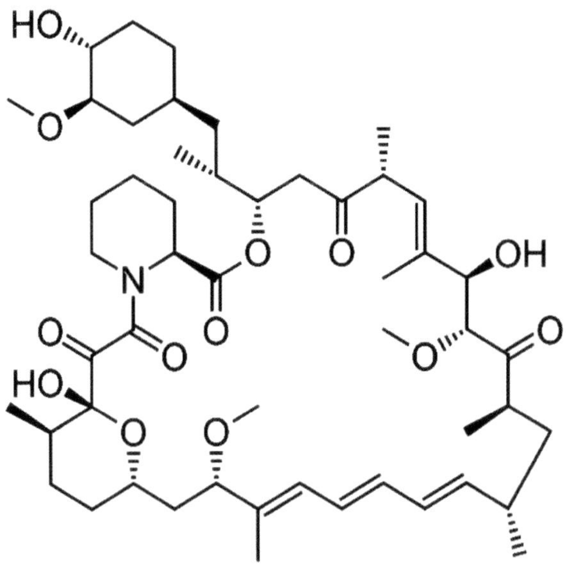

Figure1. Structure of Sirolimus (Rapamycin) molecule.

Materials and Methods

Chemicals

Sirolimus was obtained from Poli (Lazio, Italy). Diclofenac, Naproxen, Warfarin sodium, and diazepam were provided from Sigma (Louis, MO, USA). Piroxicam was provided from Cenateur (India). Monobasic potassium phosphate (KH2PO4), sodium hydroxide, ammonium acetate, sodium lauryl sulfate (SLS) were obtained from Merck (Darmstadt, Germany). Pharmaceutical-grade human albumin 20% was purchased from (CSL Behring GmbH, Germany). HPLC grade solvents, such as methanol and acetonitril (ACN) were also purchased from Merck (Darmstadt, Germany). Double-distilled water was used during the procedure.

Preparation of Stock solutions and standards

The primary stock solutions of Sirolimus, Diclofenac, Piroxicam and Naproxen with a concentration of 500 μg/ml were prepared. These stock solutions were stored in glass vials at +4°C. Finally, working standard solutions for HPLC calibrations or binding experiments were prepared by serially dilution to obtain Sirolimus concentrations of 8, 10, 12, 14, 16 and 18 μg/ml in monobasic potassium phosphate buffer solution (pH=7.4). Also, for investigating of Sirolimus complexions with NSAIDs, these drugs were added to diluted concentrations in their plasma concentrations.

Preparation of buffer solution

Buffer solution was prepared by placing 50 ml of the monobasic potassium phosphate solution in a 200 ml volumetric flask and 39.1 ml of the 0.2 M sodium hydroxide solution was added to the mixture. Then purified water was added to volume and pH was adjusted to 7.4.

Protein binding investigation by ultrafiltration

Solutions containing 8, 10, 12, 14, 16 and 18 μg/ml of Sirolimus were separately exposed to 0.04 g/ml human serum albumin in glass vials for one hour to complete protein binding in pH 7.4. For enhancing the stability of Sirolimus against the light, incubations were performed at 37°C, in glass vials, away from light, for 1 hour. After 1 hour, to produce ultrafiltrates containing unbound drug, the samples were added in the ultrafiltration system (cellophane membrane with 12,000 molecular weight cut-off). Centrifugations were performed at 37°C, for 10 min at 4000 rpm, resulting in filtrate volumes of 0.3–0.4 mL. The same process was performed in the presence of NSAIDs, Diclofenac, Piroxicam and Nproxen at the concentrations of 5, 17, and 70 μg/ml respectively for investigating of complexion of these drugs with Sirolimus.

Determination of binding site of Sirolimus on HSA at pH 7.4 and 37°C

Warfarin sodium and Diazepam were used as site I and site II specific probes respectively. HSA solutions of 6×10^{-4} molar concentration (5 ml) were taken in six test tubes. Then ten ml of 3×10^{-4} M warfarin sodium solution were added to each five tube. The sixth tube was taken as control containing only HSA (6×10^{-4} M). The final protein/warfarin ratio in tubes was 1:1. Increasing concentrations of Sirolimus solution was added to four tubes of five, so as the fifth tube contained only protein and Warfarin. The samples were mixed and to ensure the maximum binding of protein and warfarin, the mixture were allowed to stand for one hour. After that, the samples were added in the ultrafiltration system and the above mentioned process was followed. The free warfarin concentration was measured using a HPLC method developed by Yung et al with UV detection at 300 nm.[16] The same protocol was followed for diazepam as site II specific marker. A simple HPLC method developed and validated by Sruthi et al with UV detection at 230 nm was used for determination of free diazepam concentration.[17] The reverse experiment with the same protocol was also performed to verify the ability of warfarin sodium and diazepam to displace Sirolimus from its binding site.

HPLC Determination of Sirolimus

The validated RP-HPLC method was used for calculating of free Sirolimus concentration in the absence and presence of the NSAIDs after ultrafiltration.[11] Briefly C8 (10 μm, 4.6 ×150 mm) column was used as analytical column. The temperature of column was set at 55°C. The mobile phase was a mixture of 70% ACN and 30% ammonium acetate buffer, containing 10 mM sodium lauryl sulfate (SLS). The ammonium acetate buffer was prepared by dissolving 0.8 g ammonium acetate in 1000 ml water, adjusted to pH 5.8 with NaOH 0.1M. Injection volume of 100 μl was injected into the column using a Hamilton injector syringe (Bonaduz, Switzerland). The flow rate was set at 1.5 ml/min. Sirolimus was detected by UV detector at 272 nm. Binding data were evaluated based on both the Scatchard plots.[18]

Data treatment

The fraction of unbound drug was calculated by measuring the ultrafilterate concentrations using HPLC analysis. The drug concentrations were plotted according to Scatchard where the abscissa represents the factor r (the number of molecules of drug bound per molecule of albumin), and the ordinate represents r/D_f (D_f=free drug concentration). The data of r and D_f were fitted by linear least squares regression analysis when number of binding sites and association constants were calculated. Results are the mean±SD of three replicates. Finally, all data were analyzed statistically. Difference was considered significant when p-value was < 0.05.

Results and Discussion

There are two main types of protein binding, such as strong affinity binding to a small number of sites (site I in subdomain IIA) and weak affinity binding to a large number of sites (site II within subdomain IIIA).[7] Drug interactions leading to pharmacokinetic changes, arise from effects on drug-protein binding in both plasma and tissues. Concurrent administration of drugs which are capable of binding to the same site on protein leads to competitive displacement. Noncompetitive or allosteric displacement may also occur due to drug-induced conformational change in binding sites.[19,20] Drugs can bind to albumin at site I or site II or both sides. In the present study based on the probe displacement method, Sirolimus binding site on albumin was investigated using warfarin sodium as a site-I-specific probe and diazepam as a site-II-specific probe. According the obtained results the free fraction of warfarin sodium increased from initial 100% to 410% with increasing Sirolimus concentration. On the other hand the same increase in Sirolimus concentration led to 2.1 times augmentation in free diazepam concentration (210% vs initial 100%). That means free fraction increment in the case of warfarin was more than that of diazepam. In the reverse experiment, the free concentration of Sirolimus was increased from initial 100% to 350% and 150% with increasing warfarin sodium and diazepam respectively. This confirms the results of previous experiment. Therefore data suggested that Sirolimus is mainly binds to site I (high-affinity binding) than site II (low affinity binding). In other words in low plasma concentrations, Sirolimus binds to site I while in higher concentration both sites are involved in drug binding. So concurrent administration of drugs having a high affinity to site I may cause rapid action or excretion of Sirolimus from the body. It may even cause drug toxicity at normal doses.

In the next step binding characteristics of Sirolimus was investigated in the presence of some anti-inflammatory drugs. For drug-protein binding data interpretation, different analysis models could be used. These models are based on various features of binding process. In the present study the most common graphical presentation of the binding data, the Scatchard plot, was employed. According to the obtained data for Sirolimus and HSA binding, Scatchard plot was drawn and the binding parameters of Sirolimus were characterized (Figure 2). As it is clear, the binding of the drug at pH 7.4 and protein concentration of 0.04 g/L (4%) provided a linear plot, suggesting the presence of single class of binding sites for Sirolimus on the protein. The calculated affinity association constant (K), the number of binding sites (ν) for Sirolimus binding to HSA, and the mean protein binding percentage were found to be 3.99×10^5, 0.06, and 91.24 ±0.41 respectively. Therefore a high protein binding level and affinity association constant for Sirolimus were exhibited. Figures 3, 4 and 5 show, respectively, the Scatchard plots for Sirolimus-HSA binding in the presence of Diclofenac, Naproxen, and Piroxicam. Table 1 lists the calculated results for protein binding level (%), binding constants (K_a), and the number of binding sites (υ) per albumin molecule, for three investigated systems. Each system were examined at three pHs and two HSA concentrations. As it is clear from the Table, the values of K_a were of the order of 10^5. This demonstrates that there was a strong binding force between HSA and Sirolimus. It was found that the mean protein binding level of Sirolimus decreased significantly ($p<0.05$) in the presence of Diclofenac, Naproxen, and Piroxicam as compared with that in the absence of NSAIDs. The decrease was more noticeable in lower HSA concentration. The decrease in protein binding level could be attributed to reduced number of binding sites and/or reduced binding affinity. Based on the data in Table 1, the values of K_a (binding constant) in the presence of Diclofenac and 2% HSA was decreased significantly ($p<0.05$) in all three pH values while in the case of 4% HSA, reduced affinity was observed only in pH 7.9. Similarly, the same significant reduction was found in the number of binding sites (υ) in the presence of Diclofenac and HSA 4% compared with that in the absence of any NSAIDs. However in systems containing 2% HSA the reduced number of binding sites was only seen in low pH of 6.9. The results indicated that the presence of Diclofenac decreased the binding capability of sirolimus with HSA, which was raised from the replacement of sirolimus by Diclofenac from site I on HSA. Based on the obtained results, in most cases, both reduced binding constant and number of binding sites were responsible for the replacement. Therefore Diclofenac could change free sirolimus concentration in plasma. Considering the data obtained in systems containing Naproxen and Piroxicam, it seems that in most cases, reduction in number of binding sites is the predominant reason for reduced protein binding of Sirolimus. The non-steroidal anti-inflammatory drugs selected in the present study, Naproxen (pKa 4.38), Diclofenac (pKa 4.08) and Piroxicam (pKa 5.1), are in their anionic form in the investigated pH range of 6.9-7.9. Since HSA has the strongest affinities for anionic drugs, therefore displacement of Sirolimus by these NSAIDs were expected. Our results are in consistence with the observations of Jose´ Pe´rez-Urizar that demonstrated experimental hypoalbuminemia could increase free plasma tolmetin concentration by not only changing the number of available sites.[21] In a study by Rahman et al it was suggested that NSAIDs with a carboxyl group (like Diclofenac and Naproxen) and without a carboxyl group (like Piroxicam) are able to displace probes from site II and I on albumin molecule.[22] Our results demonstrated relatively higher displacement of sirolimus (site I binding drug) by Piroxicam compared with two other NSAIDs confirming the above mentioned finding.[22] Other processes like alterations in drug affinity to its binding site could also be considered. These changes may be a consequence of conformational changes in the albumin molecule. However in the body, pathophysiological conditions in hypoalbuminema and the probable generated metabolites could give further explanation for the observation. This is in agreement with our finding that the level of protein binding in systems containing 2% HSA, resembling hypoalbuminemia, were lower compared with those containing 4% HSA. Sirolimus is essentially unionized at all investigated pH values. On the other hand, as mentioned earlier, according to the results of the present study, pH changes resulted in alteration of Sirolimus-HSA binding. Since there is no known changes in physicochemical properties of Sirolimus in the pH Ranges of 6.9-7.9, the observed pH-dependent alterations must be due to conformational changes in HSA molecule.[23]

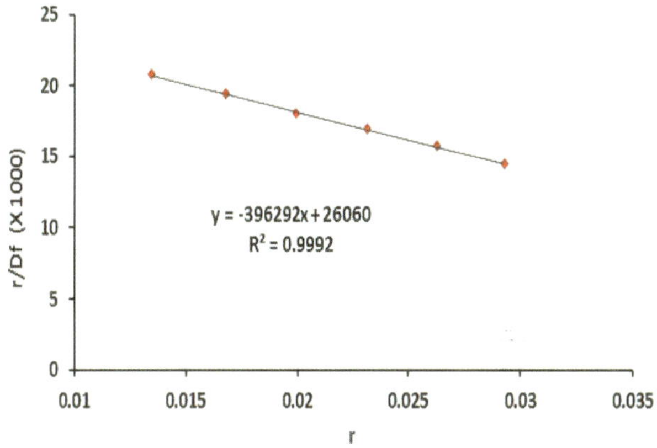

Figure 2. The Scatchard plot for Sirolimus-HSA binding (pH=7.4, HSA 4%). The abscissa represents the factor r (the number of molecules of drug bound per molecule of albumin), and the ordinate represents r/D_f (D_f=free drug concentration)

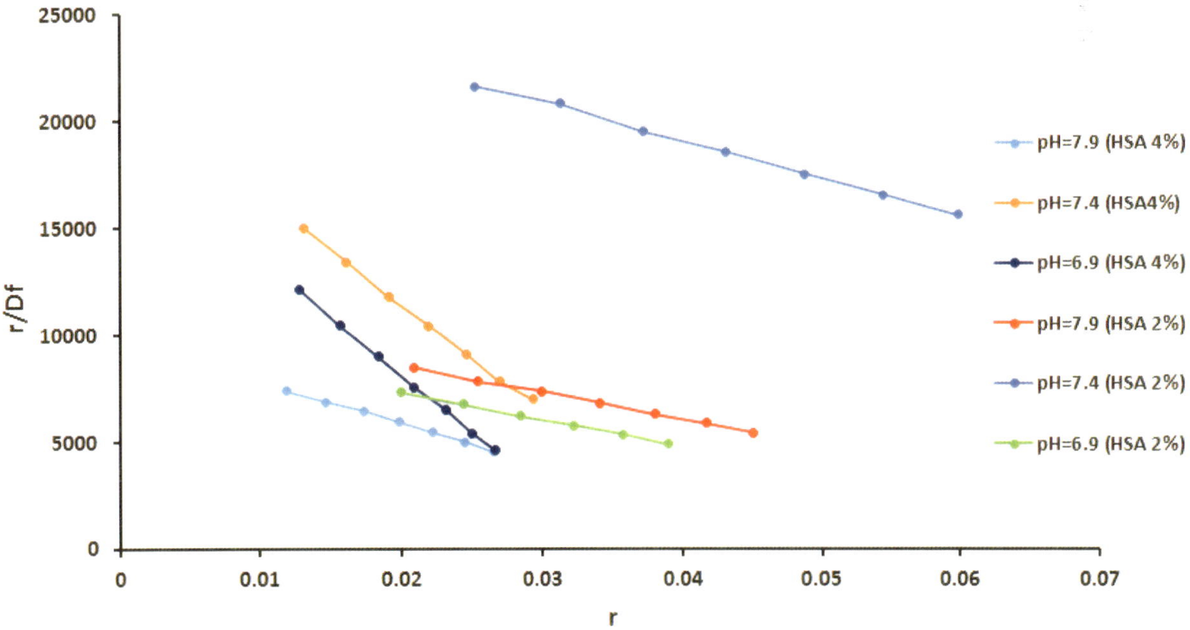

Figure 3. Scatchard plots for Sirolimus binding in the presence of Diclofenac at three different pHs (6.9, 7.4, 7.9) and two different HSA concentration (2% and 4%). Diclofenac concentration was 5 μg/ml. The abscissa represents the factor r (the number of molecules of drug bound per molecule of albumin), and the ordinate represents r/D_f (D_f=free drug concentration)

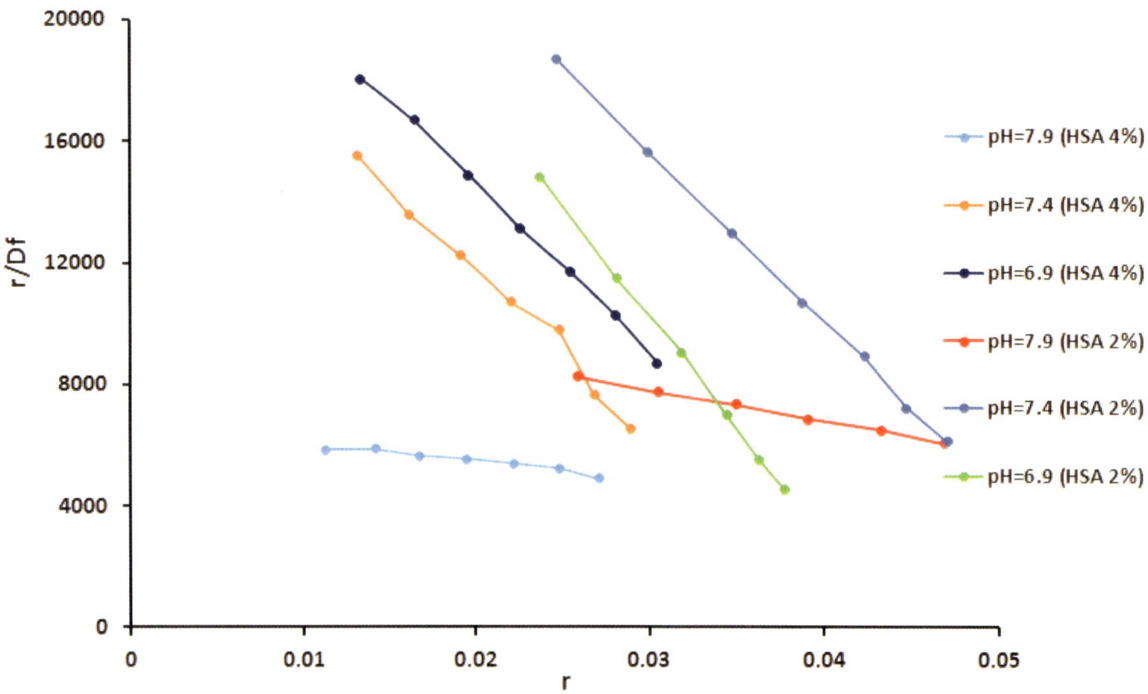

Figure 4. Scatchard plots for Sirolimus binding in the presence of Naproxen at three different pHs (6.9, 7.4, 7.9) and two different HSA concentration (2% and 4%). Naproxen concentration was 70 µg/ml. The abscissa represents the factor r (the number of molecules of drug bound per molecule of albumin), and the ordinate represents r/D_f (D_f=free drug concentration)

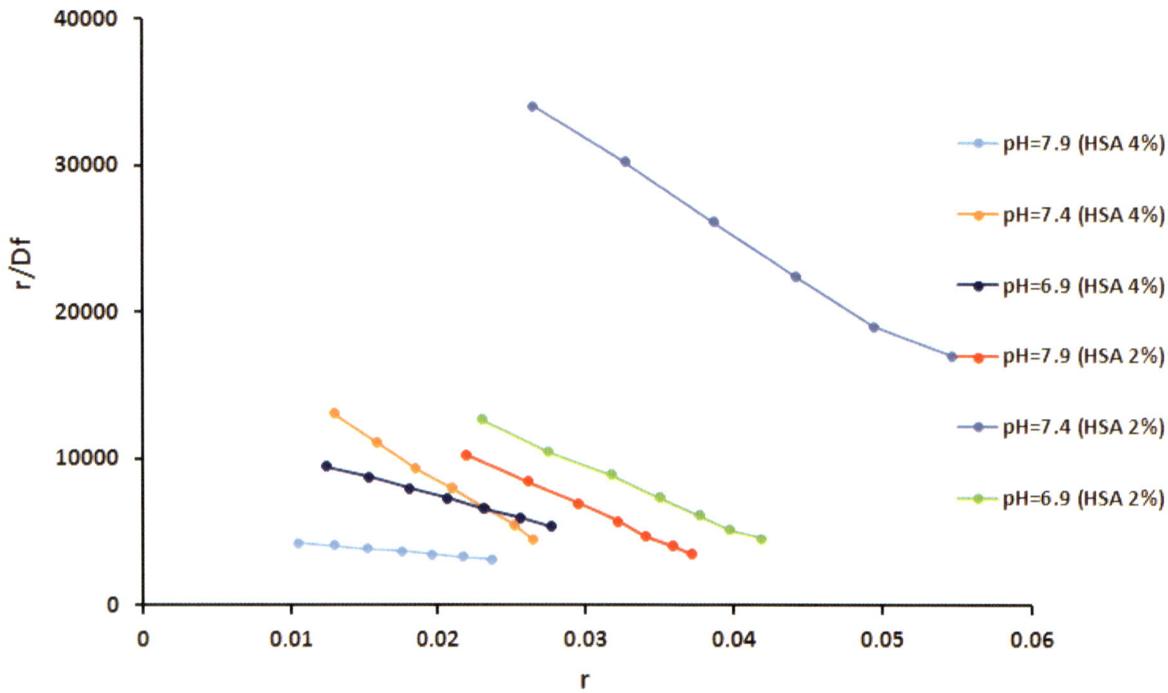

Figure 5. Scatchard plots for Sirolimus binding in the presence of Piroxicam at three different pHs (6.9, 7.4, 7.9) and two different HSA concentration (2% and 4%). Piroxicam concentration was 17 µg/ml. The abscissa represents the factor r (the number of molecules of drug bound per molecule of albumin), and the ordinate represents r/D_f (D_f=free drug concentration)

Conclusion

According to the results obtained presence of anti-inflammatory drugs Diclofenac, Piroxicam and Naproxen, could significantly decrease the percentage of sirolimus protein binding. This may lead to a higher apparent clearance and shorter half-life of drug. The Binding reduction was the most in the presence of Piroxicam. Therefore in patients under sirolimus regimen, concurrent administration of these NSAIDs (especially Piroxicam) is not recommended. Moreover Sirolimus-NSAIDs interactions were increased in higher pH values while in lower pH conditions, such as acidosis, less interactions were observed. It was also concluded that sirolimus-NSAIDs interactions were more considerable in low albumin concentrations and more considerations in co-administration of NSAIDs and sirolimus for patients with hypoalbumiemia is recommended. Therefore, extrapolating our results to the clinical situation, a higher level of sirolimus displacement could be expected in patients administering NSAIDs concomitantly and also in diseases involving hypoalbuminemia. However, further in vivo studies are needed to explore the biological significance of the above mentioned interaction.

Table 1. Mean of protein binding level (PB%), association constant (K), and number of equivalent binding sites (ν) of Sirolimus-HSA complex at three different pHs (6.9, 7.4, 7.9) and two different HSA concentration (2% and 4%)

Systems	HSA Concentration (%)	pH	Mean PB% ± SD	K	ν
HSA-Sirolimus + Diclofenac	4%	7.9	78.60±0.61	1.94×10^5	0.05
		7.4	86.67±0.11	5.01×10^5	0.04
		6.9	82.83±0.13	5.40×10^5	0.03
	2%	7.9	67.91±0.82	1.25×10^5	0.08
		7.4	85.09±0.12	1.77×10^5	0.14
		6.9	64.31±0.71	1.25×10^5	0.07
HSA-Sirolimus + Naproxen	4%	7.9	77.05±0.22	5.78×10^4	0.11
		7.4	86.97±0.11	5.51×10^5	0.04
		6.9	68.16±0.20	5.46×10^5	0.04
	2%	7.9	69.79±1.27	1.03×10^5	0.10
		7.4	77.46±0.74	5.62×10^5	0.05
		6.9	71.36±2.77	7.34×10^5	0.04
HSA-Sirolimus + Piroxicam	4%	7.9	69.28±0.37	8.38×10^4	0.06
		7.4	83.43±0.25	6.23×10^5	0.03
		6.9	81.94±0.20	2.67×10^5	0.04
	2%	7.9	65.44±0.73	4.50×10^5	0.04
		7.4	78.66±3.06	6.24×10^5	0.03
		6.9	70.51±0.55	4.34×10^5	0.05

Acknowledgments

This work was supported by Drug Applied Research Center, Tabriz University of Medical Sciences.

Ethical Issues

Not applicable.

Conflict of Interest

The Authors report no conflict of interests in the present study.

References

1. Yang XX, Hu ZP, Chan SY, Zhou SF. Monitoring drug-protein interaction. *Clin Chim Acta* 2006;365(1-2):9-29. doi: 10.1016/j.cca.2005.08.021
2. Singh SS, Mehta J. Measurement of drug-protein binding by immobilized human serum albumin-hplc and comparison with ultrafiltration. *J Chromatogr B Analyt Technol Biomed Life Sci* 2006;834(1-2):108-16. doi: 10.1016/j.jchromb.2006.02.053
3. Vuignier K, Schappler J, Veuthey JL, Carrupt PA, Martel S. Drug-protein binding: A critical review of analytical tools. *Anal Bioanal Chem* 2010;398(1):53-66. doi: 10.1007/s00216-010-3737-1
4. Carter DC, He XM, Munson SH, Twigg PD, Gernert KM, Broom MB, et al. Three-dimensional structure of human serum albumin. *Science* 1989;244(4909):1195-8.
5. Jr TP. Ligand binding by albumin. All about albumin. San Diego: Academic Press; 1995.
6. Ghuman J, Zunszain PA, Petitpas I, Bhattacharya AA, Otagiri M, Curry S. Structural basis of the drug-binding specificity of human serum albumin. *J Mol Biol* 2005;353(1):38-52. doi: 10.1016/j.jmb.2005.07.075
7. Rahman M, Prianka F, Shohel M, Mazid MA. Interaction of palmitic acid with metoprolol succinate at the binding sites of bovine serum albumin. *Adv Pharm Bull* 2014;4(4):379-83. doi: 10.5681/apb.2014.056
8. Wanke R, Harjivan SG, Pereira SA, Marques MM, Antunes AM. The role of competitive binding to human serum albumin on efavirenz-warfarin interaction: A nuclear magnetic resonance study. *Int J Antimicrob Agents* 2013;42(5):443-6. doi: 10.1016/j.ijantimicag.2013.06.023
9. Valizadeh H, Mohammadi G, Ehyaei R, Milani M, Azhdarzadeh M, Zakeri-Milani P, et al. Antibacterial activity of clarithromycin loaded PLGA nanoparticles. *Pharmazie* 2012;67(1):63-8.
10. Zakeri-Milani P, Valizadeh H, Ghanbarzadeh S, Nemati M. Pharmacokinetics and comparative

bioavailability study of two clarithromycin suspensions following administration of a single oral dose to healthy volunteers. *Arzneimittel-Forsch* 2009;59(8):429-32. doi: 10.1055/s-0031-1296419
11. Islambulchilar Z, Ghanbarzadeh S, Emami S, Valizadeh H, Zakeri-Milani P. Development and validation of an hplc method for the analysis of sirolimus in drug products. *Adv Pharm Bull* 2012;2(2):135-9. doi: 10.5681/apb.2012.021
12. Molnar-Kimber KL. Mechanism of action of rapamycin (sirolimus, rapamune). *Transplant Proc* 1996;28(2):964-9.
13. Sehgal SN. Rapamune (rapa, rapamycin, sirolimus): Mechanism of action immunosuppressive effect results from blockade of signal transduction and inhibition of cell cycle progression. *Clin Biochem* 1998;31(5):335-40.
14. Chen KH, Tsai MK, Lai IR, Lin Wu FL, Hu RH, Lee PH. Favorable results of concomitant tacrolimus and sirolimus therapy in taiwanese renal transplant recipients at 12 months. *J Formos Med Assoc* 2008;107(7):533-9.
15. Jones K, Saadat-Lajevard S, Lee T, Horwatt R, Hicks D, Johnston A, et al. An immunoassay for the measurement of sirolimus. *Clin Ther* 2000;22 Suppl B:B49-61.
16. Yung An C, Wan Zaidah A, Siew Hua G. Development of a high-performance liquid chromatography method for warfarin detection in human plasma. *Turk J Med Sci* 2012;42(5):930-41.
17. Sruthi A, Tejaswi P, Thanuja N, Sudheer Kumar D, Vivek Sagar P. Simple rp-hplc method for estimation of diazepam in tablet dosage form. *J Pharm Res* 2013;6:140-4.
18. Bolandnazar S, Divsalar A, Valizadeh H, Khodaei A, Zakeri-Milani P. Development and application of an HPLC method for erlotinib protein binding studies. *Adv Pharma Bull* 2013;3(2):289-93. doi: 10.5681/apb.2013.047
19. Liu BM, Zhang J, Bai CL, Wang X, Qiu XZ, Wang XL, et al. Spectroscopic study on flavonoid-drug interactions: Competitive binding for human serum albumin between three flavonoid compounds and ticagrelor, a new antiplatelet drug. *J Luminescence* 2015;168:69-76.
20. Ashrafi-Kooshk MR, Ebrahimi F, Ranjbar S, Ghobadi S, Moradi N, Khodarahmi R. Comparative studies on drug binding to the purified and pharmaceutical-grade human serum albumins: Bridging between basic research and clinical applications of albumin. *Biologicals* 2015;43(5):333-43. doi: 10.1016/j.biologicals.2015.07.003
21. Perez-Urizar J, Flores-Murrieta FJ, Castaneda-Hernandez G. Effect of experimental hypoalbuminemia on the plasma protein binding of tolmetin. *Life Sci* 2002;71(9):1015-22.
22. Rahman MH, Yamasaki K, Shin YH, Lin CC, Otagiri M. Characterization of high affinity binding sites of non-steroidal anti-inflammatory drugs with respect to site-specific probes on human serum albumin. *Biol Pharm Bull* 1993;16(11):1169-74.
23. Esmaeilzadeh S, Valizadeh H, Zakeri-Milani P. The effects of PH, temperature and protein concentration on the in vitro binding of flutamide to human serum albumin. *Pharm Dev Technol* 2016:1-10. doi: 10.3109/10837450.2016.1163392

Aggregated Nanotransfersomal Dry Powder Inhalation of Itraconazole for Pulmonary Drug Delivery

Mehdi Hassanpour Aghdam[1], Saeed Ghanbarzadeh[2,3], Yousef Javadzadeh[4], Hamed Hamishehkar[3]*

[1] *Research Center for Pharmaceutical Nanotechnology, and Students' Research Committee, Tabriz University of Medical Sciences, Tabriz, Iran.*

[2] *Zanjan Pharmaceutical Nanotechnology Research Center, and Department of Pharmaceutics, Faculty of Pharmacy, Zanjan University of Medical Sciences, Zanjan, Iran.*

[3] *Drug Applied Research Center, Tabriz University of Medical Sciences, Tabriz, Iran.*

[4] *Biotechnology Research Center and Department of Pharmaceutics, Faculty of Pharmacy, Tabriz University of Medical Sciences, Tabriz, Iran.*

Keywords:
- Pulmonary drug delivery
- Dry powder inhaler
- Transfersome
- Itraconazole
- DPI

Abstract

Purpose: Local therapy is a valuable and strategic approach in the treatment of lung associated diseases and dry powder inhalation (DPI) formulations play the key role in this plan. Transfersome has been introduced as a novel biocompatible vesicular system with potential for administration in pulmonary drug delivery. The present study was designed to prepare Itraconazole-loaded nanotrantransfersomal DPI formulation.

Methods: Itraconazole-loaded nanotransfersomes with three different types of surfactant in varying concentrations were prepared and characterized in the point of particle size distribution and morphology by laser light scattering and scanning electron microscopy (SEM) methods. The optimized transferosomal formulations were co-spray dried with mannitol and the aerosolization efficiency and aerodynamic properties of dry powders were determined by next generation impactor using a validated HPLC technique.

Results: The volume mean diameter of optimized nanotransfersomal formulation with lecithin:Span® 60 in the ratio of 90:10 was 171 nm with narrow size distribution pattern which increased up to 518 nm after drug loading. Different types of surfactant did not influence the particle size significantly. SEM images confirmed the formation of aggregated nanoparticles in the suitable range (1-5 μm) for the pulmonary drug delivery. Aerosolization evaluation of co-spray dried formulations with different amounts of mannitol indicated that 2:1 ratio of mannitol:transfersome (w:w) showed the best aerosolization efficiency (fine particle fraction (FPF)=37%). Increasing of mannitol significantly decreased the FPF of the optimized formulations.

Conclusion: The results of this study was introduced the potential application of nanotransfersomes in the formulation of DPIs for lung delivery of various drugs.

Introduction

Itraconazole is a broad-spectrum synthetic triazole antifungal agent which is active against a broad spectrum of fungal species including *Cryptococcus, Candida, Aspergillus, Blastomyces* and *Histoplasma capsulatum.*[1] The lungs are suitable for both local and systemic drug delivery due to the presence of a large alveolar surface area with high permeability owing to their thin epithelial layer.[2] Development of drug delivery systems for pulmonary application had received considerable attention and high patient compliance in the last three decades due to be a noninvasive method of drug administration. Furthermore, the possibility to locally and more site-specific drug delivery at high concentrations into the diseased lung by avoiding the first-pass metabolism and reduced systemic doses would lead to maximum therapeutic efficiency and minimum side effects, respectively.[3-6] The use of liposomes as drug carriers for pulmonary delivery has been reported for different kinds of therapeutics.[7,8] The utilization of lipidic vesicular systems for pulmonary drug delivery has many potential advantages over aerosol delivery of the corresponding non-encapsulated drug, including carrier suitability for most lipophilic drugs, compatibility and reducing local irritation of lung tissue, prolonging local and systemic therapeutic drug levels and finally facilitating intracellular drug delivery especially to alveolar macrophages, tumor cells or epithelial cells.[9] Intensive research over the past 25 years led to the introduction and development of a new class of highly deformable liposomes resembling the natural cell vesicle, named transferosomes.[10-12] Transfersomes are composed of phospholipids like phosphatidylcholine and edge

***Corresponding author:** Hamed Hamishehkar, Email: Hamishehkarh@tbzmed.ac.ir activators which self assembles into lipid bilayer in aqueous environment and closes to form a vesicle.[13,14] An edge activator is often a single-chain surfactant with a high radius of curvature that destabilizes the lipid bilayers of the vesicles and increases the deformability of the bilayers.[15] Spray drying has been considered as a simple one-step process for producing small particles for pulmonary administration, that can be easily scaled up.[16-18] Pressurized metered-dose inhalers (MDI), nebulizers, and dry powder inhalers (DPI) are the three main delivery systems used for aerosol inhalation in humans. Among these, DPI appears to be the most promising for future use. They are propellant-free, portable, easy to operate and low-cost devices with improved stability of the formulation as a result of the dry state.[19,20] According to our literature review, there is no report about the application of nanotransfersomes in pulmonary drug delivery. Therefore, the primary aim of this study was to introduce transfersomes as a carrier for pulmonary delivery in the form of dry powder inhalation formulation.

Materials and Methods

Materials

Acetonitrile, Tween® 80, Ursodiol, Chloroform and Ortho-phosphoric acid were purchased from Merck Chemicals Co. (Germany). Soybean phosphatidylcholine (SPC, purity >99%) was purchased from Lipoid GmbH (Ludwigshafen, Germany). Itraconazole was supplied from Cipla Company (India). Span® 60 and Span® 80 were supplied from Sigma Company (USA) and BDH laboratory (UK), respectively. D-Mannitol and ethyl alcohol were obtained from Fluka (Germany) and JATA (Iran) Companies, respectively.

Methods

Preparation of nanotransfersomes

Transfersomes were prepared by the thin film hydration method. Briefly, desired amounts of SPC (100 mg), Itraconazole (5 mg) and surfactant (5, 10, and 15 mg) were dissolved in an appropriate volume of organic solvent (Table 1). The container tightly closed, protected from light and maintained at room temperature for one day to make sure of formation of complete and homogeneous solution. The mixture was transformed to a round-bottomed flask for solvent removal using a rotary evaporator (Heidolph, Germany) at reduced pressure and above phase transition temperature of lecithin (60 °C). The dried film was hydrated for one hour at 60 °C and then sonicated using a prob sonicator (Sonix, Vibracell), with 0.5 sec on and 0.5 sec off intervals, for a total period of 15 min.[12,21]

Table 1. Composition of various nanotransfersome formulations. Data was presented as mean ± standard deviation (n=3).

Formulation code	Type of Surfactant	Surfactant (mg)	Itraconazole (mg)	VMD[a] (nm)	Span
T1	Span® 80	10	0	360 ± 21	1.18 ± 0.03
T2	Span® 80	5	5	556 ± 29	1.44 ± 0.04
T3	Span® 80	10	5	526 ± 31	1.74 ± 0.03
T4	Span® 80	15	5	598 ± 34	1.70 ± 0.06
T5	Span® 60	10	0	171 ± 28	1.03 ± 0.03
T6	Span® 60	5	5	535 ± 22	1.33 ± 0.03
T7	Span® 60	10	5	518 ± 23	1.07 ± 0.03
T8	Span® 60	15	5	534 ± 30	2.16 ± 0.14
T9	Ursodiol	5	5	545 ± 22	1.17 ± 0.04
T10	Ursodiol	10	5	522 ± 27	1.04 ± 0.04
T11	Ursodiol	15	5	594 ± 41	1.66 ± 0.04

[a] Volume median diameter

Spray drying process

For producing DPI formulations, different amounts of mannitol powder (100, 200, 300 and 600 mg named as F1, F2, F3 and F4, respectively) was co-spray dried with the nanotransfersomal dispersion (100 mg) with desired characteristics using a mini spray dryer at an inlet temperature of 100 ± 5 °C, outlet temperature of 60 ± 5 °C, aspiration setting of 90% and spray flow of 400 NL/h. Immediately after powder collection from the cyclone of spray dryer, spray-dried particles were packed into the tightly closed container wrapped in aluminum foil and desiccated over silica gel at room temperature until further studies.

Particle size analysis

The particle size and particle size distribution of prepared nanotransfersomal dispersions were determined by particle size analyzer (Wing SALD 2101, Japan). The size distribution was expressed by the volume median diameter (VMD) and span value. The smaller span values correspond to narrower size distribution. Span value calculated using following equation:

$$\text{Span} = \frac{D(v90\%) - D(v10\%)}{D(v50\%)}$$

Where D(v,90), D(v,10) and D(v,50) are the equivalent volume diameters at 90, 10 and 50% cumulative volume, respectively.[22,23]

Scanning electron microscopy (SEM)

The shape and surface morphology of the particles were studied by the scanning electron microscope (LEO 1430 VP, UK & Germany). Prior to scanning, the samples were coated with a thin layer of gold, using a direct current sputter technique (Emitechk450X, England).

In vitro aerosolization assessment

The *in vitro* aerodynamic parameters including aerodynamic diameter, aerosolization efficiency, dispersion and deposition characteristics of optimized Itraconazole-loaded nanotransfersomal dry powders were assessed by an aerolizer connected to the next generation impactor (NGI) with pre-separator and USP induction port (Copley Scientific, Nottingham, UK).[24] The NGI was assembled and operated in accordance with USP General Chapter 601 to assess the drug delivered. An appropriate number of hard gelatin capsules (N = 3) were filled with 10 mg of spray dried powder. To ensure efficient particle capture and prevent inter-stage losses due to particle bounce, the particle collection surface of each stage was coated with Tween® 80. For this purpose, every eight collection cups of the NGI were soaked into Tween® 80 ethanolic solution (1%) and placed under the fume hood until the complete evaporation of ethanol. The cups were placed into the apertures in the cup tray and the cup tray was located into the bottom frame and lowered into place. The impactor lid was closed with the sealed body attached and the handle was operated to lock the impactor together. Capsules were gathered after actuation for the study of remained powder. The content uniformity test was carried out for 10 mg of each formulation in 5 repetitions. The coefficient variation percentage (CV%) were less than 6% for all spray-dried powders. The batches that showed CV% above 6% were excluded from the study. The induction port was connected to the first stage of the NGI. The flow rate was calibrated using a flow meter (DFM 2000, Copley Scientific, Nottingham, UK) and fixed at 60 L/min. Fine particle fraction (FPF), mass median aerodynamic diameter (MMAD), and geometric standard deviation (GSD) indexes were calculated using the Copley Inhaler Testing Data Analysis Software (CITDAS, version 3.10). The MMAD is defined as the diameter at which 50% of the particles by mass are larger and 50% are smaller. FPF represents the percentage of emitted particles with an MMAD of 5 µm or less estimating the fraction of particles expected to deposit deep within the lungs. The emission was defined as the mass of drug delivered from the inhaler (i.e., total amount excluding the inhaler device and capsule), expressed as a percentage of the total amount of Itraconazole collected. Dispersibility was defined as the ratio of FPF per emission. Each value was expressed as the mean ± standard deviation.[25]

Chloroform as a solvent that can dissolve both SPC and Itraconazole was used as the washing solvent to rupture the transfersomes and extract Itraconazole. The whole process of washing was performed under the fume hood. The capsule shells, pre-separator, USP induction port and NGI stages were washed with suitable amount of chloroform. Chloroform containing extracted drug was moved into the test tubes. The test tubes were kept under nitrogen flow for complete removal of organic solvent. The tubes were filled with certain amount of acetonitrile, vortexed and sonicated for a few minutes to dissolve the extracted Itraconazole completely. 500 µl of acetonitrile was moved into the micro tubes and centrifuged at 13000 rpm for 10 minutes to separate the undissolved transfersome compositions and capsule residuals to yield a particle free solution suitable for HPLC analysis. After deposition onto the stages of the NGI, the mass deposited on each of the impactor pieces was collected and the total mass of drug was quantified by a validated HPLC system.

High performance liquid chromatography analysis

The Itraconazole content of each NGI stage was analyzed using a Knauer apparatus HPLC system (Germany) consisted of a model 1000 HPLC pump and a model 2600 tunable absorbance detector, with the following condition: Column: C-18 (150 × 4.6mm, 10 µm, 125 A°) (Germany) protected by a C-18 guard column, mobile phase: acetonitrile: water (90:10), flow rate: 1 mL/min, wave length: 263 nm and injection volume: 20 µl. The run time for Itraconazole appearance following the sample injection was approximately 3 min. The area under the curve (AUC) that demonstrates the Itraconazole concentration was calculated through the machine software (Chromgate® V3.3.1). An excess amount of sample was injected into the injector to make sure that the loop has been completely filled with the sample. Calibration curve was leaner in the range of 1.25 to 25 µg/mL (r^2=0.997).

Statistical analysis

Data are expressed as a mean value ± standard deviation (SD). Statistical analysis was performed using a one-way analysis of variance (ANOVA) with multiple comparisons between deposition data using a Tukey-Kramer HSD test by SPSS software (version 13.0, Chicago, IL, USA). A P value <0.05 was considered statistically significant.

Results

Preparation of Itraconazole-loaded nanotransfersomes

The effect of different kinds of surfactants and their concentration on the size of transfersomes are shown in Table 1. The size of blank transfersomes (T1 and T5) were smaller than drug-loaded transfersomes (T3 and T7) with the same compositions. Both drug free and drug-loaded transfersomes showed relatively narrow size distribution pattern (Figure 1). Although there are no statistically difference among the formulations composed of different type and amount of surfactants, formulations containing 10 mg of Span® 60 (T7) was selected for further experiments due to its lowest size and narrowest size distribution (Table 1). Results also showed that preparation of nanotransfersomal formulations with 10 mg of all types of surfactants resulted in the lowest size compared to using 5 and 15 mg of surfactant.

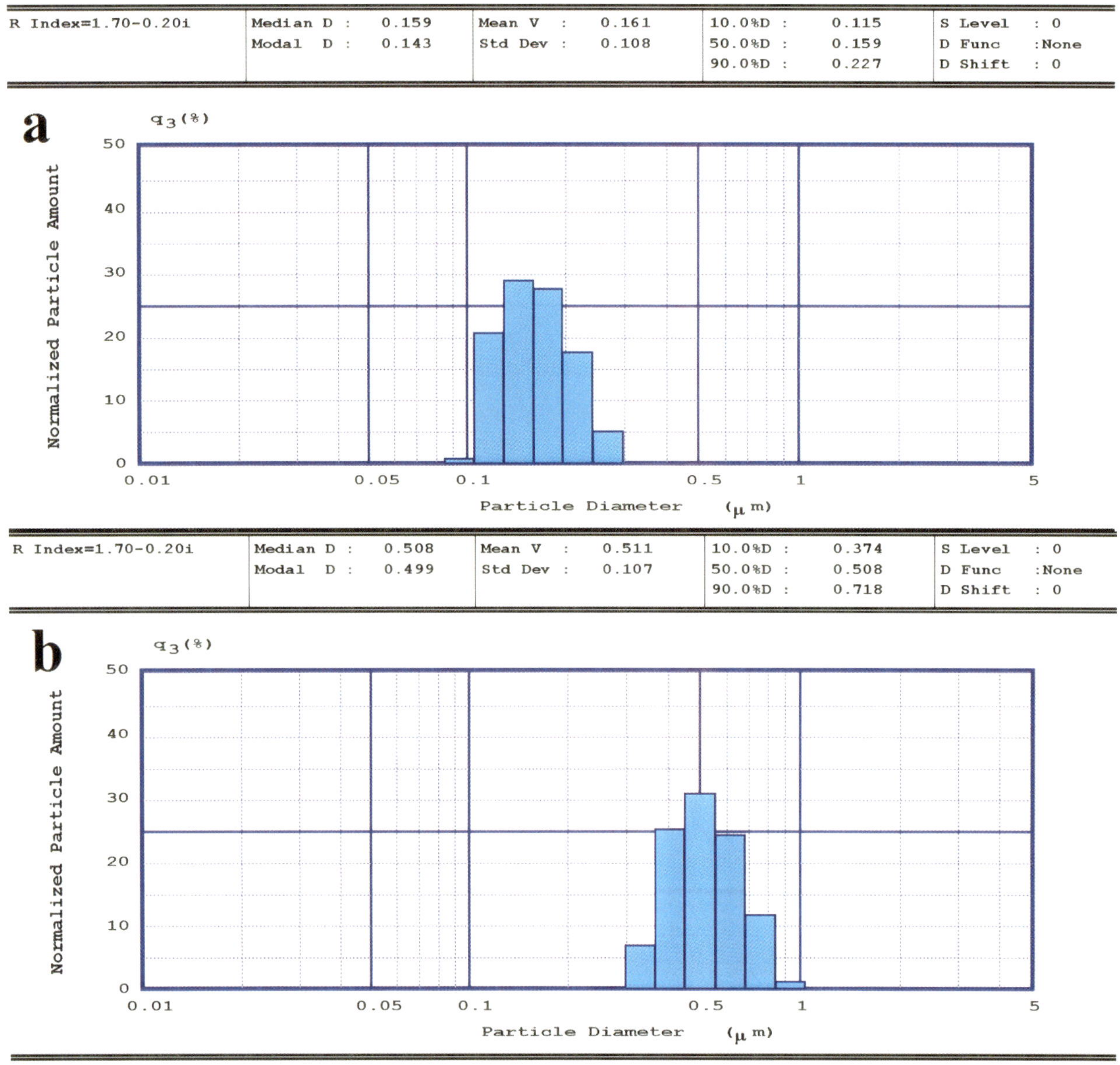

Figure 1. The size distribution pattern of a) drug free nanotransfersomes (T2) and b) drug loaded nanotransfersome (T7) formulations.

Preparation of DPI formulation

DPI formulations containing aggregated Itraconazol-loaded nanotransfersomes were prepared by various ratios of transfersomes to mannitol. The formulation F1 was not collected from the cyclone of the spray dryer and mostly adhered to the inner wall of heating chamber. It was reported that lecithin forms a viscous isotropic phase from 88 to 109 °C (the inlet temperature of spray dryer in our experiment) which may be responsible for the formulation adhesion to the spray dryer's chamber. The rest of the formulations with higher amounts of mannitol provided the suitable amounts of powder which were collected from the cyclone (yield value around 50 %) and assessed by NGI for determination of their aerosolization efficacy. Figures 2a and 2b show SEM images of the spray- dried particles (F2), confirmed the formation of aggregated nanoparticles in the suitable range for pulmonary drug delivery.

In vitro deposition

The amount of Itraconazole in each stage of NGI device was analyzed by HPLC method and illustrated in Figure 3. The in vitro parameters which were calculated according to the results of Figure 3 including FPF, MMAD and GSD are shown in Table 2. F2 showed the highest FPF and dispersibility, therefore, was selected as the optimized formulation. Although F4 had the best emission and GSD indicating its suitable flowability and aerodynamic size distribution, respectively, the main aerosolization indexes (FPF and dispersibility) are lower than other formulations.

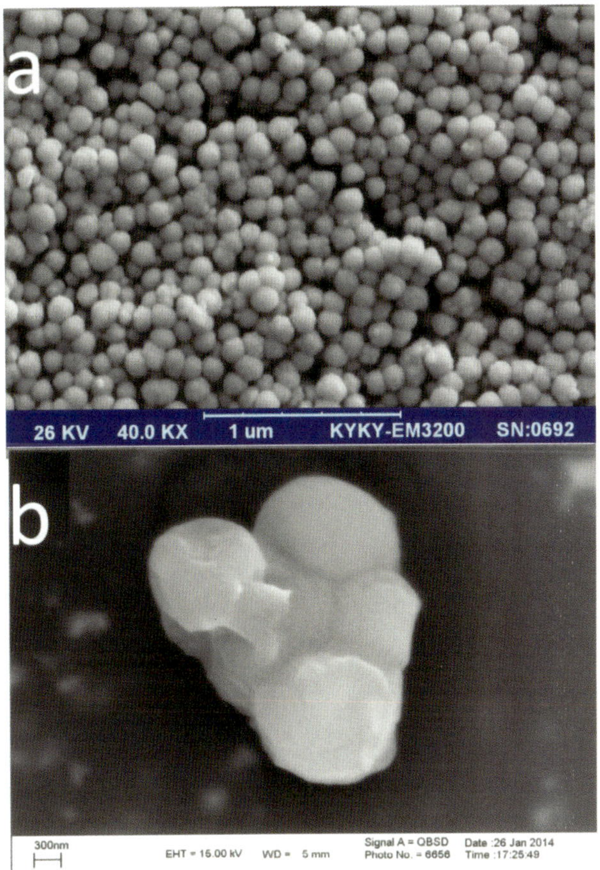

Figure 2. Scanning electron micrographs of a) Itraconazole-loaded nanotransfersomes (formulation T7) and b) those co-spray dried with mannitol (formulation F2).

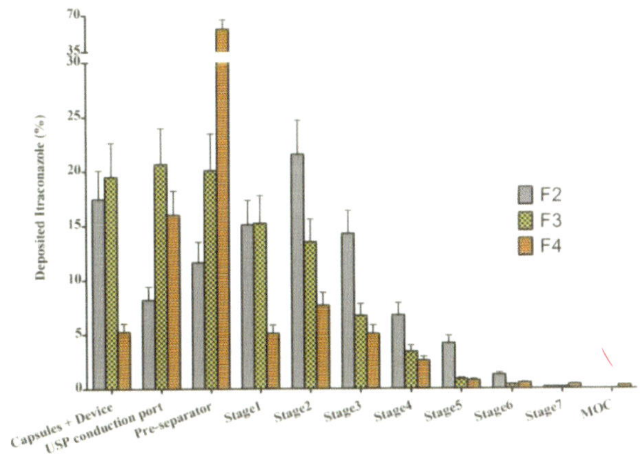

Figure 3. The percentage of Itraconazole from formulations F2, F3 and F4, deposited in various stages of NGI. Data was presented as mean ± standard deviation (n=3).

Table 2. Aerosolization efficiency indexes of selected Itraconazole-loaded nanotransfersomal dry powders measured by the NGI (mean ± SD, n= 3).

Parameters	[d]F2	F3	F4
[a]FPF (%)	37.3 ± 3.1	17.8 ± 2.9	10.4 ± 1.4
[b]MMAD (µm)	5.1 ± 0.7	6.5 ± 1	5.2 ± 0.9
[c]GSD	2.1 ± 0.2	2.1 ± 0.1	1.9 ± 0.1
Emission (%)	82.7 ± 2.6	80.5 ± 3.1	94.8 ± 0.8
Dispersibility	45.23 ± 2.9	22.11 ± 3.0	10.9 ± 1.1

[a] Fine Particle Fraction, [b] Mass Median Aerodynamic Diameter, [c] Geometric Standard Deviation, [d] F2, F3 and F4 were prepared by co-spray drying of 100 mg nanotransfersome and 200, 300 and 600 mg of mannitol, respectively

Discussion

Itraconazole is a poorly soluble drug that has displayed a low and variable oral absorption following oral administration. Absolute bioavailability of the oral Itraconazole capsule is 40% lower in the non-fed state compared to the fed state. To obtain a therapeutic level of drug at the site of lung infections, a high oral or intravenous dose must be administered which consequently increases the incidence of unwanted side effects associated with a high drug serum concentration.[26] In addition, gastrointestinal side effects have been reported in recipients of the oral solution up to 25% in a randomized trial and are the major reason for patient incompliance.[27] Local targeting of the drug at the usual site of infection (the lungs) means that less total drug may be required for dosing and therefore, the potential for side effects may be minimized due to a much reduced systemic concentration.[28] It has been reported that pulmonary delivery of nanoparticulate Itraconazole can achieve a significantly higher (more than 10-fold) lung tissue concentrations compared to conventional oral administration of Itraconazole. Effective and sustained lung tissue concentrations were achieved via inhalation of a nanoparticulate Itraconazole formulation.[29] Additionally, a targeted therapy may also initiate a quicker therapeutic onset and ultimately reduce the duration of treatment.[28] The utilization of lipidic vesicular systems for pulmonary drug delivery has many potential advantages over aerosol delivery of the corresponding nonencapsulated drug, including universal carrier suitability for most lipophilic drugs, compatibility and preventing local irritation of lung tissue, providing a pulmonary sustained release reservoir prolonging local and systemic therapeutic drug levels and facilitating intracellular drug delivery especially to alveolar macrophages, tumor cells or epithelial cells.[9] The present study explored a new idea for nanoparticle delivery to the lower respiratory regions of the lung using micrometer-sized carrier particles. In this investigation Itraconazole-loaded nanotransfersomes were incorporated as model drug delivery system by the lipid film hydration technique followed by sonication for size reduction. For the formulation of DPI, prepared nanotransfersomes should have a mean size below 5µm[30] to form inhalable carrier particles. This requirement was satisfied well when nanotransfersomes were co-spray dried with mannitol, a regularly used inert excipient in pulmonary drug delivery. The administered excipients (lecithin, mannitol, ursodiol, Span® 60 and Span® 80) were used because of their biocompatibility and pharmaceutical acceptability. The particle size of the transfersomes with different types of surfactant did not show a significant difference. These results indicate that the particle size of the vesicles was not significantly affected by the type of surfactant.[31] Spray drying is a low-cost, one-step pharmaceutical process that is widely used in the development of novel dry powder formulations.[3] Spray drying technique offers a number of potential advantages over lyophilization technique. Spray drying technique was utilized for stabilization of nanoliposomes and development of uniform sized particles with desired aerosolization properties for pulmonary administration to overcome constraints associated with lyophilization technique, such as formation of hard cake, need of micronization, addition of coarse carriers for aersolization, and heterogeneous size distribution pattern.[32] Once the nanotransfersome aggregates, with their large surface area, in the dry powder formulation is deposited in the aqueous lining fluid in the lung, the mannitol may quickly dissolve, resulting in the dispersion of nanotransfersomes in the respiratory tract fluids.[33] Carriers form the backbone structure of the solid particles during the spray drying process and facilitate pulmonary delivery.[32] The carrier of choice for DPI products is currently lactose monohydrate and almost all DPI products already in market are using lactose as a carrier. The advantages of lactose monohydrate are its well-investigated toxicity profile, its broad availability and its relatively low price.[19] However, it has some disadvantages that should be considered in its usage as carrier for DPIs. Lactose is incompatible with some drugs and compounds with a primary amine group. Lactose may develop a yellow brown color with browning aging that is accelerated by the process of spray drying. Lactose monohydrate is produced from bovine or with bovine-driven additives so that the Transmissible Spongiform Encephalopathy (TSE) discussion is still an issue for this compound. In addition, Lactose intolerance is a situation that requires a solution. For overcoming the above mentioned drawbacks of lactose, mannitol is a suitable substitute carrier that possesses further positive aspects.[20] For these reasons, mannitol was chosen as an excipient for co-spray drying with nanotransfersomes. Once the nanotransfersomes aggregate, with their large surface area, in the dry powder formulation is deposited in the aqueous lining fluid in the lung, the mannitol may quickly dissolve, resulting in the dispersion of nanotransfersomes in the respiratory tract fluids.[33] Due to the flexibility in use and high productivity, NGIs (a new impactor type specifically designed for testing pharmaceutical inhalers using the very newest and modern designed theory in 1997) have been used as the most popular testing machine within many inhaler research laboratories. NGI was launched in 2000 and was subsequently accepted into the European Pharmacopeia as Apparatus E and into the United States Pharmacopeia as Apparatus 5 and 6 in 2005. The ideal size for a therapeutic particle is not known exactly but it may be assumed that the MMAD should be not more than 5 μm to pass into the tracheobronchial tree and smaller airways if peripheral deposition is required.[34] Formulation F2 exhibited an MMAD of 5.1 ± 0.7 μm, and a higher FPF in comparison to the other formulations. In this study, it was shown that increase in mannitol ratio in the spray dried formulations caused a decrease in aerosolization efficiency (Table 2). Maximum FPF of 37.35 ± 3.1% was observed in formulation F2 containing 200 mg of mannitol as compared with F3 (300 mg of mannitol) of 17.8 ± 2.9% and F4 (600 mg of mannitol) of 10.4 ± 1.4%. Previous studies have indicated that increasing the lipid concentration in the spray drying feeds can decrease the residual water content in the powder[35] which consequently may improve the aerodynamic properties of the DPI formulation. Higher ratios of mannitol improved emission of formulation F4 which may be attributed to the powder flowability improvement by addition of carrier. The findings of this investigation showed that dry powder inhalation formulation of Itraconazole-loaded nanotransfersomes prepared by co-spray drying with mannitol possessed suitable aerosolization performance. Therefore, this formulation may have a potential to deliver Itraconazole to the site of infection in the lungs in the pulmonary aspergillosis. The results highlight the need to examine the enhanced *in vivo* therapeutic effects of pulmonary drug delivery via nanotransfersomal DPI formulations. The results of this study was introduced the potential application of nanotransfersomes in the formulation of DPIs for lung delivery of various drugs.

Acknowledgments
This paper was extracted from Pharm.D. thesis No. 3662 that was submitted to the Faculty of Pharmacy of Tabriz University of Medical Sciences and financially supported by grant No. 90/92 from the Drug Applied Research Center of the same university.

Ethical Issues
Not applicable.

Conflict of Interest
The authors report no conflicts of interest.

References

1. Hong JY, Kim JK, Song YK, Park JS, Kim CK. A new self-emulsifying formulation of itraconazole with improved dissolution and oral absorption. *J Control Release* 2006;110(2):332-8. doi: 10.1016/j.jconrel.2005.10.002
2. Lu D, Hickey AJ. Liposomal dry powders as aerosols for pulmonary delivery of proteins. *AAPS PharmSciTech* 2005;6(4):E641-8. doi: 10.1208/pt060480
3. Sung JC, Pulliam BL, Edwards DA. Nanoparticles for drug delivery to the lungs. *Trends Biotechnol* 2007;25(12):563-70. doi: 10.1016/j.tibtech.2007.09.005
4. Ugwoke MI, Vereyken IJ, Luessen H. Microparticles and liposomes as pulmonary drug delivery systems: What are the recent trends? *Chapter VI* 2007:308-77.
5. Emami J, Hamishehkar H, Najafabadi AR, Gilani K, Minaiyan M, Mahdavi H, et al. Particle size design of plga microspheres for potential pulmonary drug delivery using response surface methodology. *J Microencapsul* 2009;26(1):1-8. doi: 10.1080/02652040802083900

6. Emami J, Hamishehkar H, Najafabadi AR, Gilani K, Minaiyan M, Mahdavi H, et al. A novel approach to prepare insulin-loaded poly(lactic-co-glycolic acid) microcapsules and the protein stability study. *J Pharm Sci* 2009;98(5):1712-31. doi: 10.1002/jps.21544
7. Gaspar MM, Bakowsky U, Ehrhardt C. Inhaled liposomes–current strategies and future challenges. *J Biomed Nanotechnol* 2008;4(3):245-57. doi: 10.1166/jbn.2008.334
8. Kaur IP, Agrawal R. Nanotechnology: A new paradigm in cosmeceuticals. *Recent Pat Drug Deliv Formul* 2007;1(2):171-82.
9. Chougule M, Padhi B, Misra A. Development of spray dried liposomal dry powder inhaler of dapsone. *AAPS PharmSciTech* 2008;9(1):47-53. doi: 10.1208/s12249-007-9024-6
10. Elsayed MM, Abdallah OY, Naggar VF, Khalafallah NM. Lipid vesicles for skin delivery of drugs: Reviewing three decades of research. *Int J Pharm* 2007;332(1-2):1-16. doi: 10.1016/j.ijpharm.2006.12.005
11. Singh D. Ultradeformable system: A carrier for transdermal drug delivery. *Int J Pharm Sci Res* 2013;4(11):98-104.
12. Ghanbarzadeh S, Arami S. Formulation and evaluation of piroxicam transferosomal gel: An approach for penetration enhancement. *J Drug Deliv Sci Technol* 2013;23(6):587-90. doi: 10.1016/S1773-2247(13)50089-X
13. Gharsallaoui A, Roudaut G, Chambin O, Voilley A, Saurel R. Applications of spray-drying in microencapsulation of food ingredients: An overview. *Food Res Int* 2007;40(9):1107-21. doi: 10.1016/j.foodres.2007.07.004
14. Ghanbarzadeh S, Valizadeh H, Zakeri-Milani P. Sirolimus nano liposomes. *Pharm Ind* 2013;75(8).
15. Ghanbarzadeh S, Khorrami A, Arami S. Nonionic surfactant-based vesicular system for transdermal drug delivery. *Drug Deliv* 2015;22(8):1071-7. doi: 10.3109/10717544.2013.873837
16. Faramarzi P, Haririan I, Ghanbarzadeh S, Yaqoubi S, Hamishehkar H. Development of carrier free montelukast dry powder inhalation formulation. *Pharm Ind* 2015;77(10):1535-42.
17. Rojanarat W, Changsan N, Tawithong E, Pinsuwan S, Chan HK, Srichana T. Isoniazid proliposome powders for inhalation-preparation, characterization and cell culture studies. *Int J Mol Sci* 2011;12(7):4414-34. doi: 10.3390/ijms12074414
18. Rahimpour Y, Hamishehkar H. Lactose engineering for better performance in dry powder inhalers. *Adv Pharm Bull* 2012;2(2):183-7. doi: 10.5681/apb.2012.028
19. Hamishehkar H, Emami J, Najafabadi AR, Gilani K, Minaiyan M, Mahdavi H, et al. Influence of carrier particle size, carrier ratio and addition of fine ternary particles on the dry powder inhalation performance of insulin-loaded plga microcapsules. *Powder Technol* 2010;201(3):289-95. doi:10.1016/j.powtec.2010.04.017
20. Hamishehkar H, Emami J, Najafabadi AR, Gilani K, Minaiyan M, Mahdavi H, et al. Effect of carrier morphology and surface characteristics on the development of respirable plga microcapsules for sustained-release pulmonary delivery of insulin. *Int J Pharm* 2010;389(1-2):74-85. doi: 10.1016/j.ijpharm.2010.01.021
21. Ghanbarzadeh S, Valizadeh H, Zakeri-Milani P. The effects of lyophilization on the physico-chemical stability of sirolimus liposomes. *Adv Pharm Bull* 2013;3(1):25-9. doi: 10.5681/apb.2013.005
22. Ghaderi S, Ghanbarzadeh S, Mohammadhassani Z, Hamishehkar H. Formulation of gammaoryzanol-loaded nanoparticles for potential application in fortifying food products. *Adv Pharm Bull* 2014;4(Suppl 2):549-54. doi: 10.5681/apb.2014.081
23. Hamishehkar H, Shokri J, Fallahi S, Jahangiri A, Ghanbarzadeh S, Kouhsoltani M. Histopathological evaluation of caffeine-loaded solid lipid nanoparticles in efficient treatment of cellulite. *Drug Dev Ind Pharm* 2015;41(10):1640-6. doi: 10.3109/03639045.2014.980426
24. United States Pharmacopeia 35/National Formulary 30. Rockville, MD, USA: United States Pharmacopeial Convention; 2015.
25. Yazdani A, Normandie M, Yousefi M, Saidi MS, Ahmadi G. Transport and deposition of pharmaceutical particles in three commercial spacer-mdi combinations. *Comput Biol Med* 2014;54:145-55. doi: 10.1016/j.compbiomed.2014.08.001
26. De Beule K. Itraconazole: Pharmacology, clinical experience and future development. *Int J Antimicrob Agents* 1996;6(3):175-81.
27. Alvarez CA, Wiederhold NP, McConville JT, Peters JI, Najvar LK, Graybill JR, et al. Aerosolized nanostructured itraconazole as prophylaxis against invasive pulmonary aspergillosis. *J Infect* 2007;55(1):68-74. doi: 10.1016/j.jinf.2007.01.014
28. McConville JT, Overhoff KA, Sinswat P, Vaughn JM, Frei BL, Burgess DS, et al. Targeted high lung concentrations of itraconazole using nebulized dispersions in a murine model. *Pharm Res* 2006;23(5):901-11. doi: 10.1007/s11095-006-9904-6
29. Vaughn JM, McConville JT, Burgess D, Peters JI, Johnston KP, Talbert RL, et al. Single dose and multiple dose studies of itraconazole nanoparticles. *Eur J Pharm Biopharm* 2006;63(2):95-102. doi: 10.1016/j.ejpb.2006.01.006
30. Joshi M, Misra A. Dry powder inhalation of liposomal ketotifen fumarate: Formulation and characterization. *Int J Pharm* 2001;223(1-2):15-27.
31. Duangjit S, Opanasopit P, Rojanarata T, Ngawhirunpat T. Characterization and in vitro skin permeation of meloxicam-loaded liposomes versus transfersomes. *J Drug Deliv* 2011;2011:418316. doi: 10.1155/2011/418316

32. Chougule M, Padhi B, Misra A. Nano-liposomal dry powder inhaler of tacrolimus: Preparation, characterization, and pulmonary pharmacokinetics. *Int J Nanomedicine* 2007;2(4):675-88.
33. Yang W, Tam J, Miller DA, Zhou J, McConville JT, Johnston KP, et al. High bioavailability from nebulized itraconazole nanoparticle dispersions with biocompatible stabilizers. *Int J Pharm* 2008;361(1-2):177-88. doi: 10.1016/j.ijpharm.2008.05.003
34. Newman SP, Clarke SW. Therapeutic aerosols 1--physical and practical considerations. *Thorax* 1983;38(12):881-6.
35. Rowe RC, Sheskey PJ, Owen SC, editors. Pharmaceutical Press and American Pharmacists Association. Handbook of pharmaceutical excipients. 4th ed. London: Pharmaceutical Press; 2006.

Studying the Effect of Sertraline in Reducing Aggressive Behavior in Patients with Major Depression

Alireza Farnam, Arezoo MehrAra*, Hossein Dadashzadeh, Golamreza Chalabianlou, Salman Safikhanlou

Research Center of Psychiatry and Behavioral Sciences, Razi Hospital, Tabriz University of Medical Sciences, Tabriz, Iran.

Keywords:
- Depression
- Aggression
- Sertraline
- STAXI-II

Abstract

Purpose: Depression causes dysfunction in various spheres of individual and social life, which is now considered as the fourth-leading cause of the global disease burden. Given that violence and aggression associated with depression in the community cause serious damage to the family, the prediction, early detection and effective treatment of aggressive and violent behavior are essential. The present study compared the severity of aggression before and after treatment with sertraline in patients with major depression.

Methods: This is an intervention type study and the study population consisted of patients with depression and aggression. The sampling included 23 eligible patients. Data were obtained by SCID-I, SCID-II, STAXI-II, BDI-II and was also analyzed using SPSS 23 software.

Results: The results showed that depression, anger mood, desire to verbally express anger, controlling anger and anger control before treatment was reduced but the desire for physical expression of anger increased.

Conclusion: Obtained results in this research support the effect of Sertraline on reduction of severity of depression, reduction of severity of symptoms of aggression and anger (state of anger, anger feeling, and the tendency to express anger verbally), increased controlling external anger and significantly controlling internal anger. Hence, Sertraline can be found effective in the treatment of patients with depression and aggressive behaviors. Also Sertraline increases tend to cause physical representation of anger, then this issue supports the increase in the euthanasia behavior in primary days of treatment with SSRI that requires more assessments.

Introduction

Mental disorder is an illness with psychological and behavioral protests which cause considerable confusion in the different functional areas and is developed as a result of biological, social, psychological, genetic, physical or chemical disorders. According to the revised version of the fourth edition of the Diagnostic and Statistical book of DSM-IV-TR, mental disorders contain 17 main categories (children's disorders, mood etc) and 375 disorders (major depression and schizophrenia etc.).[1]

It can be said that mental disorders are the greatest public health problems of the current era, such that depression has exceeded forecasts and has become the biggest cause of the disease.[2]

Depression occurs in about one of five women and one in ten men in a lifetime.[3]

In addition to the problems caused by depression, there is an idea that aggression plays a major role in depression development which has been fused in psychiatric thinking composition.[4]

Emotion and aggressive behavior is a common element of a whole hypersensitivity in response to any threat and tend to attack.[5]

Emotion and aggressive behaviors include a spectrum such that their common elements are hypersensitivity in response to any threat and tend to attack. In the mildest case, the spectrum starts with hypersensitivity and the increasing severity of the threats, verbal intimidation, physical violence and bullying is also followed by murder in the other side of the spectrum and sometimes lead to violence and sadism.[5]

Aggressive and violent behaviors are usually observed as symptoms of many psychiatric diseases. For example, violence has been seen in patients with substance abuse, personality disorders as well as mood and anxiety disorders.[6]

One of the most important adverse effects of violence and aggression in society is harm to families. Depending on what was noted, prediction, early detection and effective treatment of aggressive and violent behavior are essential. The first step in this direction is recognition of the nature, causes, symptoms and phenomena associated with aggression and violence.

In the conducted studies, the probability of domestic violence against women in Canada was 51% and the prevalence of purely physical violence against women in various cities is estimated between 2.7 to 18.6%.[7-9]

According to Fava and Rosenbaum (1998), anger, hostility and irritability are generally observed in patients

***Corresponding author:** Arezoo MehrAra, Email: safikhanlous@tbzmed.ac.ir with depressive disorder. Almost 1/5 (one fifth) of outpatient depressed patients are referred with symptoms of attack. Anger periods are usually associated with activation of the autonomic systems such as tachycardia, sweating, hot flash and compression of the chest. Depressed patients are considerably anxious and exhibit hostile rage with anger attacks than non-depressed and are more likely to have refrained criteria, dependent, narcissistic or antisocial and borderline personality disorder. In several studies, it was suggested that anger attacks significantly decrease with anti-depressant treatment. Anger attacks in 53 to 71% of outpatient depression treated with anti-depressants such as Fluoxetine, sertraline and imipramine disappeared. Moreover, the amount of anger attacks after treatment with Fluoxetine (7 to 6%) have no difference with the observed data after treatment with sertraline (8%) and imipramine (10%) and these values are less than the incidence associated with placebo (20%). Finally, since the serotonergic neurotransmitter system is involved in the regulation of aggressive behavior in humans and animals, it can be assumed that anti-depressants affective on this system can be effective in depressed patients with dramatic aggression.[10] In their previous study, Mezza et al. revealed the reduction of HR and HRV which confirms vagal activity in aggressive patients.[11] In one study, it was found that there is a relationship between decrease in DBP, SBP and HR and increase in the aggressive behavior of preschool children.[12] It was also found that SCL was higher in patients with a greater score of aggression, also anger triggers driving under the influence at the time of placement.[12]

In another study in 2013, Baker et al. concluded that reduction of skin conductance activity (SCA) in babies predict aggressive behavior at 3 years of age.[13] Dibajnia and Moghadasin reported that numerous studies show the association between experience and expression of anger, depression, anxiety and stress.[14] Researchers also reported that based on Pearson correlation coefficient and stepwise regression analysis of previous results the state of anger, trait of anger and internalized anger expression are the best predictors of depression. The scale of internal rage mood and anger expression respectively is the best predictor for anxiety and Trait Anger Scale, inner expression of anger and rage mode are also the best predictors of stress.[14]

Few studies have been conducted on aggression but according to their results, in an acceptable rate it can be concluded that low excitation of the autonomic nervous system is a biomarker of aggression.

Materials and Methods

This study is an interventional type with a population of depressed patients having aggressive behaviors, referred to psychiatric clinics affiliated with the University of Medical Sciences during 2015 to 2016. The method used was simple random sampling and it included 23 samples.

Inclusion criteria

This includes the following:

1) Diagnosis of depression with any degree and severity was based on the clinical evaluation of specialists and structured interviews based on the DSM-IV-TR criteria as well as the Beck and SCID questionnaires.[15-17]

2) Patients in the first period of depression or who previously did not receive any anti-depressant drug treatment.

3) The presence of a history of aggressive behaviors or physical examination was based on Trait Anger Expression Inventory (Anger scale score of 8 to 32).

4) Patients tend to use higher quality drugs, albeit with a higher cost.

5) Drug therapy using a Selective Serotonin Reuptake Inhibitor (SSRI) Asentra film-coated tablets (ACTOVERCO Pharmaceutical factory, Karaj, Iran, under license of KAKA, Slovenia) which started with a dose of 50 mg daily which increased to a dose of 100 mg daily later.

6) Having Iranian nation.

7) The age range of 20 to 40 years (due to the continuing development of CNS up to about 19 years old).

8) Patient agreement to participate in the study by signing an informed consent.

Exclusion criteria

1) The existence of any current psychiatric disease or a history of depression exception.
2) The use of any drugs affecting the CNS or PNS other than anti-depressants.
3) The existence of any of these diseases: amyloidosis, acute porphyria, cardiovascular diseases, respiratory, endocrine, nervous system, malnutrition, abuse of alcohol and drugs, multiple sclerosis, amyotrophic lateral sclerosis (ALS) and other diseases such as primary and secondary autonomic conflict.
4) Pre-menstruation period for women.
5) The history of these diseases were also considered in patients and in the case of strong suspicion of a genetic or environmental predisposition, the patient was not enrolled.
6) It is noteworthy that during studying each individual who had lost one of the conditions and criteria or has one of the criteria or for whatever reason is not willing to continue to participate in the study or becomes unavailable is excluded and their data were not used in the statistical analysis.

Results

The average age of participants was 33.91 with a standard deviation of 14.8 and the minimum and maximum ages of 21 and 40 years respectively. Mean age was 34.63 years with a standard deviation of 8.06 and the average age of men was 30.50 years old with a standard deviation of 8.81.

Among the age ranges of women and men, the difference was not significant (F=0.30, T=0.87, Df=4.13, P=0.44). As well as between women and men

in terms of education, the difference was not significant (Chi-Sq=3.69, Df=1, P=0.06).
Table 1 shows the severity of depression before and after the drug treatment such that the severity of symptoms was reduced.

Table 1. Paired t-test for assessing changes in depression symptoms after treatment as compared to before treatment.

Variable	Stage	Average	SD	t	P-Value
Beck depression	Before treatment	25.32	10.20	3.34	0.003
	After treatment	18.39	10.22		

Additionally, classification of the patients in terms of severity of depression before and after treatment using sertraline was demonstrated in Table 2.

Table 2. Severity of depression symptoms in treatment stages, according to Beck.

-	Before treatment		After treatment	
Depression level	Number	%	Number	%
Normal	0	0	6	26.1
Slight	8	34.8	9	39.1
Mild	6	26.1	4	17.4
Severe	9	39.1	4	17.4

According to Table 2, depression severity after starting sertraline decreased significantly such that from 23 patients, 6 patients reported themselves with no depression symptom and others were also adjusted from extreme level to mid-level and upper-middle class moderate to mild level. The Wilcoxon test at 0.02 levels was significantly achieved and represented the loss of these symptoms and severity of depression.
Results of Table 3 showed the state of anger, feelings of anger, a desire to verbally express anger, control anger and internal anger control before starting the drug and after that was significant so that the severity of symptoms are reduced and anger control is also increased.

Table 3. Paired t-test for the difference between variables Trait Anger before and after the treatment of depression.

Variable	Stage	Average	SD	t	P- Value
Anger state	Before treatment	34.65	10.83	3.32	0.003
	After treatment	26.04	10.10		
Anger feeling	Before treatment	14	3.45	4.18	000
	After treatment	10.61	3.33		
Tend to represent verbal anger	Before treatment	12.30	4.73	3.01	0.01
	After treatment	8.78	4.13		
Anger trait	Before treatment	28	5.62	0.96	0.35 NS
	After treatment	26.65	5.74		
Aggressive behavior	Before treatment	11.09	3.80	1.53	0.14 NS
	After treatment	10.22	3.23		
Aggressive reaction	Before treatment	16.91	3.30	0.52	0.61 NS
	After treatment	16.43	3.69		
Presence of external anger	Before treatment	19.65	5.06	1.55	0.14 NS
	After treatment	18	4.95		
The presence of internal anger	Before treatment	20.74	3.29	1.17	0.25 NS
	After treatment	19.61	3.60		
Control on external anger	Before treatment	17.30	4.19	-4.44	000
	After treatment	21.87	4.51		
Control on internal anger	Before treatment	16.26	4.66	-4.06	0.001
	After treatment	21.70	4.88		

Since the variable, tendency to represent anger physically in the Kolmogorov- Smirnov test was significant and had no normal distribution, the Wilcoxon test was used. Results of Table 4 revealed that the tendency to represent anger physically in order to increase scores before starting the drug and after that was significant. It can be interpreted that although Sertraline reduced verbal anger representation effectively, it also increased the willingness to represent anger physically.

On the other hand, there was a significant positive correlation between anger state, anger trait, aggressive behavior, aggressive feeling, tend to represent anger verbally, and aggressive reaction.
Results of the multivariable regression in Table 4 demonstrated that aggressive feeling with correlation coefficient of R=0.43 and determination coefficient of R^2=0.18 predicts that about %14 of the changes is related to the severity of symptoms of depression.

Table 4. Wilcoxon test for studying before- and after- test variable tending to represent anger physically.

Model	Entered variables	Multidimensional correlation coefficient	Determination coefficient of R^2	Adjusted R	Scale error	Beta standard	t	Significance level
1	Aggressive feeling	0.43	0.18	0.14	9.48	0.43	2.16	0.04

Discussion

Our research confirmed the study of Fava and Rosenbum (1998) who concluded that Sertraline was effective in the reduction of aggressive attacks and controlling the anger and increased it significantly.[10]

On the other hand, according to Dibajnia and Moghadasian[14] and Khakbaz et al[15] a significant relationship between depression and aggression was observed.

Similar to the research of Fan et al.,[16] our study also emphasized that Sertraline led to a reduction of depression symptoms and also anger after 8 weeks of treatment.

Strik and et al. [17] in their study concluded that Fluoxetine was effective in reducing the symptoms of depression and anger in patients with severe depression and we also found the same results using Sertraline.

Dibajnia and Moghadasian[14] in their study reported anger state, internal anger expression and anger trait as the best predictors of depression and our study also revealed that anger feeling could predict 14% of depression.

Conclusion

Obtained results in this research support the effect of Sertraline on reduction of severity of depression, reduction of severity of symptoms of aggression and anger (state of anger, anger feeling, and the tendency to express anger verbally), increased control of external anger and significantly increased control of internal anger. Hence, Sertraline can be found effective in the treatment of patients with depression and aggressive behaviors.

According to analysis, Sertraline increases tend to cause physical representation of anger, then this issue supports the increase in the euthanasia behavior in primary days of treatment with SSRI that requires more assessments.

Limitations of the study include small sample size and short period of treatment.

Acknowledgments

All participants and subjects who helped in the collection and codification of this article are acknowledged.

Ethical Issues

Not applicable.

Conflict of Interest

The authors declare no conflict of interests.

References

1. Sadock BJ, Sadock VA. Kaplan and Sadock's Pocket Handbook of Clinical Psychiatry. 5th ed. Tehran: Teimourzadeh publication; 2010.
2. Wittchen HU, Jacobi F, Rehm J, Gustavsson A, Svensson M, Jonsson B, et al. The size and burden of mental disorders and other disorders of the brain in europe 2010. *Eur Neuropsychopharmacol* 2011;21(9):655-79. doi: 10.1016/j.euroneuro.2011.07.018
3. Desai HD, Jann MW. Major depression in women: A review of the literature. *J Am Pharm Assoc (Wash)* 2000;40(4):525-37.
4. Kendell RE. Relationship between aggression and depression. Epidemiological implications of a hypothesis. *Arch Gen Psychiatry* 1970;22(4):308-18.
5. Sadock BJ, Sadock VA. Kaplan & Sadock's Comprehensive Textbook of Psychiatry. 9th ed. Tehran: Teimourzadeh publication; 2009.
6. Harford TC, Yi HY, Grant BF. Other- and self-directed forms of violence and their relationships to dsm-iv substance use and other psychiatric disorders in a national survey of adults. *Compr Psychiatry* 2013;54(7):731-9. doi: 10.1016/j.comppsych.2013.02.003
7. Nouhjah S, Latifi SM. Variation in the prevalence of domestic violence between neighboring areas. *Int Sch Res Notices* 2014;2014:721951. doi: 10.1155/2014/721951
8. Bodaghabadi M. Prevalence of violence and related factors in pregnant women referring to Shahid Mobini hospital of Sabzevar. *Med J Hormozgan Univ* 2007;11(1):71-6.
9. Saberian M, Atash Nafas E, Behnam B. Prevalence of domestic violence in women referred to the heath care centers in Semnan (2003). *Koomesh* 2005; 6(2):115-22.
10. Fava M, Rosenbaum JF. Anger attacks in patients with depression. *J Clin Psychiatry* 1999;60 Suppl 15:21-4.
11. Mezzacappa E, Tremblay RE, Kindlon D, Saul JP, Arseneault L, Pihl RO, et al. Relationship of aggression and anxiety to autonomic regulation of heart rate variability in adolescent males. *Ann N Y Acad Sci* 1996;794:376-9.
12. Choi MH, Lee SJ, Yang JW, Kim JH, Choi JS, Kim HS, et al. An analysis of the correlation between young males' personal aggression and their skin conductance levels during exposure to aggression images. *Psychiatry Res* 2011;186(2-3):441-2. doi: 10.1016/j.psychres.2010.08.035
13. Baker E, Shelton KH, Baibazarova E, Hay DF, van Goozen SH. Low skin conductance activity in infancy predicts aggression in toddlers 2 years later. *Psychol Sci* 2013;24(6):1051-6. doi: 10.1177/0956797612465198

14. Dibajnia P, Moghaddasin M. Evaluation of the correlation between constructs state-trait anger expression inventory-2 (STAXI-2) and depression anxiety and stress scales (DASS), predicting psychological constructs DASS based on STAXI-2. *Pajoohandeh J 2012;* 16(7):339-46.
15. Khakbaz H, Karami H, Shafi'e-Abadi A, Malmir M, Farhadi MH. The Relationship between depression, anxiety, stress and aggression in patients with drug dependence. *Rehabil J 2014;* 14(S1):15-20
16. Fann JR, Uomoto JM, Katon WJ. Sertraline in the treatment of major depression following mild traumatic brain injury. *J Neuropsychiatry Clin Neurosci* 2000;12(2):226-32. doi: 10.1176/jnp.12.2.226
17. Strik JJ, Honig A, Lousberg R, Lousberg AH, Cheriex EC, Tuynman-Qua HG, et al. Efficacy and safety of fluoxetine in the treatment of patients with major depression after first myocardial infarction: Findings from a double-blind, placebo-controlled trial. *Psychosom Med* 2000;62(6):783-9.

Comparative Evaluation of Dexmedetomidine and Magnesium Sulphate on Propofol Consumption, Haemodynamics and Postoperative Recovery in Spine Surgery

Vinit K. Srivastava[1]*, Abhishek Mishra[1], Sanjay Agrawal[2], Sanjay Kumar[3], Sunil Sharma[1], Raj Kumar[1]

[1] *Apollo Hospitals Bilaspur, Chhattisgarh, India.*
[2] *Himalayan Institute of Medical Sciences, Dehradun, India.*
[3] *Sanjay Gandhi Postgraduate Institute of Medical Sciences, Lucknow, India.*

Keywords:
- Dexmedetomidine
- Magnesium sulfate
- Hemodynamics
- Spine surgery

Abstract

Purpose: Dexmedetomidine and magnesium sulfate have been used in anesthesia as adjuvant to provide hemodynamic stability and anesthetic agents sparing effect. We compared these effects of dexmedetomidine and magnesium sulfate in spine surgeries.

Methods: Ninety patients were randomly assigned to three groups. Group D received dexmedetomidine loading dose 1 μg/kg over a period of 15 minutes and maintenance 0.5 μg/kg/h throughout the surgery. Group M received magnesium sulfate loading dose 50 mg/kg over a period of 15 minutes and maintenance 15 mg/kg/h throughout the surgery. Group C received same volume of normal saline. Heart rate (HR) and blood pressure values were recorded at various intervals. The induction and maintenance doses of anesthetics and recovery parameters were also recorded.

Results: Heart rate in group D and group M were significantly decreased ($p<0.05$) during the whole intraoperative period compared to preoperative values. There was a significant difference in HR values between group C, D and M, during the whole intraoperaive period ($p<0.05$). Blood pressure values were statistically significantly lower in the group D and group M compared to group C after intubation and all time observations of surgery ($p<0.05$). Both drugs reduced the anesthetic agent's requirement during surgery. However, the recovery parameters were statistically significant increase with magnesium sulphate compared to dexmedetomidine and control groups.

Conclusion: Dexmedetomidine is more effective than magnesium sulfate for maintaining the hemodynamic stability in spine surgeries. Both these drugs also reduce the requirements of anesthetic agents. Recovery from dexmedetomidine is as rapid as control group compared to magnesium sulfate.

Introduction

Spine surgery poses challenges to anesthesiologists due to its specific needs of stable hemodynamics, relatively dry operative field, the need for intraoperative somatosensory or motor evoked potential as well as perioperative position. These factors warrant the use of medications to maintain adequate depth of anesthesia as well as specific need of the surgery.

The use of perioperative magnesium sulfate,[1,2] dexmedetomidine,[3,4] beta blocker (esmolol),[5] opioids,[6] gabapentin, pregabalin,[7] and clonidine[8] have been reported to provide beneficial effects during general anesthesia, however with varying success rate.

Magnesium sulfate ($MgSO_4$) is a non-competitive N-methyl- D-aspartate (NMDA) receptor antagonist with antinociceptive effects.[9,10] Numerous clinical investigations have demonstrated that Mg infusion during general anesthesia reduced anesthetic requirement and postoperative analgesic consumption.[1,2]

Perioperative use of alpha-2 adrenoceptor agonists decreases sympathetic tone, attenuates the stress responses to anesthesia and surgery, sedation and postoperative analgesia. Dexmedetomidine is a highly specific alpha-2 adrenergic receptor agonist.

Few studies in the literature demonstrate the effectiveness of dexmedetomidine and magnesium sulfate individually for providing intraoperative hemodynamic stability, decrease anesthetic requirements and improved postoperative recovery in general anesthesia.[1,2,3,4] This present prospective, randomized, placebo-controlled, double blind study was designed to evaluate and compare the pharmacological effects of the use of dexmedetomidine and magnesium sulfate on propofol consumption, hemodynamics and postoperative

***Corresponding author:** Vinit K. Srivastava, Email: drvinit_srivastava@apollohospitals.com recovery in patients undergoing spine surgery under general anesthesia.

Materials and Methods

This prospective, randomized, placebo-controlled study was conducted after approval from the Institutional Ethics Committee and written informed consent from the patients. The study was registered at Clinical Trials.gov www.ctri.nic.in (ref: CTRI/2013/08/003939).

A total of 106 patients 20-60 years of age, ASA physical status I or II, of either sex, and scheduled for elective spine surgery under general anesthesia were included in this study. Patients with a history of preoperative neuromuscular disease, hepatic, renal, endocrinal, hematological disorder or cardiovascular dysfunction, any degree of heart block, BMI>30 kg/m^2, patients receiving magnesium supplementation, drugs known to have a significant interaction with NMDAs, chronic use of opioids and current treatment with a β-blocker or calcium channel blocker were excluded from the study. The 90 patients were randomly allocated to three groups of 30 each with the help of a computer generated table of random numbers.

Group D – Dexmedetomidine loading dose 1 μg/kg before induction over a period of 15 min and maintenance 0.5 μg/kg/h throughout the surgery.

Group M – Magnesium sulfate loading dose 50 mg/kg before induction over a period of 15 min and maintenance 15 mg/kg/h throughout the surgery.

Group C (Control group) - The same volume of normal saline was administered

In the operating room, preloading was done with 10 ml/kg of normal saline. Routine monitoring of electrocardiography (ECG), pulse oximetry and blood pressure were established before starting study drug. Radial artery cannulation was performed under local anesthesia. Electrodes were applied to the patient's forehead for monitoring the bispectral index (BIS) of the electroencephalogram. Neuromuscular transmission was monitored using train-of-four (TOF) supramaximal stimulations (2 Hz, 50 mA; TOF Watch SX, Organon Ltd, Dublin, Ireland).

All the drugs were prepared by an independent anesthesiologist not involved in the study, in identical syringes and infused with infusion pump (Perfusor Compact, B Braun, Germany). The loading doses of the drugs were administered 20 min prior to induction. Induction of anesthesia in all the groups was started 5 minutes after termination of the loading dose of study drug.

Anesthesia was induced with inj. midazolam 0.03 mg/kg, inj. fentanyl 1 μg/kg and inj. propofol 10 mg every 5 seconds until the BIS below 60 followed by vecuronium 0.1 mg/kg body weight and intubation completed with appropriate size cuffed endotracheal tube. Anesthesia was maintained with oxygen: nitrous oxide (O_2:N_2O; 40:60), and propofol infusion to achieve a target BIS between 40 and 60. Ventilation was adjusted to maintain an end-tidal carbon dioxide (ETCO2) between 35 and 40 mmHg. Propofol consumption was noted every hour. Presence of hypertension (mean arterial pressure > 20% from baseline) or tachycardia with maintaining BIS between 40 and 60 was treated with a bolus dose of fentanyl 0.5 μg/kg. TOF supramaximal neuromuscular stimulation (2 Hz, 50 mA) was measured at 5 min intervals to the end of surgery. Vecuronium (0.015 mg/kg) was administered when TOF count exceeded 2 until 10 min before the end of surgery. After skin closure, all infusion drugs were stopped and neuromuscular blockade was reversed with inj. neostigmine (40 μg/kg) and inj. glycopyrolate (10 μg/kg) when T4/T1 ratio reached 75% or higher followed by tracheal extubation. The time elapsed between stoppage of propofol infusion and a BIS value of 80 was considered as the recovery time. The time of cessation of anesthetics to tracheal extubation, response to verbal commands and orientation were also recorded.

Heart rate (HR), systolic blood pressure (SBP), diastolic blood pressure (DBP), mean arterial pressure (MAP) and BIS were recorded at preoperative, after study drug administration, after induction, after intubation, intraoperative period at 20 min intervals, after surgery and after extubation.

Any hypotension (MAP <30% baseline) was managed with a fluid bolus of 200 ml of normal saline. If hypotension did not respond to fluid administration, inj. mephentermine 5 mg i.v. was administered. If hypotension did not respond to 2 repeat doses of mephentermine then other means were sought as per the need. Any incidence of bradycardia (HR <50/min) was treated with inj. atropine 0.6 mg i.v.

The sample size was calculated by power analysis, using a two-sample *t* test, with a two sided type I error of 5% (α=0.05) and power at 80.37 (α=0.19). Therefore 25 patients in each group were needed to detect an intergroup difference of at least 20% in blood pressure and heart rate. We enrolled 30 patients in each group to account for potential dropouts or protocol violations.

Statistical analysis was performed using the Graph pad prism 6.0 statistical software. Patient characteristic data were analyzed with one way analysis of variance (ANOVA) for continuous variables and Chi square test for categorical variables. Intergroup comparison of hemodynamic parameters were done with one way analysis of variance (ANOVA), followed by an unpaired t test. Repeated measure analysis of variance (ANOVA) with the *post hoc* Tukey test was used to compare means for hemodynamic variables in intragroup comparison to baseline parameters. A P value of <0.05 was considered statistically significant.

Results

A total of one hundred six patients were assessed for eligibility, out of which ninety patients were included in the study after randomization and eighty four patients (93.33%) completed the study (Figure 1). Sixteen patients were excluded in this study on account of patient's refusal (four patients), not meeting inclusion criteria (six patients), pregabalin consumption (four patients) and analgesic consumption (two patients). Six patients were not included in this study on account of ventricular ectopic (one patient in group M), hypotension in group D (two patients), bradycardia (one patient in group D) and blood loss (two patients, one in group M and one in group C) which require blood transfusion. Their data has been included in the comparison of demographic profile; however, they were not subjected to further statistical analysis.

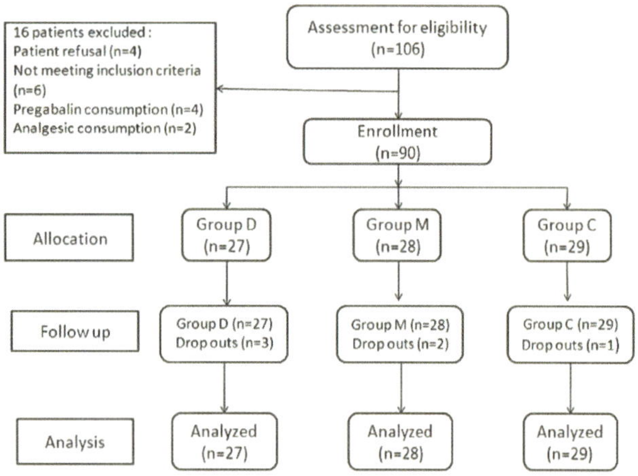

Figure 1. Study Design

There was no significant difference amongst the groups with regard to demographic variables (P>0.05) (Table 1). Propofol induction dose and maintenance dose were significantly lower in the group D and group M than in the group C (P<0.05). Vecuronium and fentanyl maintenance doses were also significantly lower in the group D and group M than in the group C (P<0.05) (Table 2).

Table 1. Demographic data

-	Group C (n=30)	Group D (n=30)	Group M (n=30)	P Value
Mean age (yrs)	46.57 ±8.73	45.93±9.19	48.30±7.70	0.543
Weight (Kg)	62.27±10.19	60.37 ±7.20	64.70 ±8.12	0.153
Male/Female	16/14	18/12	17/13	0.873
Spine surgery Cervical/Lumbar	10/20	8/22	11/19	0.713
Duration of surgery (hrs)	2.73±0.62	2.62±0.59	2.41±0.48	0.087

Data are presented as either mean values ± SD or by absolute numbers

There was no significant difference in preoperative hemodynamic parameters between the groups. After administration of the study drugs, there was a significant decrease in heart rate in group D (p<0.05). After induction, there was no change in HR in group M only. There was no significant increase in HR in group D after intubation (p>0.05). HR in group D and group M were significantly decreased (p<0.05) during the whole intraoperative period except 20 min in group M, however, this decrease was not seen in group C, compared to preoperative values. There was no significant change in HR after surgery and extubation in all groups except in group D after surgery (p<0.05). There was a significant difference in HR values between group C, D and M, during the whole intraoperaive period (p<0.05) (Figure 2).

Table 2. Induction dose of propofol and maintenance dose of propofol, vecuronium and fentanyl

Variable	Group C (n=29)	Group D (n=27)	Group M (n=28)	P value		
				C vs D	C vs M	D vs M
Propofol Induction dose (mg)	106.03±20.93	74.07±12.41	95.35±12.54	<0.001	<0.05	<0.001
Propofol Maintenance dose (mg/hr)	213.41±47.82	155.60±34.63	180.34±29.63	<0.001	<0.01	<0.05
Vecuronium Maintenance dose (mg/hr)	2.21±0.82	1.82±0.48	1.40±0.40	<0.05	<0.001	<0.05
Fentanyl Maintenance dose (µg/hr)	44.38±10.40	25.07±8.03	34.93±8.44	<0.001	<0.001	<0.001

Data are presented as mean values ± SD

SBP and DBP values were statistically significantly lower in the group D after study drug administration. Intubation caused significant increased in SBP and DBP values in group C only, compared to preoperative value. SBP values were statistically significantly lower in all three groups at all time observations of surgery compared to preoperative values. In group C there was no statistically significant change in DBP values after 40 min to all times of observations. These values were statistically significantly lower in the group D and group M after intubation and all time observations of surgery, when compared with the group C (p<0.05). There was no significant difference of SBP and DBP values between group C and group M after surgery (p>0.05). After extubation, there was no significant difference in SBP values only between group C and group M (Figure 3).

MAP values were statistically significantly lower in the group D and group M comparative to group C after intubation and all time observations of surgery (p<0.05). There was a significant decrease in MAP in all groups, compared to preoperative values at all time intervals of surgery (p<0.05). There was no significant difference in MAP after surgery between the group C and M (p=0.237). MAP values difference were more when compared the group D with group C (p<0.001), than group M with group C (p<0.05) (Figure 3).

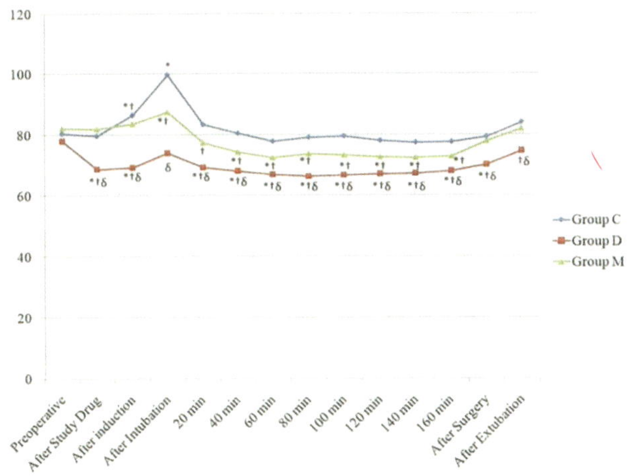

Figure 2. Changes in the heart rate (HR) observed in the three groups during the study period. *P<0.05 within group (vs baseline value), † P < 0.05 compared with group C, δ P < 0.05 group D vs group M.

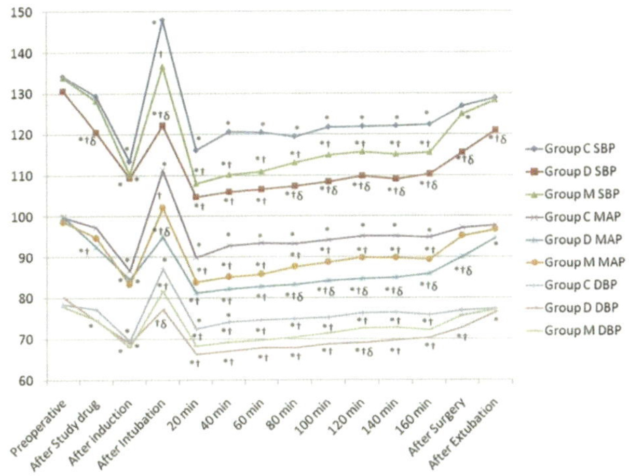

Figure 3. Changes in the blood pressure (SBP, DBP and MAP) observed in the three groups during the study period. *P<0.05 within group (vs baseline value), † P < 0.05 compared with group C, δ P < 0.05 group D vs group M.

Extubation time, response to verbal command and orientation time were significantly delayed in group M when compared with group C and D (p<0.05) (Table 3). In group M, serum magnesium levels increased from the pre-operative level 1.59±0.17 mg/dl to 2.10±0.26 mg/dl (postoperative value).

Hypotension was observed in only two patients (6.66%) in group D, which responded to administration of 2 doses of mephentermine 5 mg i.v. and one patient (3.33%) in group D developed bradycardia, which required atropine 0.6 mg i.v. One patient in the group M developed ventricular ectopic during the intraoperative period (serum Mg 3.0 mg/dl) without change in HR and blood pressure.

Discussion

In spine surgery hemodynamic stability is most important as sudden intraoperative hypertensive episodes causes intraoperative bleeding and it impairs quality of vision of the surgical field leading to an increased rate of complications. Therefore, improving the visibility of the surgical field by reducing bleeding during spine surgery is an important issue for anesthesiologists. In spine surgery, agents providing controlled hypotension and total intravenous anesthesia have emerged with the purpose of surgical field clarity. Therefore, we tested the superiority of two agents, magnesium sulfate and dexmedetomidine, against each other for maintaining hemodynamic stability and consumption of anesthetic agents.

Our study demonstrated that perioperative use of dexmedetomidine and magnesium sulfate is associated with hemodynamic stability as well as reduced anesthetic consumption. The degree of decrease of perioperative consumption of propofol and fentanyl was 20% more with dexmedetomidine compared to magnesium.

Table 3. Recovery parameter

Variable	Group C	Group D	Group M	P Value		
				C vs D	C vs M	D vs M
Extubation time (min.)	10.78±2.98	11.19±3.55	13.39±3.65	0.633	<0.05	<0.05
Response to verbal command (min.)	9.82±2.59	10.34±3.11	12.68±3.29	0.496	<0.01	<0.05
Orientation time (min)	11.81±2.86	12.57±3.65	14.68±3.19	0.386	<0.01	<0.05

Data are presented as mean values ± SD

Dexmedetomidine was associated with a higher incidence of hypotension and bradycardia and this effect is dose related. We chose to study a dose of 1μg/kg over 15 min duration and maintenance 0.5 μg/kg/h and this dose are supported by various studies.[3,4,11] Magnesium sulfate is also safe to use as an adjuvant. There have been cases of magnesium toxicity leading to cardiac arrest and death.[12] However, magnesium toxicity begins at serum concentrations of 2.5–5.0 mmol/litre, which is much higher than the highest level in Group M in this study. Goral N, et al[13] also noted that toxic level of serum magnesium concentration is not reached even after using magnesium sulfate in the dose of bolus (50mg/kg) and continuous infusion (20 mg/kg/hr). In the present study, we administered magnesium sulfate bolus dose (50 mg/kg), and the maintenance dose (15 mg/kg/hr) based on previous studies.[1,2,14]

In the present study dexmedetomidine group achieved a 20% more decrease in propofol and fentanyl requirements comparison of magnesium group with the control group. This reduction in dexmedetomidine group is due to the hypnotic, sedative, analgesic and anesthetic sparing effect of dexmedetomidine. The interaction of α2-adrenoreceptors and opioids lead to decrease in the dose of fentanyl. The α2 adrenoceptors have an effect on the spinal cord, especially α2A and α2C as well as modulating the descending noradrenergic pathways leading to 30% to 50% reduction in the requirements of opioids.[15] Our study is in accordance with other studies[16,17] Magnesium could modulate anesthesia by several mechanisms. The mechanism of analgesic effect of magnesium is due to interference with calcium channels and antagonism of the NMDA receptor in the CNS. The first possibility is based on the observation that calcium channel blockers have an antinociceptive action and enhance opiate analgesia in patients with cancer chronically treated with morphine. Magnesium blocks NMDA-induced currents in a voltage-dependent manner by blocking the receptor channel effects,[9] second possible explanation for the analgesic action of magnesium. Telci et al[18] and Choi et al[19] demonstrated significant reductions in infusion rates of propofol and opioids, titrated to maintain BIS between 45 and 60 by using a magnesium infusion throughout the operations. These results are similar to our study.

It is well known that magnesium sulfate prolongs and potentiates neuromuscular block by non-depolarizing neuromuscular blocking agents. Consistent with previous studies[1,20,21] our study also showed that lower vecuronium requirements with magnesium use. Fuchs-Buder et al[22] reported that an intravenous infusion of magnesium at 40 mg/kg significantly potentiated the neuromuscular blockade of vecuronium, and plasma magnesium concentrations increased significantly from a baseline after the magnesium sulfate infusion, but no symptoms of muscle weakness were observed in any patients. In addition, Baraka and Yazigi[23] found no clinical or electromyographic signs of muscle weakness, even at slightly higher plasma magnesium concentrations (1.7–2.5 mmol/L).

In the present study, both the study drugs (dexmedetomidine and magnesium sulfate) have better hemodynamic stability with minimum fluctuations during whole intraoperative period. Dexmedetomidine group has been associated with a greater decrease in HR, in part because of the sympatholytic effects of this drug, but also because of a vagal mimetic effect. From postintubation to the end of surgery, MAP remained at a significantly lower level in dexmedetomidine and magnesium sulfate treated subjects than in controls; this probably indicates that the analgesic properties of dexmedetomidine and magnesium sulfate reduce sympathetic stimulation. Magnesium produces vasodilatation by directly acting on the blood vessels and by interfering with a wide range of vasoconstrictor substances. In addition to its direct effects on the vessel wall, raised serum magnesium levels may also reduce peripheral vascular tone by a number of other mechanisms, including sympathetic blockade and inhibition of catecholamine release. Dexmedetomidine also is known to decrease sympathetic outflow and circulating catecholamine levels and would therefore be expected to cause a decrease of MAP similar to those of magnesium. The hypotension and bradycardia that occurred in the dexmedetomidine group were predictable from the known properties of α2 agonists, and have been confirmed from previous studies.[24,25]

Similar to our results, Ryu, et al[21] showed lower trends of hemodynamic parameters with attenuation of stress response to intubation and surgery in the magnesium group. Our study is also supported by previous other studies of magnesium sulfate use as an adjuvant. Soliman RN, et al[26] used the same dose of dexmedetomidine in craniotomy patients and showed that it maintained the hemodynamic stability, reduced sevoflurane and fentanyl requirements and improved significantly the outcomes. Turgat N, et al[6] used dexmedetomidine 0.6 μg/kg as bolus before induction and 0.2 μg/kg/hr by infusion during spine surgery and found that MAP values were better controlled in dexmedetomidine treated patients except after intubation comparison to fentanyl group and we felt this result may be due to low dose of dexmedetomidine. In our study, we used different doses of dexmedetomidine in spine patients and found that MAP is better controlled at all points of the observations. The major problem with dexmedetomidine is its hemodynamic effects, as the drug often causes hypotension and bradycardia. In our study, hypotension (6.66%) and bradycardia (3.33%) were also noted and it was also found in other studies.[27,28]

In the present study, patients received magnesium sulfate were associated with significantly longer recovery time, this effect was also reported in previous studies when they added magnesium sulfate to anesthetic regimen.[8,18,22] Few studies also observed that there was a no significant increase in the recovery parameter in magnesium sulfate treated patients when monitored through TOF.[20,21] We also monitored TOF but we have given vecuronium until 10 min. prior to the end of surgery, because some of our patients are in the prone position and this causes hemodynamic derangements during change of position.

There are some limitations of this study. First, the use of nitrous oxide might confound the interpretation of BIS. Second, we determine the serum magnesium concentration before and after surgery in only group M due to cost factor. So the relationship between serum magnesium and analgesic effect could not be evaluated. Third, we used fixed doses of study drugs. Therefore, further experiments on the different doses of study to minimize adverse effects of drug are needed.

Conclusion

Dexmedetomidine and magnesium sulfate led to a significant reduction of propofol, fentanyl, vecuronium requirements and maintained the haemodynamic stability during intubation and surgery. Dexmedetomidine was associated with bradycardia and hypotension and magnesium sulfate caused a delay in recovery.

Acknowledgments
The authors thank Mr. Teku Ram Kashyap, Mr Jogendra Kumar and the surgical staff for all their assistance and suggestions during the current study.

Ethical Issues
Not applicable.

Conflict of Interest
The authors report no conflicts of interest.

References
1. Seyhan TO, Tugrul M, Sungur MO, Kayacan S, Telci L, Pembeci K, et al. Effects of three different dose regimens of magnesium on propofol requirements, haemodynamic variables and postoperative pain relief in gynaecological surgery. *Br J Anaesth* 2006;96(2):247-52. doi: 10.1093/bja/aei291
2. Na HS, Lee JH, Hwang JY, Ryu JH, Han SH, Jeon YT, et al. Effects of magnesium sulphate on intraoperative neuromuscular blocking agent requirements and postoperative analgesia in children with cerebral palsy. *Br J Anaesth* 2010;104(3):344-50. doi: 10.1093/bja/aep379
3. Bekker A, Sturaitis M, Bloom M, Moric M, Golfinos J, Parker E, et al. The effect of dexmedetomidine on perioperative hemodynamics in patients undergoing craniotomy. *Anesth Analg* 2008;107(4):1340-7. doi: 10.1213/ane.0b013e3181804298
4. Kang WS, Kim SY, Son JC, Kim JD, Muhammad HB, Kim SH, et al. The effect of dexmedetomidine on the adjuvant propofol requirement and intraoperative hemodynamics during remifentanil-based anesthesia. *Korean J Anesthesiol* 2012;62(2):113-8. doi: 10.4097/kjae.2012.62.2.113
5. Hosseinzadeh H, Eidy M, Ghaffarlou M, Ghabili K, Golzari SE. Esmolol: A unique beta-blocker in maintaining cardiovascular stability following neurosurgical procedures. *Adv Pharm Bull* 2012;2(2):249-52. doi: 10.5681/apb.2012.038
6. Turgut N, Turkmen A, Gokkaya S, Altan A, Hatiboglu MA. Dexmedetomidine-based versus fentanyl-based total intravenous anesthesia for lumbar laminectomy. *Minerva Anestesiol* 2008;74(9):469-74.
7. Khurana G, Jindal P, Sharma JP, Bansal KK. Postoperative pain and long-term functional outcome after administration of gabapentin and pregabalin in patients undergoing spinal surgery. *Spine (Phila Pa 1976)* 2014;39(6):E363-8. doi: 10.1097/BRS.0000000000000185
8. Altan A, Turgut N, Yildiz F, Turkmen A, Ustun H. Effects of magnesium sulphate and clonidine on propofol consumption, haemodynamics and postoperative recovery. *Br J Anaesth* 2005;94(4):438-41. doi: 10.1093/bja/aei070
9. Clarke RJ, Glasgow NG, Johnson JW. Mechanistic and structural determinants of nmda receptor voltage-dependent gating and slow mg2+ unblock. *J Neurosci* 2013;33(9):4140-50. doi: 10.1523/JNEUROSCI.3712-12.2013
10. Wu L, Huang X, Sun L. The efficacy of n-methyl-d-aspartate receptor antagonists on improving the postoperative pain intensity and satisfaction after remifentanil-based anesthesia in adults: A meta-analysis. *J Clin Anesth* 2015;27(4):311-24. doi: 10.1016/j.jclinane.2015.03.020
11. Akkaya A, Tekelioglu UY, Demirhan A, Bilgi M, Yildiz I, Apuhan T, et al. comparison of the effects of magnesium sulphate and dexmedetomidine on surgical vision quality in endoscopic sinus surgery: Randomized clinical study. *Rev Bras Anestesiol* 2014;64(6):406-12. doi: 10.1016/j.bjan.2014.01.008
12. Morisaki H, Yamamoto S, Morita Y, Kotake Y, Ochiai R, Takeda J. Hypermagnesemia-induced cardiopulmonary arrest before induction of anesthesia for emergency cesarean section. *J Clin Anesth* 2000;12(3):224-6.
13. Goral N, Ergil J, Alptekin A, Ozkan D, Gurer B, Dolgun H, et al. Effect of magnesium sulphate on bleeding during lumbar discectomy. *Anaesthesia* 2011;66(12):1140-5. doi: 10.1111/j.1365-2044.2011.06898.x
14. Bhatia A, Kashyap L, Pawar DK, Trikha A. Effect of intraoperative magnesium infusion on perioperative analgesia in open cholecystectomy. *J Clin Anesth* 2004;16(4):262-5. doi: 10.1016/j.jclinane.2003.08.012
15. Fairbanks CA, Stone LS, Kitto KF, Nguyen HO, Posthumus IJ, Wilcox GL. Alpha(2c)-adrenergic receptors mediate spinal analgesia and adrenergic-opioid synergy. *J Pharmacol Exp Ther* 2002;300(1):282-90.
16. Unlugenc H, Gunduz M, Guler T, Yagmur O, Isik G. The effect of pre-anaesthetic administration of intravenous dexmedetomidine on postoperative pain in patients receiving patient-controlled morphine. *Eur J Anaesthesiol* 2005;22(5):386-91.
17. Bajwa SJ, Kaur J, Singh A, Parmar S, Singh G, Kulshrestha A, et al. Attenuation of pressor response and dose sparing of opioids and anaesthetics with pre-operative dexmedetomidine. *Indian J Anaesth* 2012;56(2):123-8. doi: 10.4103/0019-5049.96303
18. Telci L, Esen F, Akcora D, Erden T, Canbolat AT, Akpir K. Evaluation of effects of magnesium sulphate in reducing intraoperative anaesthetic requirements. *Br J Anaesth* 2002;89(4):594-8.
19. Choi JC, Yoon KB, Um DJ, Kim C, Kim JS, Lee SG. Intravenous magnesium sulfate administration reduces propofol infusion requirements during maintenance of propofol-n2o anesthesia: Part i: Comparing propofol requirements according to hemodynamic responses: Part ii: Comparing bispectral index in control and magnesium groups. *Anesthesiology* 2002;97(5):1137-41.

20. Lee DH, Kwon IC. Magnesium sulphate has beneficial effects as an adjuvant during general anaesthesia for caesarean section. *Br J Anaesth* 2009;103(6):861-6. doi: 10.1093/bja/aep265
21. Ryu JH, Kang MH, Park KS, Do SH. Effects of magnesium sulphate on intraoperative anaesthetic requirements and postoperative analgesia in gynaecology patients receiving total intravenous anaesthesia. *Br J Anaesth* 2008;100(3):397-403. doi: 10.1093/bja/aem407
22. Fuchs-Buder T, Wilder-Smith OH, Borgeat A, Tassonyi E. Interaction of magnesium sulphate with vecuronium-induced neuromuscular block. *Br J Anaesth* 1995;74(4):405-9.
23. Baraka A, Yazigi A. Neuromuscular interaction of magnesium with succinylcholine-vecuronium sequence in the eclamptic parturient. *Anesthesiology* 1987;67(5):806-8.
24. Talke P, Chen R, Thomas B, Aggarwall A, Gottlieb A, Thorborg P, et al. The hemodynamic and adrenergic effects of perioperative dexmedetomidine infusion after vascular surgery. *Anesth Analg* 2000;90(4):834-9.
25. Ebert TJ, Hall JE, Barney JA, Uhrich TD, Colinco MD. The effects of increasing plasma concentrations of dexmedetomidine in humans. *Anesthesiology* 2000;93(2):382-94.
26. Soliman RN, Hassan AR, Rashwan AM, Omar AM. Prospective, randomized study to assess the role of dexmedetomidine in patients with supratentorial tumors undergoing craniotomy under general anaesthesia. *Middle East J Anaesthesiol* 2011;21(3):325-34.
27. Sakaguchi Y, Takahashi S. dexmedetomidine. *Masui* 2006;55(7):856-63.
28. Bekker A, Sturaitis MK. Dexmedetomidine for neurological surgery. *Neurosurgery* 2005;57(1 Suppl):1-10; discussion 1-.

Bacteriophage Isolated from Sewage Eliminates and Prevents the Establishment of *Escherichia Coli* Biofilm

Karla Veloso Gonçalves Ribeiro[1,2], Cleberson Ribeiro[2], Roberto Sousa Dias[2], Silvia Almeida Cardoso[3], Sérgio Oliveira de Paula[2], Jose Cola Zanuncio[4], Leandro Licursi de Oliveira[2]*

[1] *Núcleo de Microscopia e Microanálise, Universidade Federal de Viçosa, 36570-900, Viçosa, Minas Gerais, Brasil.*
[2] *Departamento de Biologia Geral, Universidade Federal de Viçosa, 36570-900, Viçosa, Minas Gerais, Brasil.*
[3] *Departamento de Medicina e Enfermagem, Universidade Federal de Viçosa, 36570-900, Viçosa, Minas Gerais, Brasil.*
[4] *Departamento de Entomologia, Universidade Federal de Viçosa, 36570-900, Viçosa, Minas Gerais, Brasil.*

Keywords:
- Biocontrol
- Biofilm
- *E. coli*
- Phage

Abstract

Purpose: Biofilm growth exerts a negative impact on industry and health, necessitating the development of strategies to control. The objective of this work was study the lytic activity of the phage isolated from the sewage network in the formation and degradation of *Escherichia coli* biofilms.

Methods: *E. coli* cultures were incubated in 96-well polystyrene microplates under controlled conditions to evaluate the biofilm formation. The *E. coli* cultures and established biofilms were treated with the suspensions of the vB_EcoM-UFV017 (EcoM017) bacteriophage obtained from sewage for 24 hours. The *E. coli* bacterial density was measured using absorbance at 600 nm and the biofilms were measured by crystal violet staining. Polystyrene coupons were used as support for Scanning Electron Microscopy and Confocal Microscopy to evaluate biofilm formation.

Results: The *E. coli* strains formed biofilms in polystyrene microplates after 48 hours' incubation. The highest EcoM017 phage titer, in the prevention and degradation experiments, reduced the bacterial growth and the quantity of biofilm formed by *E. coli* in 90.0% and 87.5%, respectively. The minimum dose capable of reducing the biofilms of this bacterium was 10^1 PFU/mL after 24 hours. The preformed *E. coli* biofilm mass was reduced 79% post exposure to the phage in the degradation assay. Microscopic analysis confirmed the results obtained in the plates assays.

Conclusion: The EcoM017 phage prevented biofilm formation and degraded the *E. coli*-established ones. The EcoM017 phage isolated from sewage can reduce bacterial attachment and lyse the *E. coli* associated biofilm cells, offering biotechnological potential applicability for this phage.

Introduction

Escherichia coli, one of the main components of the normal flora of the digestive tract of humans and animals,[1] are usually harmless, although some strains are pathogenic and can cause intra- and extra-intestinal diseases.[2] Specific gene groups and virulence factors facilitate the colonization, multiplication and survival of this bacterium in the host body.[3]

E. coli can adhere to and be internalized in epithelial cells. The persistence of this pathogen in cattle mammary glands causes an infection called mastitis, whose recurrence may be related to biofilm formation.[4] Bovine mastitis is the most significant and expensive disease affecting the dairy industry across the world.[5] *E. coli* is the most important and frequently agent isolated from the clinical cases of environmental mastitis causing milk production losses and the death of 10% of the animals.[6,7] This organism is capable of causing clinical mastitis depending on the immunological status of animal.[8]

Biofilms are complex microbial communities found adherent to a surface and embedded in a protective extracellular matrix (ECM) of polymeric substances.[9] Biofilm formation increases resistance to antibiotics, disinfectants, phages and the host immune system, including antibodies, phagocytes and the complement system, necessitating the development of strategies to control their formation.[10] Since the 20th, phages have been proposed as antimicrobial agents.[11] However, the discovery and commercialization of antibiotics from the '40s, emergence of broad-spectrum antibiotics, lack of quality therapeutic products and less understanding of the biology delayed or resulted in minimum research done on phages.[12] Inappropriate antibiotic use increased the emergence of resistant bacteria and rekindled the interest in phage therapy.[13,14] Phages are highly specific to one or a few bacteria and are often effective against multi-drug resistant organisms. This is because they kill cells via

***Corresponding author:** Leandro Licursi de Oliveira, Email: leandro.licursi@ufv.br

different molecular mechanisms without infecting eukaryotic cells or disrupting the normal host beneficial microflora.[15,16] Therefore, these organisms have been proposed to remove or reduce bacterial biofilm.[17]
The EcoM017 phage isolated from sewage has been tested for *E. coli* biocontrol isolated from animals with mastitis, aiming at preventing biofilm formation and degrading those already established by these bacteria.

Materials and Methods

Bacterial strain

Escherichia coli 30 were isolated from cow with mastitis. This strain is part of the collection of pathogens from the Laboratory of Molecular Immunovirology (LMI) of the Departamento de Biologia Geral, Universidade Federal de Viçosa (UFV) and was obtained from Embrapa Dairy Cattle. The bacteria were grown in Luria-Bertani agar (LB) (10 g/L tryptone, 5 g/L yeast extract, 10 g/L NaCl (pH 7.2) and supplemented with 1.5% bacteriological agar) at 37°C for 16 h. One colony was isolated and transferred to the LB broth (without agar supplementation) and cultivated at 37°C under stirring (180 rpm) until an optical density of 0.7 at a wavelength of 600 nm (OD_{600}) was achieved in the microplate reader (VersaMax, Molecular Device). The bacterial culture was centrifuged (4,000 × g) for 10 min. The pellet was suspended and adjusted to OD_{600} 2.0 in 10 mM $MgSO_4$. The stocks were refrigerated at 4°C and used for titration and plating of the phage.

Phage propagation

The EcoM017 phage was isolated from the sewage network samples in Viçosa municipality, Minas Gerais state, Brazil, and used in the experiments for the prevention and degradation of the *E. coli* 30 biofilm. Phage stocks were prepared using the standard agar-overlay technique. A total of 100 µL of the bacterial stock with 2.0 OD_{600} was added to 100 µL of the viral stock. This mixture was incubated at 37°C for 30 min and added to tubes containing semi-solid agar supplemented with 0.75% bacteriological agar. The entire tube contents were transferred onto a plate with LB agar. The phages were extracted in 5 mL SM buffer (100 mM NaCl, 8 mM $MgSO_4.7H_2O$, 50 mM Tris-HCl pH 7.5, 2% gelatin w/v) at 4°C with gentle agitation for 4 h, after 24 h incubation. The SM buffer was recovered, supplemented with 1 M NaCl and maintained at 4°C for 1 h. The contaminant bacteria were removed by passage through a sterile 0.22 µm filter. The EcoM017 phage stocks were stored at 4°C for use.

Phage characterization and titration

The morphology of the phage was observed by Transmission Electron microscopy (TEM). Briefly, the purified phage sample was deposited on Formvar-coated copper grid and negative stained with 2% uranyl acetate. Visualization was performed using a Zeiss TEM EM 109 (Zeiss, Oberkochen, Germany) at an accelerating voltage of 80 kV. The phage titer was analyzed with the standard agar-overlay technique through the serial dilution of stocks and calculation of plaque-forming units (PFU) per mL (PFU/mL). First, 100 µL of the phage diluted solution was added to 100 µL of the bacterial stock with 2.0 OD_{600} and incubated in plates with LB agar as described above (Phage propagation). Plate that has between 30 and 300 lysis plaques were used to calculate Plaque Forming Units per mL, using the equation:
PFU mL^{-1} = number of lysis plaques X dilution factor / volume of diluted virus added to the plate

Quantification of biofilm formation

The detection and quantification of the *E. coli* biofilm were performed in 96-well polystyrene microplates. This bacterium was cultivated under shaking at 180 rpm at 37°C for 2 h. The OD_{600} of the *E. coli* culture was adjusted to 0.1, corresponding to approximately 10^8 colony forming units (CFU) per mL,[18,19] and the culture was diluted 1:10 in fresh LB broth and inoculated into six wells per microplate (200 µL per well). The control had wells containing sterile LB broth. The plates were incubated at 37°C for 24, 48 and 72 h respectively, to allow biofilm development to occur. Post incubation, bacterial growth (OD_{600}) was determined in the microplate reader. Planktonic cells were removed by quickly inverting the plate and each well was rinsed twice with 250 µL of phosphate buffered saline (PBS) (pH 7.2). The adherent cells were stained with 250 µL of 0.1% crystal violet (CV) at room temperature for 30 min. The wells were washed four times with 250 µL distilled water and air dried for 1 h. The CV was solubilized in 200 µL of acetone-ethanol 20:80 at room temperature. The amount of CV extracted was measured by optical density at 595 nm (OD_{595}) in the microplate reader.

Biofilm prevention with phage

A total of 20 µL of bacterial culture with 0.1 OD_{600} and 20 µL phage suspension at different concentrations (concentrated solution and nine decimal dilutions in SM buffer) were added to 160 µL of the LB broth in the wells of the 96-well polystyrene microplates. The control contained the LB broth, LB plus phage and LB plus bacterial suspension. The plate was incubated at 37°C for 24 h. Post incubation, the OD_{600} was determined and the biofilm was stained with CV, as described above. The relative biofilm mass was determined by normalizing the absorbance of the positive control at 100%.

Biofilm degradation with phage

Initially 20 µL of the bacterial culture with 0.1 OD_{600} of was added to 180 µL of the LB broth in the wells of a 96-well polystyrene microplate. The control contained LB and LB plus bacterial suspension. The microplates were incubated at 37°C for 24 h. The wells were washed twice with PBS and 20 µL of the phage solution at different concentrations (concentrated solution and nine decimal dilutions in SM buffer) and 180 µL of the LB broth were added. The controls contained the LB broth, LB plus phage and LB plus bacterial suspension. The microplates were incubated at 37°C for 24 h. The OD_{600} was determined in the microplate reader and the CV stained wells as described above. The relative biofilm mass was determined by normalizing the absorbance of the positive control at 100%.

Preparation of polystyrene coupons

Polystyrene pieces (coupons) (1.0 × 1.0 × 0.1 cm) were used as the support for the biofilm formation. Each coupon was brushed with detergent, rinsed in distilled water, sterilized by immersion in 1% sodium hypochlorite and 70% ethanol for 15 min, and placed under ultraviolet light for 30 min, on each side.

Biofilm formation

The coupons were placed in 15 mL Falcon tubes containing 125 µL of the bacterial culture with 0.1 OD_{600} and 1,125 µL of the LB broth (coupons at the air-liquid interface). The control coupons were immersed in LB alone. The tubes were incubated at 37°C without shaking for 24, 48 and 72 h, and prepared for analysis by Scanning Electron Microscopy (SEM).

Phage effect on biofilm formation

The coupons were placed in 15 mL Falcon tubes containing 125 µL of the bacterial culture with 0.1 OD_{600}, 1 mL LB broth and 125 µL of the phage solution with three titers: high (10^{10} PFU/mL), medium (10^4 PFU/mL) and low (10^1 PFU/mL). The control coupons were immersed in the LB broth, LB plus SM buffer and LB plus bacterial suspension. The tubes were incubated at 37°C without stirring for 24 h. The coupons were prepared for analysis by the SEM (coupons treated with three phage titers) and Confocal Laser Scanning Microscopy (CLSM) (coupons treated with high and low titers) as described below.

Phage effect on the biofilm

The coupons were placed in 15 mL Falcon tubes with 125 µL of bacterial culture with 0.1 OD_{600} and 1,125 µL LB broth. The control coupons were immersed in the LB, LB plus SM buffer and LB plus bacterial suspension. The tubes were incubated at 37°C without stirring for 24 h. After establishment of the biofilm, the coupons were washed twice with PBS (pH 7.2) and transferred to the tubes containing 125 µL of phage solution with high (10^{10} PFU/mL), medium (10^4 PFU/mL) and low (10^1 PFU/mL) and 1,125 µL of LB. The tubes were incubated at 37°C without agitation for 24 h and the coupons prepared for analysis by SEM (coupons treated with three phage titers) and CLSM (coupons treated with high and low titers).

Scanning Electron Microscopy (SEM)

The coupons were washed in PBS (pH 7.2), fixed with 2.5% glutaraldehyde v/v in 0.05 M cacodylate buffer (pH 7.2) for 2 h and treated with 1% (w/v) osmium tetroxide solution in 0.05 M cacodylate buffer (pH 7.2) at room temperature for 1 h. After cell fixation, the samples were rinsed thrice in 0.05 M cacodylate buffer and immersed in an increasing ethanol gradient (30, 50, 70, 80 and 90% in water) for 10 min per concentration. Finally, the samples were immersed thrice in 100% ethanol for 10 min, and then dehydrated, dried in a dryer critical point (CPD Bal-tec 030) with liquid CO_2 and covered with gold (15 nm thick approximately) in a sputter (Balzers, FDU 010). The coupons were examined in a Scanning Electron Microscope (Leo 1430VP) with an accelerating voltage of 20 kV.

Confocal Laser Scanning Microscopy (CLSM)

The coupons were washed twice in PBS (pH 7.2) and incubated in a mixture of propidium iodide (IP) 20 µg/mL and fluorescein isothiocyanate 2 µg/mL in PBS (pH 7.2), for 15 min in the dark.[20] Post staining, the coupons were washed in PBS and examined under the Laser Scanning Confocal Microscope (Zeiss LSM 510 Meta) with argon laser excitation at 488 and 514 nm. The live bacteria with intact membranes would stain green, whereas dead and membrane-damaged ones would stain red or yellow.

Statistical analysis

The results of three independent experiments performed in sextuplicate were subjected to variance analysis (ANOVA) and Tukey test using the GraphPad Prism Software, Inc. Statistical significance was accepted if $P \leq 0.05$.

Results

Phage Characterization

The phage isolated from the sewage was processed for Transmission electron microscopy (TEM), the phage revealed an isometric head (~ 89 nm in length and ~78 nm in width) and contractile tails (~ 55 nm) with a basal tuft attached (Figure1). Based on these morphological characteristics, phage was assigned to the family Myoviridae according to the classification system of Ackermann[21] and named vB_EcoM-UFV017. Myoviridae phages typically possess double-stranded (ds) DNA as their genomic nucleic acid. In addition, the genome size of phage was approximately 44 kb (unpublished data).

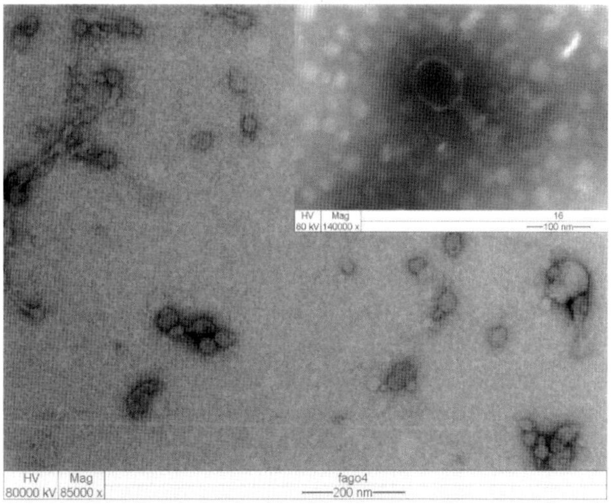

Figure 1. Transmission Electron micrograph of bacteriophage vB_EcoM-UFV017. The phage showing an isometric head structure with ~ 89 nm in length and ~78 nm in width and a tail of ~55 nm. The morphology of vB_EcoM-UFV017 corresponds to the Myoviridae family. The insert show details of phage morphology (head, tail, base plate and tail fibers). Virion particles were negatively stained with uranyl acetate for EM.

Biofilm formation

Escherichia coli formed biofilm on the polystyrene microplate in the LB medium at 37°C under static conditions for 24 and 48 hours, with a two-fold increase between these periods. At 72 hours, the biofilm mass was 5.4 times lower than that of the one at 48 hours (Figure 2) possibly due to nutrient depletion and other factors (see Discussion). The scanning electron microscopy showed similar results to those of colorimetric quantitative assays (Figure 3).

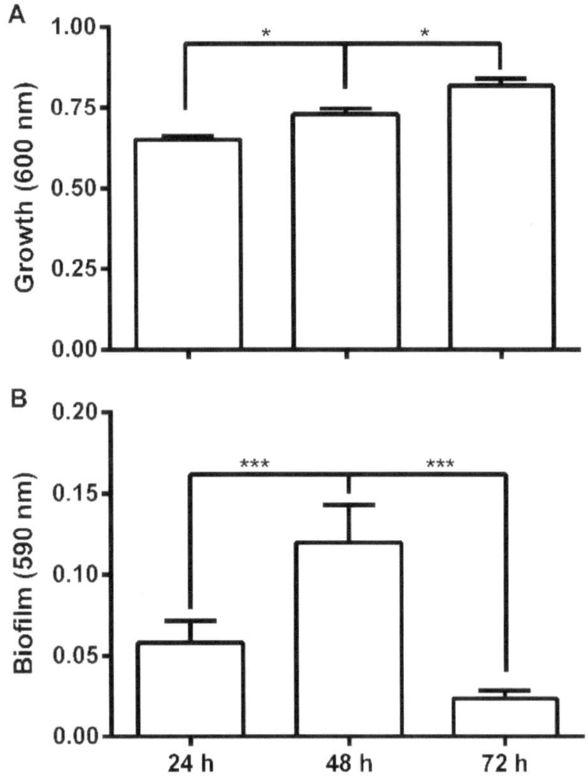

Figure 2. Bacterial growth (A) and biofilm quantification (B) of *Escherichia coli* 30 in polystyrene microplates after incubation in LB at 37 °C under static conditions for 24, 48 and 72 hours. * $P < 0.05$ and *** $P < 0.001$.

Effect of the phage on biofilm formation

The different phage titers decreased the *E. coli* population and those with 10^2 to 10^9 PFU/mL reduced the bacterial growth and biofilm formation. The highest titer (10^9 PFU/mL) reduced the growth and biofilm formation in 90.0 and 87.5%, respectively, while the 10^0 and 10^1 PFU/mL biofilms showed no difference from control (Figure 4).

Escherichia coli formed biofilm on the polystyrene coupon with large cell groups, a small amount of ECM and the prevalence of viable cells (green color) when incubated at 37°C under static conditions for 24 hours (Figures 5A, 5B and 6A).

Medium and high titer treatments decreased the biofilm formation of *E. coli*, showing a dose-dependent effect. Single cells and small clusters containing large numbers of dead cells (red staining) were observed in the treatment with the highest titer. Cell debris was also observed in both treatments (Figures 5C-5F and 6B).

Debris and a greater number of dead cells were observed near the biofilm in the presence of low titer of the phage (10^1 PFU/mL) (Figures 5G, 5H and 6C).

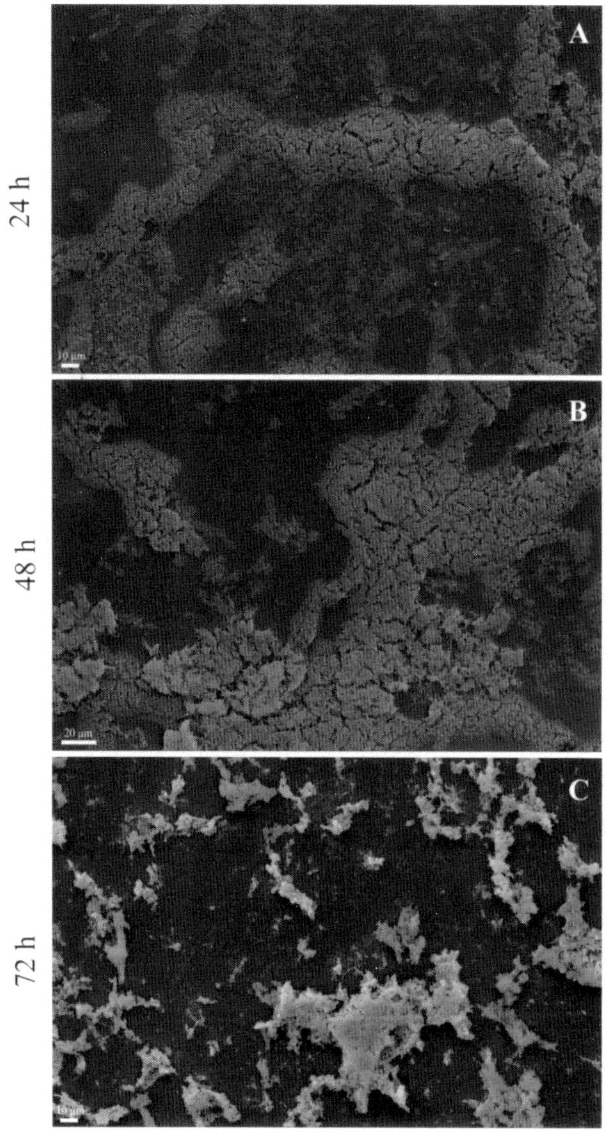

Figure 3. Scanning electron microscopy of *Escherichia coli* 30 biofilm grown on the polystyrene surface under static conditions at 37 °C for 24, 48 and 72 hours.

Effect of the phage on biofilm degradation

The minimum dose capable of reducing the *E. coli* 30 biofilm was found to be 10^1 PFU/mL. The biofilm formation dropped to 79.0% in the treatment with the highest phage titer (10^9 PFU/mL) (Figure 7)

E. coli grown in the absence of the phage yielded a complex biofilm with a predominance of viable cells (Figures 8A, 8B and 9A). The medium and high phage titers destroyed the architecture of the *E. coli* biofilm in a dose-dependent manner, revealing a predominance of dead cells (Figures 8C-8F and 9B). The low titer of the phage (10^1 PFU/mL) exerted no effect on the mature biofilm of *E. coli* (Figures 8G, 8H and 9C).

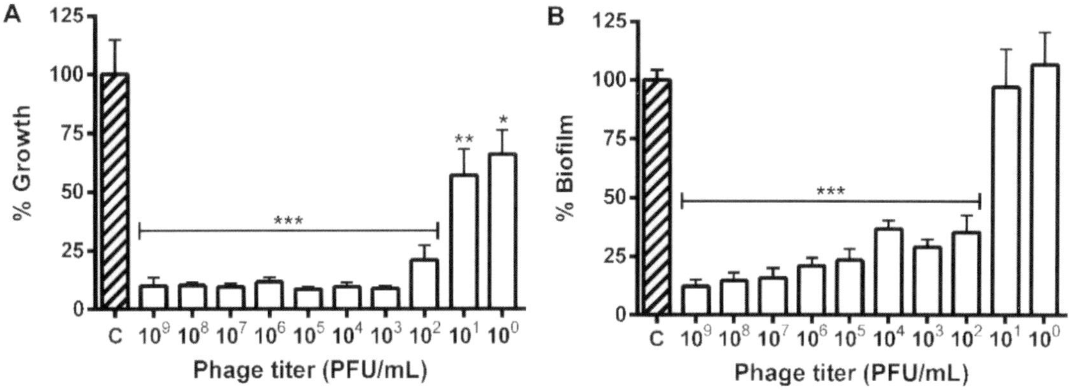

Figure 4. Prevention of the growth (A) and biofilm formation (B) of *Escherichia coli* 30 in polystyrene microplates after 24 hours of exposure to different phage titers (10^0 to 10^9 PFU/mL). * $P \leq 0.05$, ** $P \leq 0.01$ and *** $P \leq 0.001$ compared to the control.

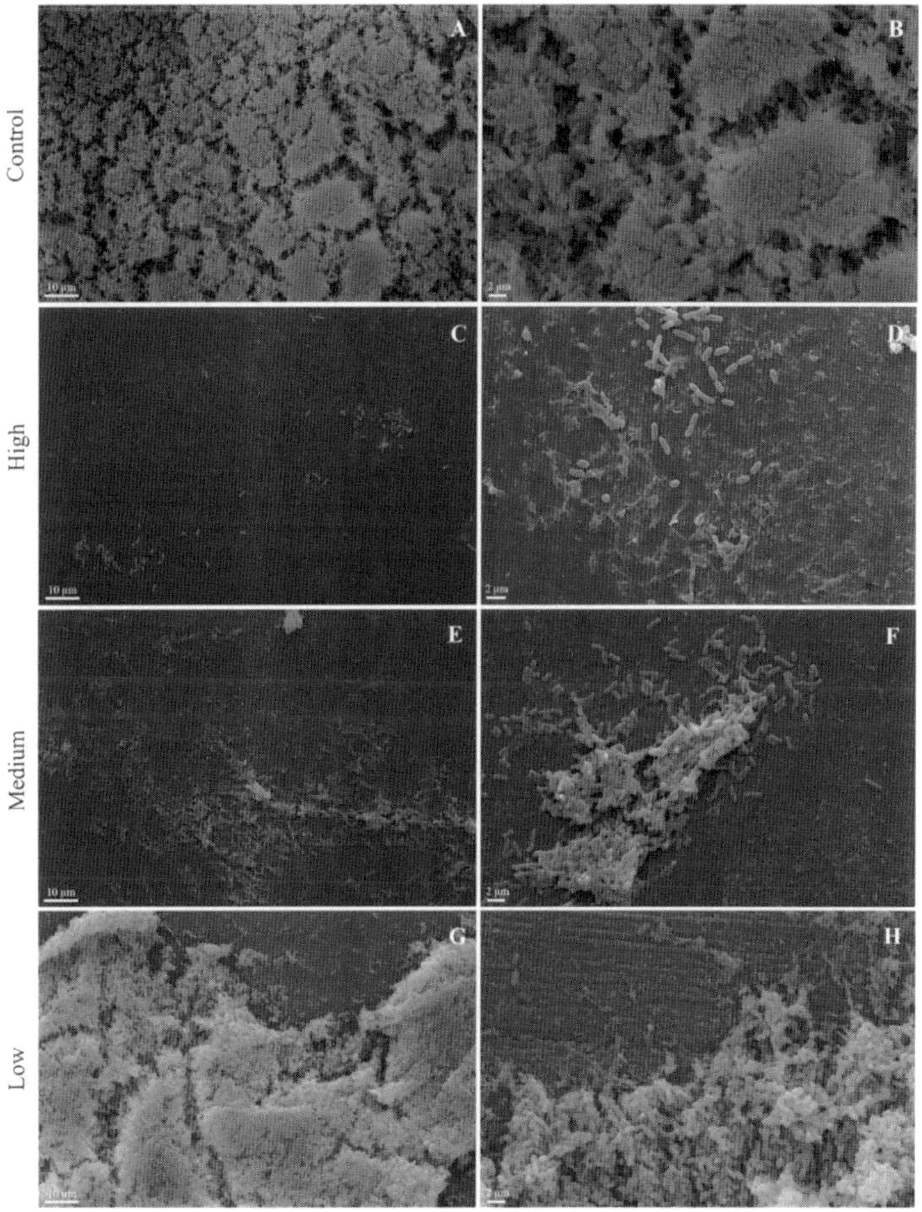

Figure 5. Scanning electron microscopy of *Escherichia coli* 30 biofilm grown on the polystyrene surface under static conditions at 37 °C for 24 hours. Control untreated (A and B). Treatment with phage with a high titer (10^9 PFU/mL) (C and D), medium titer (10^4 PFU/mL) (E and F) and low titer (10^0 PFU/mL) (G and H).

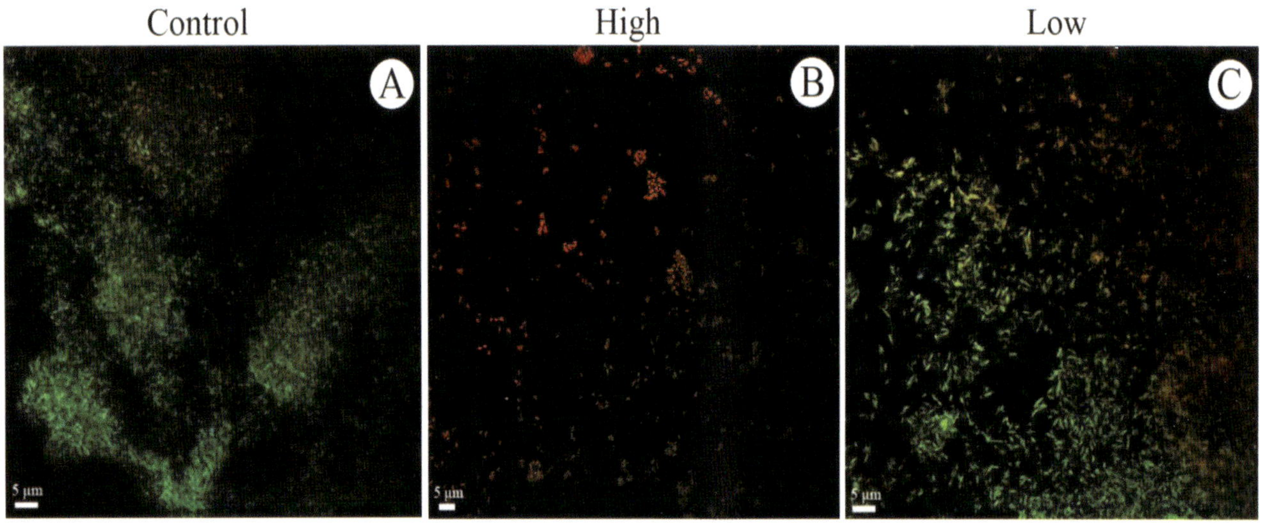

Figure 6. Confocal microscopy of *Escherichia coli* 30 biofilm grown on the polystyrene surface under static conditions at 37 °C for 24 hours. Prevention experiment: (A) Control untreated, (B) Treatment with phage solution with a high titer (10^9 PFU/mL) and (C) low titer (10^0 PFU/mL).

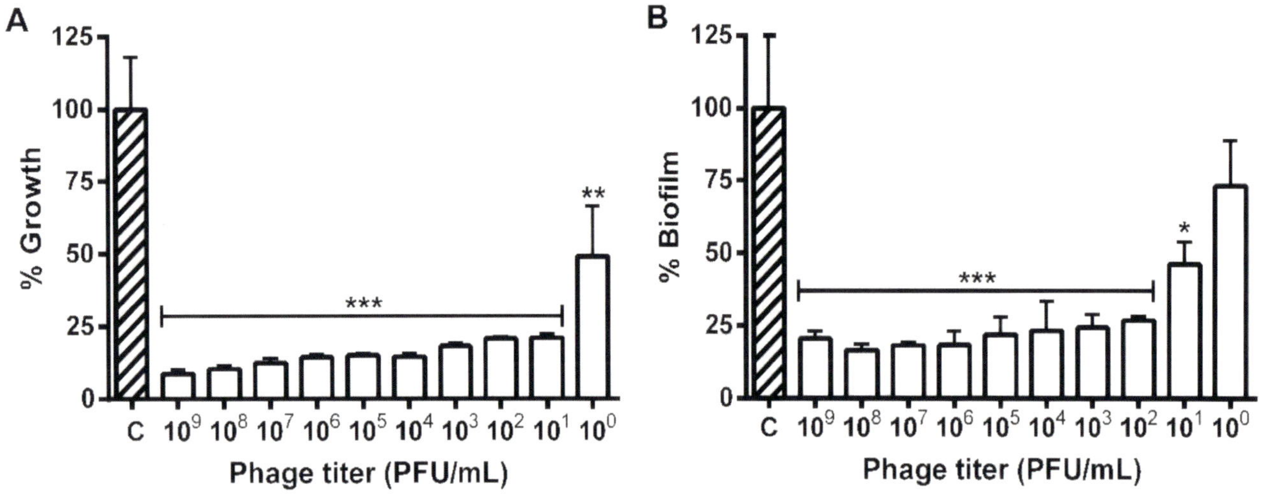

Figure 7. Growth of cell attached (A) and degradation of preformed biofilm (24h) (B) of *Escherichia coli* 30 in polystyrene microplates after 24 hours of exposure to different phage titres (10^0 to 10^9 PFU/mL). * $P \leq 0.05$, ** $P \leq 0.01$ and *** $P \leq 0.001$ compared to the control.

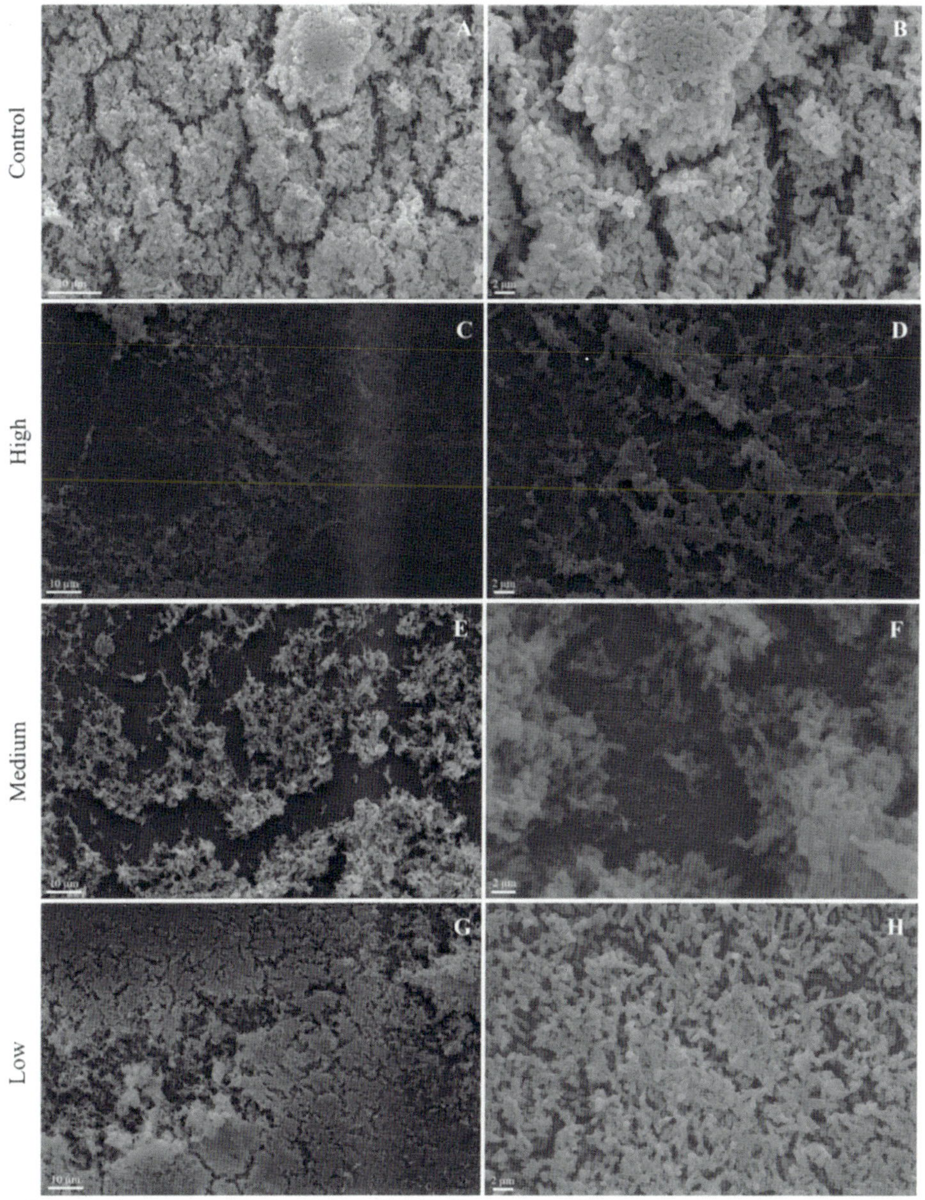

Figure 8. Scanning electron microscopy of *Escherichia coli* 30 biofilm grown on the polystyrene surface under static conditions at 37 °C for 24 hours. Control untreated (A and B). Treatment with phage with a high titer (10^9 PFU/mL) (C and D), medium titer (10^4 PFU/mL) (E and F) and low titer (10^0 PFU/mL) (G and H).

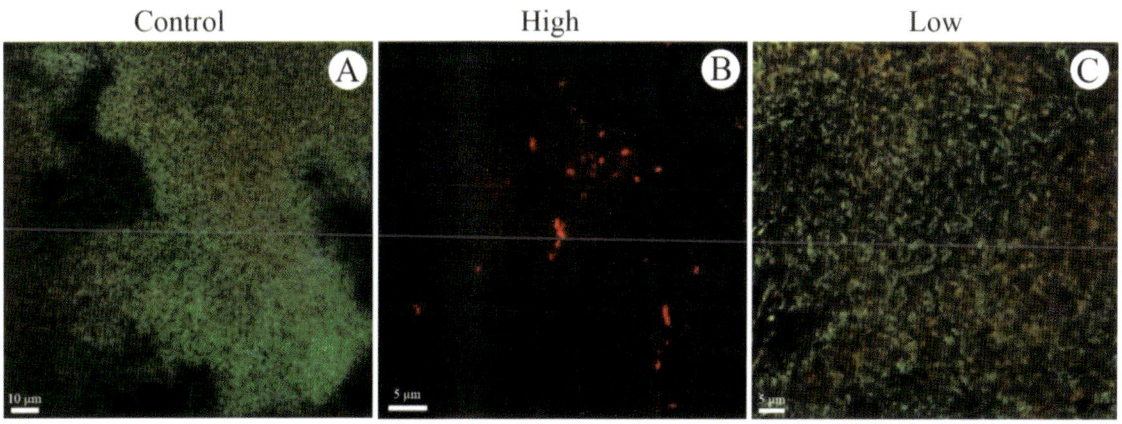

Figure 9. Confocal microscopy of *Escherichia coli* 30 biofilm grown on the polystyrene surface under static conditions at 37 °C for 24 hours. Degradation experiment: (A) Control untreated, (B) Treatment with phage solution with a high titer (10^9 PFU/mL), and (C) low titer (10^0 PFU/mL).

Discussion

The increasing inefficiency of antibiotic therapy to eliminate biofilm-associated infections has accelerated the search for alternative therapeutic agents, including phages.[22] Moreover, it has been shown that *E. coli* 30 can form more biofilm when grown in media with enrofloxacin, which is commonly used in the treatment of *E. coli* bovine mastitis, showing the importance to develop alternatives to the treatment of mastitis caused by this isolate.[23]

There is remarkable variation in biofilm formation by *E. coli* isolates *in vitro*.[24] The biofilm formation by *E. coli* 30 on the polystyrene after 24 hours' incubation is related to the ability of these bacteria to adhere to biotic and abiotic surfaces by physicochemical, molecular and cellular interactions. This action is mediated by the bacterial cell wall appendages, such as fimbriae type 1 and conjugative pili under different temperatures, pH, aerations and nutrient conditions.[25] The high production of biofilm by the *E. coli* 30 strain may be related to nutrient-rich-medium (LB) that ensure the necessary nutrients for cell proliferation and matrix production whereas in nutritionally-limited R2A medium, *E. coli* formed small clusters composed of isolated cells.[26]

Bacteria grown with renewal of media forms a big amount of biomass mature biofilm in microtiter plate.[27] The reduction in the *E. coli* 30 biofilm mass in the 72-hour period may be associated with cell death caused by a drop in the nutrient availability, lack of aeration and metabolite accumulation, resulting in the detachment of the biofilm from the substrate due no media renewal.[28,29] The stress precipitated by hypoxia and nutrient limitation promotes the expression of those genes involved in biofilm dispersion, essential for the bacteria to escape the unfavorable conditions and colonize a new environment.[30,31]

Qualitative analysis of scanning electron microscopy results confirmed the results obtained for quantitative analyses and showed that *E. coli* 30 formed structured biofilm for 48h and *unstructured* biofilm composed of isolated cell clusters after 72h. This shows that SEM is a good quality control of biofilm formation on different surfaces.[32]

Some studies have demonstrated the significant potential of phages to reduce and/or eliminate biofilms.[33] This was reported for a phage mixture where *Escherichia coli* O157:H7 biofilms formed on different surfaces, times and temperatures showed pronounced decrease in its biofilm after addition of phage mixture.[34] In our experiments the EcoM017 phage was able reduce significantly the cell growth and biofilm formed on polystyrene surface. The reduction is due to phage capacity of adsorbing on the bacterial cell surface, inject its genetic material and use the metabolic machinery of the host to multiply, resulting in cell lysis and releasing new particles inside biofilm.[35]

The greatest reduction in the bacterial growth with respect to the biofilm was observed in the highest titer of the phage (10^9 PFU/mL). This is related to the higher susceptibility of the planktonic cells (free) to the phage that are metabolically more active than biofilm cells.[36]

The low quantity of ECM observed can be linked to the *E. coli* growth under inadequate conditions of oxygen (no agitation) and matrix removal during coupon preparation for SEM and can facilitate phage penetration into biofilm.[37] It has been shown that cells at the air-biofilm interface are more evenly spaced and often not surrounded by a fibrous extracellular matrix.[38] The predominance of the viable cells in the hydrated biofilm analyzed by Confocal Microscopy shows a natural balance between the living and dead cells within the biofilm, in which the first stained green (FITC) and the second red (IP penetrated through the damaged membranes).

The presence of single cells and small cell groups along with the dead ones, besides the cellular debris in the biofilms formed when the high titer of the EcoM017 phage was used, is due to phage multiplication-induced pronounced cell lysis. Phage multiplication in biofilms can limit spread of biofilm and maintain cells at density low enough to clear the infection by immune response; however, *E. coli* biofilms treated over several days can develop phage resistance.[39] Alternatively, suspensions that are more concentrated could be used to eliminate the biofilm in a shorter time. Similar efficiency in preventing colonization of the surfaces was observed for *Escherichia coli* K12 and *Pseudomonas aeruginosa* with specific lytic phages.[40,41]

Cellular debris found in the biofilm edges during the low phage titer treatment is due the beginning of cell lysis at the ends of the biofilm as reported for *Pseudomonas fluorescens* grown in stainless steel coupons in the presence of the phage-phiIBB PF7A.[42]

The reduced biofilm formation can be related to the capacity of the EcoM017 phage to access the biofilm and infect the bacteria within causing cell death and degrading the established biofilms.[43] The phage isolated from the sewage also curtailed the biofilm formation by *E. coli* O157: H7 in steel coupons, although the phage concentration used was 10^6 times higher.[44]

The high degradation of the biofilm (79%) with the highest phage titer can be explained by the affinity of this last treatment for the bacterium and the low quantity of ECM present; it has also been reported that the use of the lytic phage in the catheter prevented *E. coli* biofilm formation associated with urinary tract infections.[45] Similar results were observed in *Klebsiella* sp. biofilms treated with the phage isolated from sewage.[46]

Our findings reveal that EcoM017 phage can destroy biofilm architecture due to the aqueous channels found between the cell groups facilitating access to the surface of the bacteria, penetrating even to the deeper layers. So EcoM017 phage to lyse the bacteria at different layers and detach parts of the biofilm in the liquid medium. The detached cells after being released from the groups to the planktonic phase are more susceptible to phage attack.[47] Dead cells and cell debris were also observed in the *Pseudomonas aeruginosa* biofilm treated with the phage isolated from sewage; however, the biofilm architecture revealed fewer alterations.[48]

Phages can be applied to inhibit the adhesion of bacteria, lysing them and favoring the action of antibiotics. EcoM017 phage suspension may be applied in inoculation via the teat canal similarly to treatment with antibiotics to reduce the bacterial attachment and lyse the cells associated with *E. coli* 30 biofilm and accordingly can be used to control of bovine mastitis.

Acknowledgments

The authors would like to thanks the 'Fundação de Amparo à Pesquisa do Estado de Minas Gerais - FAPEMIG' and 'Núcleo de Microscopia e Microanálise - NMM' of the Universidade Federal de Viçosa.

Ethical Issues

Not applicable.

Conflict of Interest

Authors declare no conflict of interest in this study

References

1. Lim JY, Yoon J, Hovde CJ. A brief overview of escherichia coli o157:H7 and its plasmid o157. *J Microbiol Biotechnol* 2010;20(1):5-14.
2. Croxen MA, Finlay BB. Molecular mechanisms of escherichia coli pathogenicity. *Nat Rev Microbiol* 2010;8(1):26-38. doi: 10.1038/nrmicro2265
3. Milanov D, Prunić B, Velhner M, Todorović D, Polaček V. Investigation of Biofilm Formation and Phylogenetic Typing of Escherichia Coli Strains Isolated from Milk of Cows with Mastitis / Ispitivanje Formiranja Biofilma I Filogenetska Tipizacija Sojeva Escherichia Coli Izolovanih Iz Mleka Krava Sa Mastitisom. *Acta Vet Brno* 2015;65(2):202-16. doi: 10.1515/acve-2015-0017
4. Costa JC, Espeschit Ide F, Pieri FA, Benjamin Ldos A, Moreira MA. Increased production of biofilms by escherichia coli in the presence of enrofloxacin. *Vet Microbiol* 2012;160(3-4):488-90. doi: 10.1016/j.vetmic.2012.05.036
5. Thomas V, de Jong A, Moyaert H, Simjee S, El Garch F, Morrissey I, et al. Antimicrobial susceptibility monitoring of mastitis pathogens isolated from acute cases of clinical mastitis in dairy cows across europe: Vetpath results. *Int J Antimicrob Agents* 2015;46(1):13-20. doi: 10.1016/j.ijantimicag.2015.03.013
6. Chaneton L, Tirante L, Maito J, Chaves J, Bussmann LE. Relationship between milk lactoferrin and etiological agent in the mastitic bovine mammary gland. *J Dairy Sci* 2008;91(5):1865-73. doi: 10.3168/jds.2007-0732
7. Bradley AJ, Green MJ. Factors affecting cure when treating bovine clinical mastitis with cephalosporin-based intramammary preparations. *J Dairy Sci* 2009;92(5):1941-53. doi: 10.3168/jds.2008-1497
8. Contreras GA, Rodriguez JM. Mastitis: Comparative etiology and epidemiology. *J Mammary Gland Biol Neoplasia* 2011;16(4):339-56. doi: 10.1007/s10911-011-9234-0
9. Abee T, Kovacs AT, Kuipers OP, van der Veen S. Biofilm formation and dispersal in gram-positive bacteria. *Curr Opin Biotechnol* 2011;22(2):172-9. doi: 10.1016/j.copbio.2010.10.016
10. Burmolle M, Thomsen TR, Fazli M, Dige I, Christensen L, Homoe P, et al. Biofilms in chronic infections - a matter of opportunity - monospecies biofilms in multispecies infections. *FEMS Immunol Med Microbiol* 2010;59(3):324-36. doi: 10.1111/j.1574-695X.2010.00714.x
11. d'Herelle F. Bacteriophage as a treatment in acute medical and surgical infections. *Bull N Y Acad Med* 1931;7(5):329-48.
12. Sulakvelidze A. Using lytic bacteriophages to eliminate or significantly reduce contamination of food by foodborne bacterial pathogens. *J Sci Food Agric* 2013;93(13):3137-46. doi: 10.1002/jsfa.6222
13. Davies J, Davies D. Origins and evolution of antibiotic resistance. *Microbiol Mol Biol Rev* 2010;74(3):417-33. doi: 10.1128/mmbr.00016-10
14. Dini C, De Urraza PJ. Isolation and selection of coliphages as potential biocontrol agents of enterohemorrhagic and shiga toxin-producing e. Coli (ehec and stec) in cattle. *J Appl Microbiol* 2010;109(3):873-87. doi: 10.1111/j.1365-2672.2010.04714.x
15. Liao KS, Lehman SM, Tweardy DJ, Donlan RM, Trautner BW. Bacteriophages are synergistic with bacterial interference for the prevention of pseudomonas aeruginosa biofilm formation on urinary catheters. *J Appl Microbiol* 2012;113(6):1530-9. doi: 10.1111/j.1365-2672.2012.05432.x
16. Bhattacharjee AS, Choi J, Motlagh AM, Mukherji ST, Goel R. Bacteriophage therapy for membrane biofouling in membrane bioreactors and antibiotic-resistant bacterial biofilms. *Biotechnol Bioeng* 2015;112(8):1644-54. doi: 10.1002/bit.25574
17. Lee Y-D, Kim J-Y, Park J-H. Characteristics of coliphage ECP4 and potential use as a sanitizing agent for biocontrol of Escherichia coli O157:H7. *Food Control* 2013;34(2):255-60. doi:10.1016/j.foodcont.2013.04.043.
18. Sieuwerts S, de Bok FA, Mols E, de vos WM, Vlieg JE. A simple and fast method for determining colony forming units. *Lett Appl Microbiol* 2008;47(4):275-8. doi: 10.1111/j.1472-765X.2008.02417.x
19. Thomas P, Sekhar AC, Upreti R, Mujawar MM, Pasha SS. Optimization of single plate-serial dilution spotting (sp-sds) with sample anchoring as an assured method for bacterial and yeast cfu enumeration and single colony isolation from diverse samples. *Biotechnol Rep (Amst)* 2015;8:45-55. doi: 10.1016/j.btre.2015.08.003
20. Calich VL, Kipnis TL, Mariano M, Neto CF, Dias da Silva WD. The activation of the complement system

by paracoccidioides brasiliensis in vitro: Its opsonic effect and possible significance for an in vivo model of infection. *Clin Immunol Immunopathol* 1979;12(1):21-30.
21. Ackermann HW. Bacteriophage taxonomy. *Microbiol Aust* 2011;32(2):90-4. doi:10.1071/MA11090.
22. Kelly D, McAuliffe O, Ross RP, Coffey A. Prevention of staphylococcus aureus biofilm formation and reduction in established biofilm density using a combination of phage k and modified derivatives. *Lett Appl Microbiol* 2012;54(4):286-91. doi: 10.1111/j.1472-765X.2012.03205.x
23. Silva VO, Soares LO, Silva Junior A, Mantovani HC, Chang YF, Moreira MA. Biofilm formation on biotic and abiotic surfaces in the presence of antimicrobials by escherichia coli isolates from cases of bovine mastitis. *Appl Environ Microbiol* 2014;80(19):6136-45. doi: 10.1128/aem.01953-14
24. Beloin C, Roux A, Ghigo JM. Escherichia coli biofilms. *Curr Top Microbiol Immunol* 2008;322:249-89.
25. Reisner A, Krogfelt KA, Klein BM, Zechner EL, Molin S. In vitro biofilm formation of commensal and pathogenic escherichia coli strains: Impact of environmental and genetic factors. *J Bacteriol* 2006;188(10):3572-81. doi: 10.1128/jb.188.10.3572-3581.2006
26. Culotti A, Packman AI. Pseudomonas aeruginosa promotes escherichia coli biofilm formation in nutrient-limited medium. *PLoS One* 2014;9(9):e107186. doi: 10.1371/journal.pone.0107186
27. Lebeaux D, Chauhan A, Rendueles O, Beloin C. From in vitro to in vivo models of bacterial biofilm-related infections. *Pathogens* 2013;2(2):288-356. doi: 10.3390/pathogens2020288
28. De Schutter K, Van Damme EJ. Protein-carbohydrate interactions as part of plant defense and animal immunity. *Molecules* 2015;20(5):9029-53. doi: 10.3390/molecules20059029
29. Karunakaran E, Mukherjee J, Ramalingam B, Biggs CA. "Biofilmology": A multidisciplinary review of the study of microbial biofilms. *Appl Microbiol Biotechnol* 2011;90(6):1869-81. doi: 10.1007/s00253-011-3293-4
30. McDougald D, Rice SA, Barraud N, Steinberg PD, Kjelleberg S. Should we stay or should we go: Mechanisms and ecological consequences for biofilm dispersal. *Nat Rev Microbiol* 2011;10(1):39-50. doi: 10.1038/nrmicro2695
31. Solano C, Echeverz M, Lasa I. Biofilm dispersion and quorum sensing. *Curr Opin Microbiol* 2014;18:96-104. doi: 10.1016/j.mib.2014.02.008
32. Sule P, Wadhawan T, Carr NJ, Horne SM, Wolfe AJ, Pruss BM. A combination of assays reveals biomass differences in biofilms formed by escherichia coli mutants. *Lett Appl Microbiol* 2009;49(3):299-304. doi: 10.1111/j.1472-765X.2009.02659.x
33. Alves DR, Gaudion A, Bean JE, Perez Esteban P, Arnot TC, Harper DR, et al. Combined use of bacteriophage k and a novel bacteriophage to reduce staphylococcus aureus biofilm formation. *Appl Environ Microbiol* 2014;80(21):6694-703. doi: 10.1128/aem.01789-14
34. Donlan RM. Preventing biofilms of clinically relevant organisms using bacteriophage. *Trends Microbiol* 2009;17(2):66-72. doi: 10.1016/j.tim.2008.11.002
35. Viazis S, Akhtar M, Feirtag J, Diez-Gonzalez F. Reduction of escherichia coli o157:H7 viability on hard surfaces by treatment with a bacteriophage mixture. *Int J Food Microbiol* 2011;145(1):37-42. doi: 10.1016/j.ijfoodmicro.2010.11.021
36. Sillankorva S, Oliveira D, Moura A, Henriques M, Faustino A, Nicolau A, et al. Efficacy of a broad host range lytic bacteriophage against E. Coli adhered to urothelium. *Curr Microbiol* 2011;62(4):1128-32. doi: 10.1007/s00284-010-9834-8
37. Suh JD, Ramakrishnan V, Palmer JN. Biofilms. *Otolaryngol Clin North Am* 2010;43(3):521-30, viii. doi: 10.1016/j.otc.2010.02.010
38. Hung C, Zhou Y, Pinkner JS, Dodson KW, Crowley JR, Heuser J, et al. Escherichia coli biofilms have an organized and complex extracellular matrix structure. *MBio* 2013;4(5):e00645-13. doi: 10.1128/mBio.00645-13
39. Kay MK, Erwin TC, McLean RJ, Aron GM. Bacteriophage ecology in escherichia coli and pseudomonas aeruginosa mixed-biofilm communities. *Appl Environ Microbiol* 2011;77(3):821-9. doi: 10.1128/aem.01797-10
40. Arya SK, Singh A, Naidoo R, Wu P, McDermott MT, Evoy S. Chemically immobilized t4-bacteriophage for specific escherichia coli detection using surface plasmon resonance. *Analyst* 2011;136(3):486-92. doi: 10.1039/c0an00697a
41. Ahiwale S, Tamboli N, Thorat K, Kulkarni R, Ackermann H, Kapadnis B. In vitro management of hospital pseudomonas aeruginosa biofilm using indigenous t7-like lytic phage. *Curr Microbiol* 2011;62(2):335-40. doi: 10.1007/s00284-010-9710-6
42. Sillankorva S, Neubauer P, Azeredo J. Pseudomonas fluorescens biofilms subjected to phage phiibb-pf7a. *BMC Biotechnol* 2008;8:79. doi: 10.1186/1472-6750-8-79
43. Xiong Y, Liu Y. Biological control of microbial attachment: A promising alternative for mitigating membrane biofouling. *Appl Microbiol Biotechnol* 2010;86(3):825-37. doi: 10.1007/s00253-010-2463-0
44. Lee Y-D, Park J-H. Characterization and application of phages isolated from sewage for reduction of Escherichia coli O157:H7 in biofilm. *LWT - Food Sci Technol* 2015;60(1):571-7. doi:10.1016/j.lwt.2014.09.017
45. Carson L, Gorman SP, Gilmore BF. The use of lytic bacteriophages in the prevention and eradication of biofilms of proteus mirabilis and escherichia coli.

FEMS Immunol Med Microbiol 2010;59(3):447-55. doi: 10.1111/j.1574-695X.2010.00696.x

46. Chai Z, Wang J, Tao S, Mou H. Application of bacteriophage-borne enzyme combined with chlorine dioxide on controlling bacterial biofilm. *LWT - Food Sci Technol* 2014;59(2):1159-65. doi:10.1016/j.lwt.2014.06.033
47. de la Fuente-Nunez C, Reffuveille F, Fernandez L, Hancock RE. Bacterial biofilm development as a multicellular adaptation: Antibiotic resistance and new therapeutic strategies. *Curr Opin Microbiol* 2013;16(5):580-9. doi: 10.1016/j.mib.2013.06.013
48. Zhang Y, Hu Z. Combined treatment of pseudomonas aeruginosa biofilms with bacteriophages and chlorine. *Biotechnol Bioeng* 2013;110(1):286-95. doi: 10.1002/bit.24630

Protective Effect of Gemfibrozil on Hepatotoxicity Induced by Acetaminophen in Mice: the Importance of Oxidative Stress Suppression

Hojatolla Nikravesh[1,2], Mohammad Javad Khodayar[1,2]*, Masoud Mahdavinia[1,2], Esrafil Mansouri[3], Leila Zeidooni[1,2], Fereshteh Dehbashi[1]

[1] *Toxicology Research Center, Ahvaz Jundishapur University of Medical Sciences, Ahvaz, Iran.*

[2] *Department of Toxicology, School of Pharmacy, Ahvaz Jundishapur University of Medical Sciences, Ahvaz, Iran.*

[3] *Cellular and Molecular Research Center, Department of Anatomical Sciences, School of Medicine, Ahvaz Jundishapur University of Medical Sciences, Ahvaz, Iran.*

Keywords:
- Acetaminophen
- Oxidative Stress
- Gemfibrozil
- Hepatoprotective
- Mice

Abstract

Purpose: Gemfibrozil (GEM) apart from agonist activity at peroxisome proliferator-activated receptor-alpha (PPAR-α) has antioxidant and anti-inflammatory properties. Accordingly, the present study was designed to investigate the protective effect of GEM on acute liver toxicity induced by acetaminophen (APAP) in mice.

Methods: In this study, mice divided in seven groups include, control group, APAP group, GEM group, three APAP groups pretreated with GEM at the doses of 25, 50 and 100 mg/kg respectively and APAP group pretreated with N-Acetyl cysteine. GEM, NAC or vehicle were administered for 10 days. In last day, GEM and NAC were gavaged 1 h before and 1 h after APAP injection. Twenty four hours after APAP, mice were sacrificed. Serum parameters include alanine aminotransferase (ALT), aspartate aminotransferase (AST) and liver tissue markers including catalase enzyme activity, reactive oxygen species (ROS), malondialdehyde and reduced glutathione (GSH) levels determined and histopathological parameters measured.

Results: GEM led to significant decrease in serum ALT and AST activities and increase in catalase activity and hepatic GSH level and reduces malondialdehyde and ROS levels in the liver tissue. In confirmation, histopathological findings revealed that GEM decrease degeneration, vacuolation and necrosis of hepatocytes and infiltration of inflammatory cells.

Conclusion: Present data demonstrated that GEM has antioxidant properties and can protect the liver from APAP toxicity, just in the same pathway that toxicity occurs by toxic ROS and that GEM may be an alternative therapeutic agent to NAC in APAP toxicity.

Introduction

Liver diseases have become one of the main causes of morbidity and mortality in around the world and hepatotoxicity because of drugs appears to be the most common causal issue.[1-3] APAP is one of the drugs that is commonly used to reduce fever and pain. This drug has few side effects at therapeutic doses[4,5] but, overdose of APAP can cause liver toxicity.[6,7] The mechanism of toxicity of this drug is because of the production of toxic metabolites, mitochondrial dysfunction and change the innate immune system.[8-11] Liver is a main critical organ that metabolizes APAP in therapeutic doses in the form of glucuronidated and sulfated metabolites and the following metabolites excreted by urine.[5] Approximately 2% excreted unchanged in the urine and 5% -10% through cytochrome P450 converted to the N-acetyl-p-benzoquinoneimine (NAPQI) which quickly reduced by GSH and excreted in the urine.[12] NAPQI is a strong electrophile oxidizing agent that normally detoxified by GSH in the liver.[13-15] But, in APAP overdose glucuronidation and sulfation pathways become to saturate and APAP metabolism by the cytochrome P450 produces a large amount of NAPQI that leads to rapid depletion of hepatic GSH levels.[16,17] NAPQI causes impairs intracellular calcium homeostasis, increased cell permeability, reduced the integrity of cells membrane.[8,15] It has been reported that released ATP, NAD and damage-associated molecular pattern (DAMP) from damaged hepatocytes can induced liver injury through P2X7 and Toll-like receptors in DAMP sensing cells.[18] According the destructive effects of APAP in overdose and poisoning, new potential therapeutics for APAP overdose are routinely investigated in preclinical studies. Many of these studies have shown that pretreatment or simultaneous treatment with diverse agents can provide protection against APAP hepatotoxicity.[19,20] Antioxidant agents have therapeutic potential in drug-induced toxicity.[21] NAC is used as present treatment for APAP toxicity, by replacing cellular GSH to prevent of cell damage by NAPQI. Administration of NAC is critical to improving the

***Corresponding author:** Mohammad Javad Khodayar, Email: khodayar-mj@ajums.ac.ir clinical effect of APAP hepatotoxicity.[22] Therefore, investigations on agents that have been therapeutic effect on APAP toxicity are attractive.

GEM is a fibrate drug that has approved for hyperlipidemia and commonly prescribed for lipid-lowering.[23,24] The most important mechanism of fibrates is considered as agonists of PPAR-α.[25] But, has recently reported that GEM has antioxidant and anti-inflammatory properties in diverse situations.[26-28] In therapy for diabetes has shown that GEM increase the level of paraoxonase activity as an antioxidant enzyme which clean up free radicals and chelate metal ions;[27,29] as well as can inhibit the pathways leading to inflammatory cytokine release,[30] and also has shown that decreased atherosclerosis in diabetes via reduction in oxidative stress and inflammation.[31] Others fibrates, have shown protective effects against inflammatory colitis,[32] inflammatory heart in autoimmune myocarditis[33] and neuroprotective effects against stroke.[34] In contrast with these studies, there is other reports that GEM weather alone or in combination with statins is associated with the highest risk of myotoxicity as well as GEM causes to increase risk of cholelithiasis and cholestatic jaundice.[35,36] Therefore, considering the importance of APAP toxicity and finding new therapeutic agents against its toxicity, GEM was selected according to its demonstrated properties. With these themes, the present study was designed to investigate the effects of GEM on acute hepatotoxicity induced by APAP in mice, mainly focusing on GEM antioxidant properties.

Materials and Methods

Animals

Experiments were performed on adult male NMRI mice aged 6-8 weeks old, weighing 23 to 27g. The animals were purchased from the Research Center and Experimental Animal House of Ahvaz Jundishapur University of Medical Sciences (AJUMS). They were retained in standard Plexiglas cages with room temperature (22-25 °C) with a 12 h light/dark cycle. During the study all animal have free access to food and water. The animals were acclimatized to the environment for three days before the initiation of research.

Drugs and chemicals

APAP, thiobarbituric acid (TBA), 5,5'-dithiobis-2-nitrobenzoic acid (DTNB) and 2',7' –dichlorofluorescin diacetate (DCFDA) were purchased from Sigma-Aldrich (St Louis, Missouri, USA). GEM was donated by Dr. Abidi pharmaceutical company (Tehran, Iran), ALT and AST activity assay kits were obtained from (Pars Azmoon, Iran). Other chemicals used were of the highest grade available.

Preparation of GEM and APAP solutions

GEM solution was prepared by wetting of GEM powder in glycerin and subsequently levigation in mortar by pestle with the addition of drinking water. APAP was dissolved in warm saline and administered (i.p.) at a dose of 400 mg/kg/10ml after 16 h overnight fasting to deplete hepatic GSH levels and thereby induce hepatotoxicity better.

Experimental protocol

The mice were divided into seven groups (seven mice in each group).

I. Received vehicle (10 ml/kg, p.o.) + a single dose of saline (10 ml/kg, i.p.)
II. Received vehicle (10 ml/kg, p.o.) + a single dose of APAP (400 mg/kg/10ml, i.p.)
III. Treated with GEM (25 mg/kg/10 ml, p.o.) + a single dose of APAP (400 mg/kg/10ml, i.p.)
IV. Treated with GEM (50 mg/kg/10 ml, p.o.) + a single dose of APAP (400 mg/kg/10ml, i.p.)
V. Treated with GEM (100 mg/kg/10 ml, p.o.) + a single dose of APAP (400 mg/kg/10ml, i.p.)
VI. Treated with NAC (100 mg/kg/10 ml, p.o.) + a single dose of APAP (400 mg/kg/10ml, i.p.)
VII. Administered GEM (100 mg/kg/10 ml, p.o.) + a single dose of saline (10 ml/kg, i.p.)

The animals treated with GEM, NAC or vehicle orally once daily for 10 days and then received a single dose APAP. In tenth day, GEM and NAC were gavaged 1 h before and 1 h after APAP. At the end of the experimental period (24 hour after APAP administration), the animals were anaesthetized and blood samples were taken from heart. The serum was separated using centrifuge at 3500 rpm for 20 min for biochemical evaluation. Liver was removed and divided into two portions, one section homogenized for liver tissue biochemical tests and another part fixed in 10% formalin for histopathological assessments.

ALT and AST activity of serum

Serum samples were used for measuring AST, ALT activity by using standard assay kits through auto analyzer (Biotechnical BT-3000 plus Chemistry Analyzer, Italy).

Preparation of homogenized liver tissue

Liver tissue was homogenized 10% (w/v) with phosphate buffer (1 mM, pH 7.4), then centrifuged at 12,000×g for 30 min at 4°C. The supernatant was used for assessment.

Determination of catalase activity in liver tissue

Catalase activity was determined by a slightly modified version. Accordingly, 500 µl of tris-HCl 0.05 mmol was added per one ml H_2O_2 and 50 µl of tissue extract (dissolved in 0.1 M, pH 7.2, phosphate buffer) were mixed and incubated for 10 min, then 500 µl Ammonium molybdate 4% was added and absorbance was measured at 410 nm. The result was expressed as U/g tissue.[37]

Lipid peroxidation measurement in liver

Lipid peroxidation in the liver was measured based on the MDA level. The reaction of MDA with TBA produces a purple color with maximum absorbance at 532 nm.[38] For this assessment, 1 ml supernatant was added to 2 ml TBA and placed in 100 °C for 15 min. After cooling, it was centrifuged (3000 RMP, 10 min) and the supernatant separated. Ultimately, the MDA level was reported as nmol/g tissue.[39]

Evaluation of GSH level in liver tissue

The GSH level was measured using the Ellman's reagent. Briefly, trichloroacetic acid 20% along with EDTA 1 mM was added to homogenate tissue. Then, it was centrifuged (10 min, 2000 rpm) and the isolated supernatant (200 µl) was added to 1.8 ml DTNB 0.1 mM. The absorbance was read at 412 nm by spectrophotometer and GSH level was reported as nmol/g tissue.[40]

ROS level in liver tissue

DCFDA was used for ROS assay in the liver tissue. Cellular peroxides convert DCFDA into highly fluorescent DCF. Briefly, 10% liver homogenate was prepared in ice-cold Tris–HCl buffer 40 mM (pH 7.4). Then homogenate tissue was mixed with 1.25 mM DCFDA in methanol for ROS evaluation. All samples were incubated for 15 min in a water bath at 37 °C. Measurement was determined based on the intensity of fluorescence at 488 nm excitation and 525 nm emission wavelength using a fluorometer (Perkin-Elmer, LS-50 B, united Kingdom) and reported as fluorescence intensity unit (FIU).[41]

Histopathological Assessments

For evaluation of microscopic changes, the liver was fixed in 10% formalin. Then, it was dehydrated through soaking in alcohol and xylol, respectively. Finally, after preparation of 5µ- tissue sections using rotary microtome, the hematoxylin and eosin (H&E) staining technique was performed. The histopathological changes were examined using light microscope.

Statistical Analysis

Statistical analyses were performed with SPSS software, version 16.0 (SPSS, Inc., Chicago, IL, US). Continuous variables are expressed as mean ± SEM. Comparison of mean value was performed by one-way analysis of variance followed by with the Tukey's post hoc test. Graphs were plotted using GraphPad Prism software. Statistical significance was set at $p < 0.05$.

Results

Effect of GEM on serum activity levels of liver enzymes

The results shown in Figure1 and Figure 2. The overdose of APAP can alter the serum liver enzymes activities. Serum ALT and AST levels indicate a measure of hepatic function. When mice were exposed to APAP, ALT and AST serum levels significantly increased compared with control group ($p<0.001$). GEM in doses of 25, 50 and 100 mg/kg could be significantly decrease ALT and AST serum activity levels compared with APAP untreated group ($p<0.001$). NAC also significantly decreased ALT and AST serum levels when compared with APAP group ($p<0.001$).

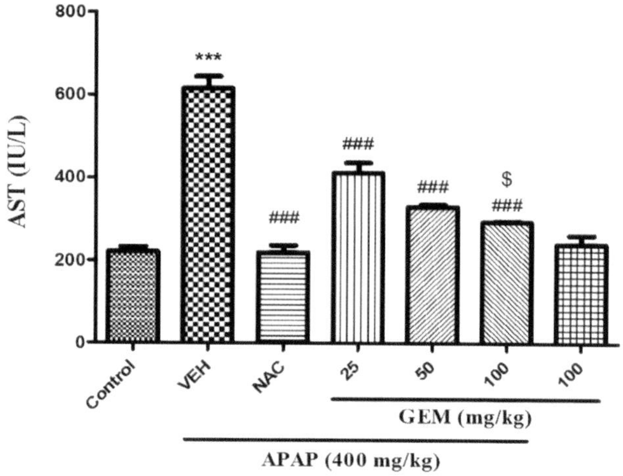

Figure 1. Effect of GEM on serum activity levels of AST in hepatotoxicity induced by APAP in mice. Data presented as Mean ± SEM (n=7). ***P<0.001 shows significant difference from control group, ###P<0.001 designates significant difference from APAP untreated group (VEH) and $P< 0.05 indicates significant difference from GEM 25 and 50 mg/kg.

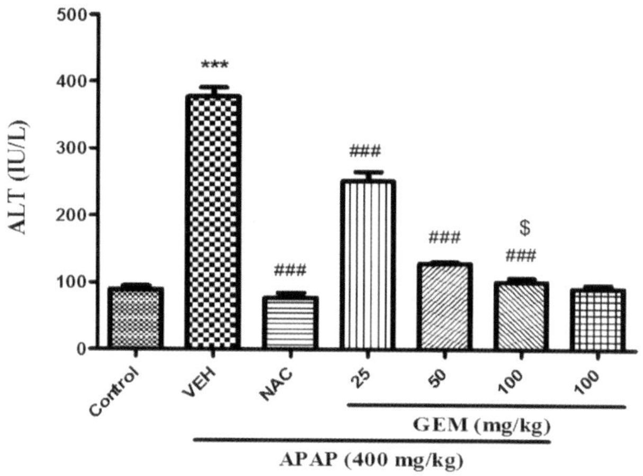

Figure 2. Effect of GEM on serum activity levels of ALT in hepatotoxicity induced by APAP in mice. Data presented as Mean ± SEM (n=7). ***P<0.001 designates significant difference from control group, ###P<0.001 defines significant difference from APAP untreated group (VEH) and $P< 0.05 designates significant difference from GEM 25 and 50 mg/kg.

Effect of GEM on liver tissue GSH level

As shown in (Figure 3) significant decrease in GSH level in liver was evident in APAP treated group when compared to control group ($p<0.001$). However, administration of GEM increased level of GSH when compared with APAP untreated group ($p<0.001$). And also NAC showed significant increase in GSH level when compared with APAP untreated group (VEH) ($p<0.001$).

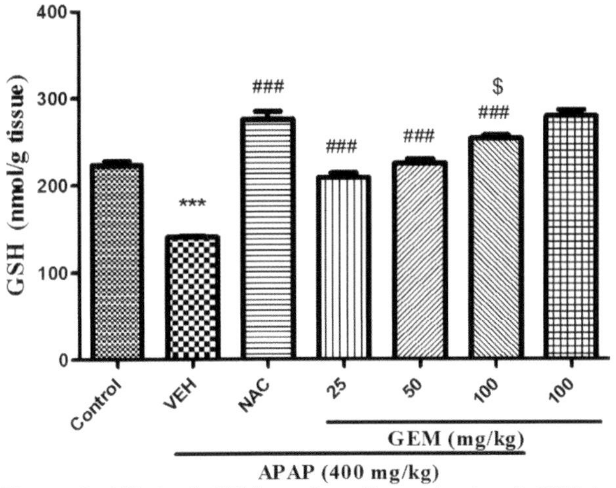

Figure 3. Effect of GEM on liver tissue levels of GSH in hepatotoxicity induced by APAP. Data presented as Mean ± SEM (n=7). ***P<0.001 designates significant difference from control group, ###P<0.001 shows significant difference from APAP untreated group (VEH) and $P< 0.05 indicates significant difference from GEM 25 and 50 mg/kg.

Effect of GEM on liver tissue thiobarbituric acid reactive substances (TBARS)

The results of lipid peroxidation in (Figure 4) showed that liver tissue MDA level in APAP treated group significantly increased when compared to control group (p<0.001). However, administration of GEM in used doses in treated animals suppressed MDA level in the liver tissue when compared with APAP group (p<0.001). And also NAC showed significant decrease in liver tissue MDA level when compared with APAP group (p<0.001).

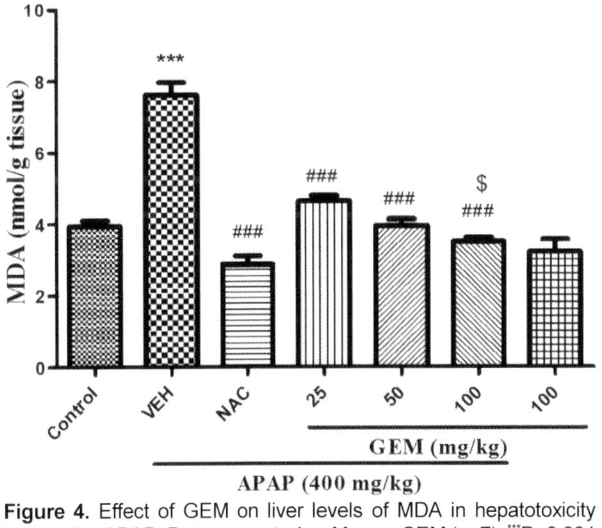

Figure 4. Effect of GEM on liver levels of MDA in hepatotoxicity induced by APAP. Data presented as Mean ± SEM (n=7). ***P<0.001 designates significant difference from control group, ###P<0.001 indicates significant difference from APAP group and $P< 0.05 designates significant difference from GEM 25 and 50 mg/kg.

Effect of GEM on liver tissue catalase activity

As shown in (Figure 5) catalase activity in APAP treated group significantly decreased when compared to control group (p<0.001). However, administration of GEM in doses of 50 and 100 mg/kg (p<0.001) and in dose 25 mg/kg (p<0.01 elevated catalase activity of liver tissue when compared with APAP untreated group. NAC showed significant increase in liver tissue catalase activity when compared with APAP group (p<0.001).

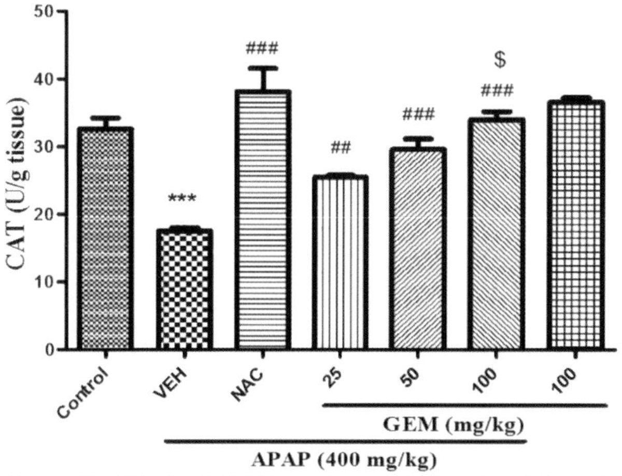

Figure 5. Effect of GEM on liver activity of catalase in hepatotoxicity induced by APAP. Data presented as Mean ± SEM (n=7). ***P<0.001 designates significant difference from control group, ##P<0.01 and ###P<0.001 show significant difference from APAP untreated group and $P< 0.05 indicates significant difference from GEM 25 and 50 mg/kg.

Effect of GEM on liver tissue ROS level

The results in (Figure 6) indicated that ROS intensity in APAP treated group significantly enhanced when compared to control group (p<0.001). However, administration of GEM in doses 50 and 100 mg/kg (p<0.001) and in dose 25 mg/kg (p<0.01) decreased intensity of ROS in the liver tissue when compared with APAP group. Furthermore, NAC showed significant increase in liver tissue ROS intensity when compared with APAP group (p<0.001).

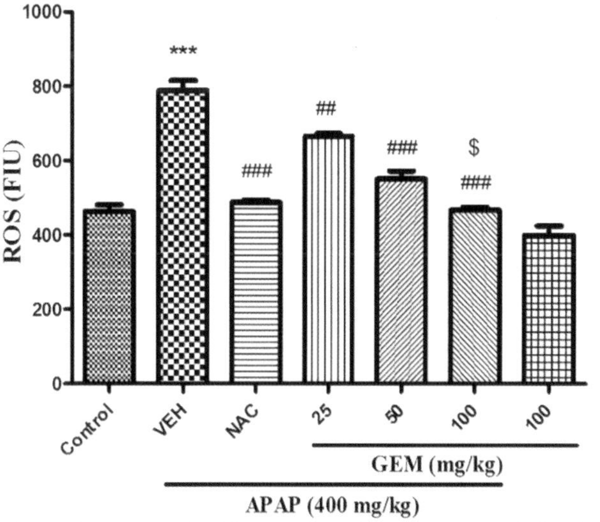

Figure 6. Effect of GEM on liver tissue levels of ROS in hepatotoxicity induced by APAP. Data presented as Mean ± SEM (n=7). ***P<0.001 designates significant difference from control group, ##P<0.01 and ###P<0.001 indicate significant difference from APAP group and $P< 0.05 indicates significant difference from GEM 25 and 50 mg/kg.

Histopathological analysis

Histopathological findings in control liver tissue indicated that hepatocyte cells, lobules and sinusoid status are normal and do not show any damage. But, in APAP group degeneration of hepatocytes, vacillation of vessels, the necrosis of hepatocytes, infiltration of inflammatory cells, and dilated sinusoids were observed (Figure 7). In mice that received APAP plus GEM 25 mg/kg liver damage can be observed but little improvement has been found. Furthermore, in mice that received APAP plus GEM 50 mg/kg, tissue damages and vacillation of vessels significantly improved, sinusoid has been almost normalized and only a small amount of damage in the form of infiltration of inflammatory cells can be seen around the central vein. Mice that received APAP plus GEM 100 mg/kg, liver tissues are normal and there was no serious damage, sinusoids and hepatic cells similar to the control group. In addition, in mice that received APAP plus NAC 100 mg/kg and mice that only received GEM 100 mg/kg, lobules of the liver tissues, cells, and sinusoids are normal and pathological changes were not observed (Figure 7). Semi quantitative scoring of hepatic damage and inflammation induced by APAP and improvement by GEM shown in Table 1.

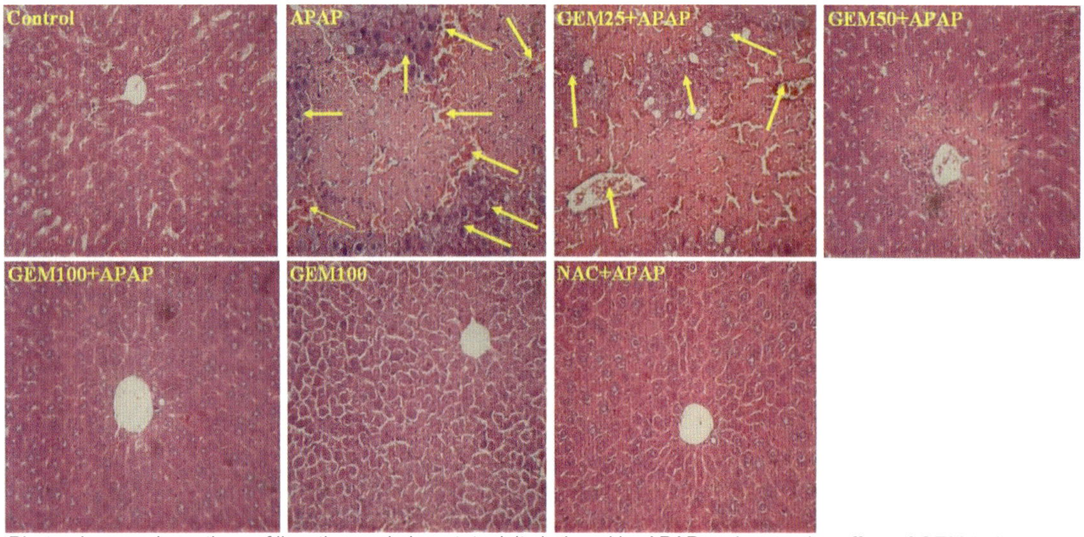

Figure 7. Photomicrograph sections of liver tissues in hepatotoxicity induced by APAP and protective effect of GEM (original magnification: x40). The mice livers: Control; Acetaminophen (APAP); APAP pretreated with GEM 25 mg/kg (GEM25 +APAP); APAP pretreated with GEM 50 mg/kg (GEM50 +APAP); APAP pretreated with GEM 100 mg/kg (GEM100 +APAP); GEM 100 mg/kg (GEM100); APAP pretreated with N-Acetyl cysteine 100 mg/kg (NAC +APAP).

Table 1. Semi quantitative scoring of histopathological examination of liver tissues. (-) indicates normal and (+) indicates mild, (++) indicates moderate, (+++) indicates severe, (++++) indicates extremely severe toxicity and damage.

Groups / Symptoms	Control	APAP	GEM25 + APAP	GEM50 + APAP	GEM100 + APAP	GEM100	NAC + APAP
Hepatocyte degeneration	-	++++	++++	++	-	-	-
Hepatocyte vacuolation	-	+++	+++	+	-	-	-
Necrosis in hepatocyte	-	++++	++++	++	-	-	-
Infiltration of inflammatory cells	-	++	++	++	+	-	-
Dilated sinusoids	-	++++	+++	-	-	-	-

Discussion

In the present study, the liver cell injury by a single dose of APAP was associated with significant increase in serum ALT and AST activities while GEM caused to significant decrease in serum ALT and AST activities. In addition, NAC at the dose 100 mg/kg significant attenuates increasing in activities of these two enzymes due to APAP intoxication. Increasing serum activity levels of transaminases (AST and ALT) have been indicated to liver tissue dysfunctions because these are normally located in the cytoplasm and leakage occurs into the circulation after cellular damage. Normalization serum activity levels of these two enzymes by GEM indicating protection of liver cells. APAP induced injury by its free radical metabolites[12,16] and the protection of liver via antioxidant activity or inhibition of the generation of free radicals are important in the protection against APAP-induced liver injury.[42] Furthermore, pretreatment of mice with GEM 25, 50 and 100 mg/kg against APAP–induced acute hepatotoxicity indicates that GEM ameliorates liver damage via augmentation of liver antioxidant function. Suppression of oxidative stress confirmed by catalase activity and ROS level as well as GSH and MDA levels in liver. It has been shown that different doses of GEM have protective effect in brain damage[43] as well as indicated that GEM has protective effect against the acute restraint stress-induced disturbances in hippocampus in male rat[44] and also demonstrated that GEM causes to decrease atherosclerosis in diabetes via reduction in oxidative stress and inflammation.[31]

GEM possess profound anti-inflammatory and antioxidant activity which, antioxidant properties dependent or independent to PPAR α/β receptors.[27]

In APAP toxicity, oxidative stress plays a key role in APAP-induced hepatotoxicity. Increased ROS levels leads to thiol oxidation that as a result decrease cellular GSH level and reduce activity of catalase enzyme function.[45] GSH is the major intracellular defense molecule against ROS and prevents of oxidative stress in cells. In APAP toxicity GSH causes to detoxifying NAPQI and prevents of oxidative damage to hepatocytes.[45-47] Therefore intracellular GSH levels are crucial in protecting from the toxic metabolite of APAP.

Present data indicated significant decrease in GSH levels 24 hours after APAP exposure. In confirming, others studies reported a significant decrease in GSH level following APAP administration.[48,49] In our study GEM at used doses caused a significant enhance in GSH level compared with APAP group. However, pretreatment with GEM showed an increase in GSH levels that likely inhibits formation of NAPQI or directly reacts with NAPQI and/or prevents of its reaction with proteins (Figure 8).

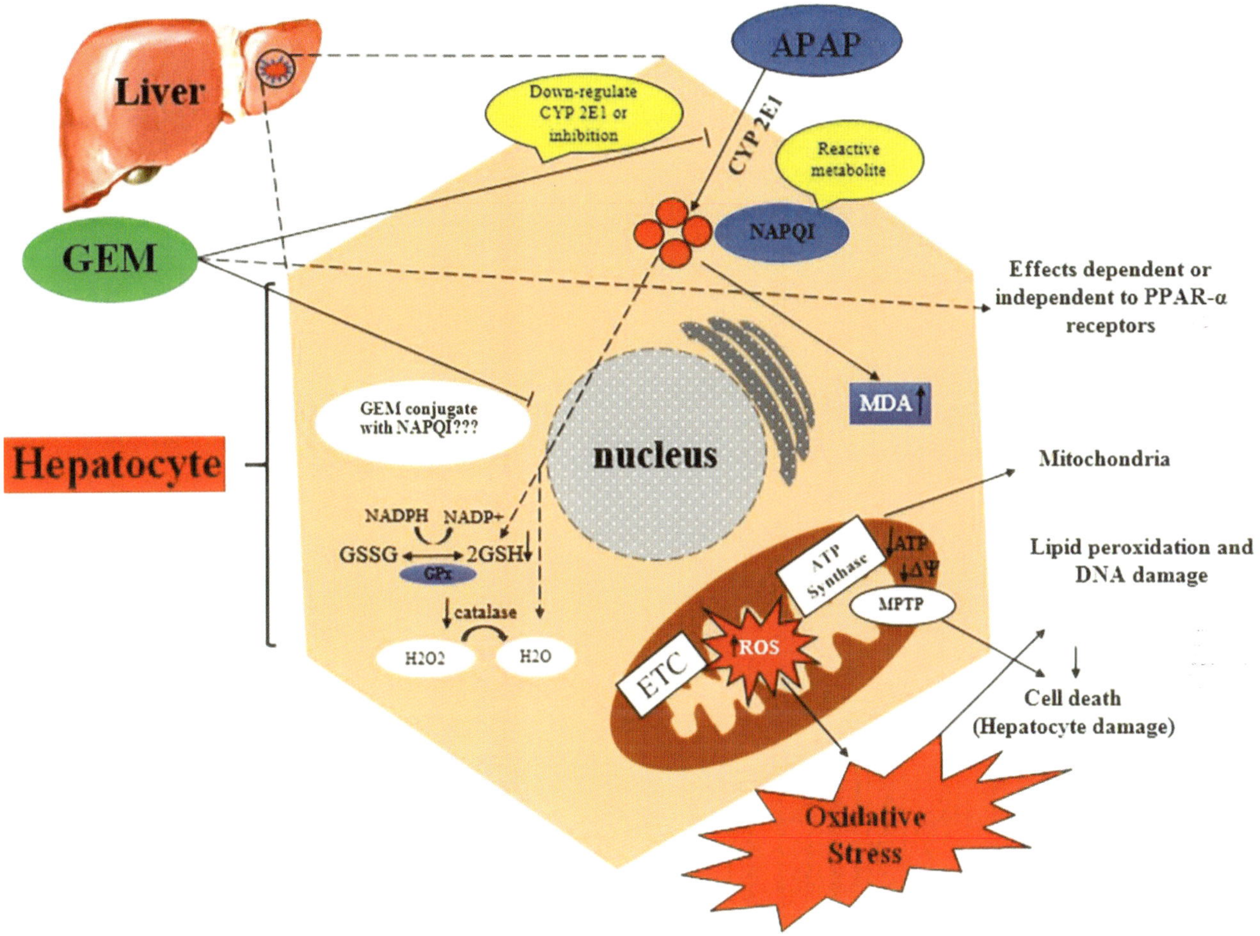

Figure 8. Graphical abstract represented regarding possible effects of GEM on liver damage induced by APAP. GEM can inhibit cytochrome P450 2E1 thus prevention the formation of NAPQI and/or that reacts with NAPQI and inhibits the action of NAPQI to liver macromolecules. GEM restore hepatocyte GSH content and catalase activity and inhibits the formation of ROS and MDA which this antioxidant properties dependent or independent to PPAR α receptors. (ETC: electron transport chain; MPTP: Mitochondrial permeability transition pore)

ROS level increased 24 hours after APAP administration in liver. In APAP overdose, increase in NAPQI level is the main cause that leads to formation of superoxide anion ($O_2 \cdot -$) and hydrogen peroxide (H_2O_2). GEM in all used doses decreased ROS level and this implies antioxidant properties of GEM (Figure 8).

Antioxidant activity of catalase is important for the removal of ROS. It has been suggested that the tissue activity of catalase may reflect ROS levels.[47] Catalase enzyme activity significantly decreased in liver 24 hours after APAP administration and GEM in all used doses increased catalase activity in APAP treated mice. This reveals increasing GSH level and alleviation ROS level by GEM (Figure 8).

ROS attacks lipid membranes and its result lipid peroxidation, impaired membrane function and generation of MDA that MDA is the end-product of lipid peroxidation and can be a indicator of oxidative stress.[50] Consequently, ROS can be calculate indirectly with the amount of MDA and the levels of some antioxidant enzyme activities like catalase in tissue.[51] In previous studies fibrates showed that decreased MDA production in diabetic rats,[52] and also pretreatment with fibrates caused to reduce in MDA level and depletion of endogenous antioxidants.[53]

In our study, the MDA level significantly enhanced in liver tissue in mice exposed to APAP and pretreatment with GEM in all used doses significantly decrease MDA level which suggests GEM may be effective in the prevention of lipid peroxidation formation (Figure 8).

Our findings indicated that GEM significantly inhibited the acute hepatotoxicity induced by high doses of APAP (400 mg/kg) in mice, as shown by a decrease in serum liver enzyme activities AST, ALT levels and also MDA and ROS levels and also increased in GSH level and catalase activity. Moreover, the liver tissue morphology and histopathology findings confirmed the protective activity of this drug against the APAP-induced hepatotoxicity. It is evident by the reversal of degenerative of hepatocytes, vacillation of vessels, the necrosis of hepatocytes, infiltration of inflammatory cells, and dilated sinusoids in hepatic parenchyma by GEM administration. Although this protective effect was dose-dependent, there was no significant difference between doses of 25 and 50. But, according to the results of biochemical and pathological, our study indicates that the highest protective effect is related to GEM at the dose 100 mg/kg. Animal received dose 100 mg/kg GEM and also NAC did not have any differences with control group based on biochemical and histopathological findings and did not cause liver damage. It has been reported that induction of PPAR-α attenuates the extent of oxidative stress in steatohepatitic mice receiving APAP and has hepatoprotective effect due to high repair of liver tissue but not due to suppression of APAP bioactivation.[54] However, application of therapeutic agents before and after APAP can associated with a chance of improvement.

Conclusion

In conclusion, we have shown that GEM has therapeutic effect along with antioxidant activity in APAP-induced hepatotoxicity. Our results propose that GEM with antioxidant properties can protect the liver from the oxidative damage induced by toxic chemicals. GEM may be an alternative therapeutic agent to NAC in APAP toxicity. However, more investigations are needed to realize the mechanism of GEM effects especially modulation and activity of PPAR-α receptors.

Acknowledgments

This paper is issued from a Master of Science thesis in Toxicology of Hojatolla Nikravesh and was financially supported by Toxicology Research Center of Ahvaz Jundishapur University of Medical Sciences, Ahvaz, Iran. (Grant No: TRC-9406).

Ethical Issues

The study was performed according to the Animal Ethics Committee guidelines of AJUMS for the use of experimental animals (code of ethics: IR.AJUMS.REC.1394.602).

Conflict of Interest

There is no conflict of interest.

References

1. Rao RB, Ely SF, Hoffman RS. Deaths related to liposuction. *N Engl J Med* 1999;340(19):1471-5. doi: 10.1056/NEJM199905133401904
2. Yuan HD, Jin GZ, Piao GC. Hepatoprotective effects of an active part from artemisia sacrorum ledeb. Against acetaminophen-induced toxicity in mice. *J Ethnopharmacol* 2010;127(2):528-33. doi: 10.1016/j.jep.2009.10.002
3. Davern TJ, Chalasani N, Fontana RJ, Hayashi PH, Protiva P, Kleiner DE, et al. Acute hepatitis e infection accounts for some cases of suspected drug-induced liver injury. *Gastroenterology* 2011;141(5):1665-72. e9.
4. Larson AM, Polson J, Fontana RJ, Davern TJ, Lalani E, Hynan LS, et al. Acetaminophen-induced acute liver failure: Results of a united states multicenter, prospective study. *Hepatology* 2005;42(6):1364-72. doi: 10.1002/hep.20948
5. Black M. Acetaminophen hepatotoxicity. *Gastroenterology* 1980;78(2):382-92.
6. Makin AJ, Williams R. Acetaminophen-induced hepatotoxicity: Predisposing factors and treatments. *Adv Intern Med* 1997;42:453-83.
7. Antoine DJ, Dear JW, Lewis PS, Platt V, Coyle J, Masson M, et al. Mechanistic biomarkers provide early and sensitive detection of acetaminophen-induced acute liver injury at first presentation to hospital. *Hepatology* 2013;58(2):777-87.
8. Lee WM. Drug-induced hepatotoxicity. *N Engl J Med* 1995;333(17):1118-27. doi: 10.1056/NEJM199510263331706
9. Hoofnagle JH, Carithers RL, Jr., Shapiro C, Ascher N. Fulminant hepatic failure: Summary of a workshop. *Hepatology* 1995;21(1):240-52.
10. Masubuchi Y, Suda C, Horie T. Involvement of mitochondrial permeability transition in acetaminophen-induced liver injury in mice. *J Hepatol* 2005;42(1):110-6. doi: 10.1016/j.jhep.2004.09.015
11. McGill MR, Williams CD, Xie Y, Ramachandran A, Jaeschke H. Acetaminophen-induced liver injury in rats and mice: Comparison of protein adducts, mitochondrial dysfunction, and oxidative stress in the mechanism of toxicity. *Toxicol Appl Pharmacol* 2012;264(3):387-94. doi: 10.1016/j.taap.2012.08.015
12. Zaher H, Buters JT, Ward JM, Bruno MK, Lucas AM, Stern ST, et al. Protection against acetaminophen toxicity in cyp1a2 and cyp2e1 double-null mice. *Toxicol Appl Pharmacol* 1998;152(1):193-9. doi: 10.1006/taap.1998.8501
13. Şener G, Şehirli AÖ, Ayanoğlu-Dülger G. Protective effects of melatonin, vitamin e and n-acetylcysteine

against acetaminophen toxicity in mice: A comparative study. *J Pineal Res* 2003;35(1):61-8.
14. Rumack BH. Acetaminophen misconceptions. *Hepatology* 2004;40(1):10-5. doi: 10.1002/hep.20300
15. Pirmohamed M, Breckenridge AM, Kitteringham NR, Park BK. Adverse drug reactions. *BMJ* 1998;316(7140):1295-8.
16. Yoon MY, Kim SJ, Lee BH, Chung JH, Kim YC. Effects of dimethylsulfoxide on metabolism and toxicity of acetaminophen in mice. *Biol Pharm Bull* 2006;29(8):1618-24.
17. Lee KJ, You HJ, Park SJ, Kim YS, Chung YC, Jeong TC, et al. Hepatoprotective effects of platycodon grandiflorum on acetaminophen-induced liver damage in mice. *Cancer Lett* 2001;174(1):73-81.
18. Hoque R, Sohail MA, Salhanick S, Malik AF, Ghani A, Robson SC, et al. P2x7 receptor-mediated purinergic signaling promotes liver injury in acetaminophen hepatotoxicity in mice. *Am J Physiol Gastrointest Liver Physiol* 2012;302(10):G1171-9. doi: 10.1152/ajpgi.00352.2011
19. Kanbur M, Eraslan G, Beyaz L, Silici S, Liman BC, Altinordulu S, et al. The effects of royal jelly on liver damage induced by paracetamol in mice. *Exp Toxicol Pathol* 2009;61(2):123-32. doi: 10.1016/j.etp.2008.06.003
20. Betto MR, Lazarotto LF, Watanabe TT, Driemeier D, Leite CE, Campos MM. Effects of treatment with enalapril on hepatotoxicity induced by acetaminophen in mice. *Naunyn Schmiedebergs Arch Pharmacol* 2012;385(9):933-43. doi: 10.1007/s00210-012-0774-7
21. Nagi MN, Almakki HA, Sayed-Ahmed MM, Al-Bekairi AM. Thymoquinone supplementation reverses acetaminophen-induced oxidative stress, nitric oxide production and energy decline in mice liver. *Food Chem Toxicol* 2010;48(8-9):2361-5. doi: 10.1016/j.fct.2010.05.072
22. Smilkstein MJ, Knapp GL, Kulig KW, Rumack BH. Efficacy of oral n-acetylcysteine in the treatment of acetaminophen overdose. Analysis of the national multicenter study (1976 to 1985). *N Engl J Med* 1988;319(24):1557-62. doi: 10.1056/NEJM198812153192401
23. Michalik L, Wahli W. Involvement of ppar nuclear receptors in tissue injury and wound repair. *J Clin Invest* 2006;116(3):598-606. doi: 10.1172/JCI27958
24. Nikkila EA, Ylikahri R, Huttunen JK. Gemfibrozil: Effect on serum lipids, lipoproteins, postheparin plasma lipase activities and glucose tolerance in primary hypertriglyceridaemia. *Proc R Soc Med* 1976;69 Suppl 2(Suppl 2):58-63.
25. Dasgupta S, Roy A, Jana M, Hartley DM, Pahan K. Gemfibrozil ameliorates relapsing-remitting experimental autoimmune encephalomyelitis independent of peroxisome proliferator-activated receptor-alpha. *Mol Pharmacol* 2007;72(4):934-46. doi: 10.1124/mol.106.033787
26. Jana M, Pahan K. Gemfibrozil, a lipid lowering drug, inhibits the activation of primary human microglia via peroxisome proliferator-activated receptor beta. *Neurochem Res* 2012;37(8):1718-29. doi: 10.1007/s11064-012-0781-6
27. Roy A, Pahan K. Gemfibrozil, stretching arms beyond lipid lowering. *Immunopharmacol Immunotoxicol* 2009;31(3):339-51. doi: 10.1080/08923970902785253
28. Kabel A, Mahmoud H, El Kholy S. Ameliorative potential of gemfibrozil and silymarin on experimentally induced nephrotoxicity in rats. *African Journal of Urology* 2013;19(4):171-8.
29. Balogh Z, Seres I, Harangi M, Kovacs P, Kakuk G, Paragh G. Gemfibrozil increases paraoxonase activity in type 2 diabetic patients. A new hypothesis of the beneficial action of fibrates? 2008.
30. Cabrero A, Laguna JC, Vazquez M. Peroxisome proliferator-activated receptors and the control of inflammation. *Curr Drug Targets Inflamm Allergy* 2002;1(3):243-8.
31. Calkin AC, Cooper ME, Jandeleit-Dahm KA, Allen TJ. Gemfibrozil decreases atherosclerosis in experimental diabetes in association with a reduction in oxidative stress and inflammation. *Diabetologia* 2006;49(4):766-74. doi: 10.1007/s00125-005-0102-6
32. Tanaka T, Kohno H, Yoshitani S-i, Takashima S, Okumura A, Murakami A, et al. Ligands for peroxisome proliferator-activated receptors α and γ inhibit chemically induced colitis and formation of aberrant crypt foci in rats1. *Cancer Res* 2001;61(6):2424-8.
33. Maruyama S, Kato K, Kodama M, Hirono S, Fuse K, Nakagawa O, et al. Fenofibrate, a peroxisome proliferator-activated receptor alpha activator, suppresses experimental autoimmune myocarditis by stimulating the interleukin-10 pathway in rats. *J Atheroscler Thromb* 2002;9(2):87-92.
34. Deplanque D, Gelé P, Pétrault O, Six I, Furman C, Bouly M, et al. Peroxisome proliferator-activated receptor-α activation as a mechanism of preventive neuroprotection induced by chronic fenofibrate treatment. *The Journal of Neuroscience* 2003;23(15):6264-71.
35. Liu A, Krausz KW, Fang Z-Z, Brocker C, Qu A, Gonzalez FJ. Gemfibrozil disrupts lysophosphatidylcholine and bile acid homeostasis via pparα and its relevance to hepatotoxicity. *Arch Toxicol* 2014;88(4):983-96.
36. Johnson TE, Zhang X, Shi S, Umbenhauer DR. Statins and pparα agonists induce myotoxicity in differentiated rat skeletal muscle cultures but do not exhibit synergy with co-treatment. *Toxicol Appl Pharmacol* 2005;208(3):210-21.
37. Sokolovic D, Djindjic B, Nikolic J, Bjelakovic G, Pavlovic D, Kocic G, et al. Melatonin reduces oxidative stress induced by chronic exposure of microwave radiation from mobile phones in rat brain. *J Radiat Res* 2008;49(6):579-86.

38. Sedlak J, Lindsay RH. Estimation of total, protein-bound, and nonprotein sulfhydryl groups in tissue with ellman's reagent. *Anal Biochem* 1968;25(1):192-205.
39. Sinha M, Manna P, Sil PC. Arjunolic acid attenuates arsenic-induced nephrotoxicity. *Pathophysiology* 2008;15(3):147-56. doi: 10.1016/j.pathophys.2008.03.001
40. Ellman GL. Tissue sulfhydryl groups. *Arch Biochem Biophys* 1959;82(1):70-7.
41. Socci D, Bjugstad K, Jones H, Pattisapu J, Arendash G. Evidence that oxidative stress is associated with the pathophysiology of inherited hydrocephalus in the h-tx rat model. *Exp Neurol* 1999;155(1):109-17.
42. Forouzandeh H, Azemi ME, Rashidi I, Goudarzi M, Kalantari H. Study of the protective effect of teucrium polium l. Extract on acetaminophen-induced hepatotoxicity in mice. *Iran J Pharm Res* 2013;12(1):123-9.
43. Guo Q, Wang G, Liu X, Namura S. Effects of gemfibrozil on outcome after permanent middle cerebral artery occlusion in mice. *Brain Res* 2009;1279:121-30. doi: 10.1016/j.brainres.2009.04.055
44. Khalaj L, Nejad SC, Mohammadi M, Zadeh SS, Pour MH, Ahmadiani A, et al. Gemfibrozil pretreatment proved protection against acute restraint stress-induced changes in the male rats' hippocampus. *Brain Res* 2013;1527:117-30. doi: 10.1016/j.brainres.2013.06.041
45. Yayla M, Halici Z, Unal B, Bayir Y, Akpinar E, Gocer F. Protective effect of et-1 receptor antagonist bosentan on paracetamol induced acute liver toxicity in rats. *Eur J Pharmacol* 2014;726:87-95. doi: 10.1016/j.ejphar.2014.01.022
46. James LP, McCullough SS, Lamps LW, Hinson JA. Effect of n-acetylcysteine on acetaminophen toxicity in mice: Relationship to reactive nitrogen and cytokine formation. *Toxicol Sci* 2003;75(2):458-67. doi: 10.1093/toxsci/kfg181
47. Bayrak O, Bavbek N, Karatas OF, Bayrak R, Catal F, Cimentepe E, et al. Nigella sativa protects against ischaemia/reperfusion injury in rat kidneys. *Nephrol Dial Transplant* 2008;23(7):2206-12. doi: 10.1093/ndt/gfm953
48. Yapar K, Kart A, Karapehlivan M, Atakisi O, Tunca R, Erginsoy S, et al. Hepatoprotective effect of l-carnitine against acute acetaminophen toxicity in mice. *Exp Toxicol Pathol* 2007;59(2):121-8. doi: 10.1016/j.etp.2007.02.009
49. Aycan IO, Tufek A, Tokgoz O, Evliyaoglu O, Firat U, Kavak GO, et al. Thymoquinone treatment against acetaminophen-induced hepatotoxicity in rats. *Int J Surg* 2014;12(3):213-8. doi: 10.1016/j.ijsu.2013.12.013
50. Tayman C, Cekmez F, Kafa IM, Canpolat FE, Cetinkaya M, Tonbul A, et al. Protective effects of nigella sativa oil in hyperoxia-induced lung injury. *Arch Bronconeumol* 2013;49(1):15-21. doi: 10.1016/j.arbres.2012.03.013
51. Pepicelli O, Fedele E, Berardi M, Raiteri M, Levi G, Greco A, et al. Cyclo-oxygenase-1 and -2 differently contribute to prostaglandin e2 synthesis and lipid peroxidation after in vivo activation of n-methyl-d-aspartate receptors in rat hippocampus. *J Neurochem* 2005;93(6):1561-7. doi: 10.1111/j.1471-4159.2005.03150.x
52. Olukman M, Sezer ED, Ulker S, Sozmen EY, Cinar GM. Fenofibrate treatment enhances antioxidant status and attenuates endothelial dysfunction in streptozotocin-induced diabetic rats. *Exp Diabetes Res* 2010;2010:828531. doi: 10.1155/2010/828531
53. Boshra V, Moustafa AM. Retracted article: Effect of preischemic treatment with fenofibrate, a peroxisome proliferator-activated receptor-α ligand, on hepatic ischemia–reperfusion injury in rats. *J Mol Histol* 2011;42(2):113-22.
54. Donthamsetty S, Bhave VS, Mitra MS, Latendresse JR, Mehendale HM. Nonalcoholic steatohepatitic (NASH) mice are protected from higher hepatotoxicity of acetaminophen upon induction of pparα with clofibrate. *Toxicol Appl Pharmacol* 2008;230(3):327-37. doi: 10.1016/j.taap.2008.02.031

Teucrium polium Extract Enhances the Anti-Angiogenesis Effect of Tranilast on Human Umbilical Vein Endothelial Cells

Fatemeh Sheikhbahaei[1], Mozafar Khazaei[2], Seyed Noureddin Nematollahi-Mahani[3]*

[1] *Department of Anatomy, Afzalipour School of Medicine, Kerman University of Medical Sciences, Kerman, Iran.*
[2] *Fertility and Infertility Research Center, Kermanshah University of Medical Sciences, Kermanshah, Iran.*
[3] *Physiology Research Center, Institute of Neuropharmacology, Kerman University of Medical Sciences, Kerman, Iran.*

Keywords:
- Angiogenesis
- Apoptosis
- *Teucrium polium*
- Tranilast
- Human Umbilical Vein Endothelial Cells (HUVECs)

Abstract

Purpose: Angiogenesis plays an important role in numerous pathophysiological events like cancer. As a result of this, tranilast as an anti-fibrotic drug induces the promising antitumor activities through the inhibition of angiogenesis. Further, *Teucrium polium* (*TP*) is a herbal medicine (family *Lamaceae)* with antitumor properties. This study was conducted to investigate the combination effects of tranilast and *T. polium* on human umbilical vein endothelial cells (HUVECs) viability and apoptotic genes expression.

Methods: The HUVECs line was treated using different doses of tranilast and *T. polium* alone or their combination. The cell cytotoxicity was evaluated using MTT and LDH assays; apoptosis was examined using acridine orange/ethidium bromide staining, nitric oxide (NO) production was evaluated using Griess reaction and the expression of *BAX* and *BCL-2* genes were detected using real-time RT-PCR. One-way analysis of variance (ANOVA) test was used to compare the data in different groups.

Results: The survival rate of HUVECs was significantly reduced ($p<0.05$) in a dose dependent manner by tranilast and *T. polium*. However, *T. polium* and tranilast combination significantly ($p<0.001$) reduced cell viability and increased apoptotic cells as compared to each drug alone. Also, HUVECs treated with Tranilast / *T. polium* combination showed a reduced level of NO as regards to cells exposed only to Tranilast or *T. polium* ($p<0.05$). Furthermore, a significant increase in *BAX* and a decrease in *BCL-2* mRNA expression were observed in combination group ($p<0.001$).

Conclusion: *T. polium* synergistically increased the antiangiogenic effect of tranilast on *in vitro* angiogenic model of HUVECs.

Introduction

Angiogenesis targeting has recently been suggested as a promising approach for anticancer therapies.[1] Branching of the vascular network and formation of new blood vessels from pre-existing vasculature identified as angiogenesis is considered as a key biological process, which involved physiologic conditions such as embryonic development, endometrial repair, ovulation, and pathologic changes including solid cancers growth, diabetic retinopathy and rheumatoid arthritis.[2] It has been suggested that angiogenesis requires the balance between the activation of stimulating and inhibitory molecules that initiate or stop this phenomenon. Owing to this, factors such as hypoxia, decreased pH, increased lactic acid, mutations in oncogene and tumor suppressor genes seem to disturb the balance in an attempt to alter the process of angiogenesis.[3] It is evident that in the absence of vascular support, apoptosis and/or necrosis may be activated in tumoral cells. When it is observed that tumor mass is required to achieve more nutrients and oxygen; angiogenesis signaling is stimulated to compensate for deprivation. Hence, inhibition of angiogenesis may be considered as an important way to combat cancer progression.[4]

Tranilast (N-[3,4-dimethoxycinnamonyl]-anthranilic acid) was first introduced by Koda *et al.* to suppress progression of homologous passive coetaneous anaphylaxis.[5] It was later used for the treatment of hypertrophic scars and keloids. Some researchers found that tranilast is able to inhibit the proliferation of fibroblasts *in vitro* and selectively suppress collagen deposition *in vivo.*[6] Also, it was developed as an anti-fibrotic and anti-allergic drug in Japan.[7] Aside these, tranilast was found to decrease the proliferation of fibroblasts from normal tissues and suppress the release of *TGF-β* from fibroblasts.[8]

In addition , its antitumor activity has been reported in some cell lines such as PC-3, LNcap-SF and LNcap (prostate cancer cell lines),[9] LN-18 and T98G (human malignant glioma cells).[10] In addition, numerous studies have shown the antigrowth effect of tranilast on breast

***Corresponding author:** Seyed Noureddin Nematollahi-Mahani, Email: nnematollahi@kmu.ac.ir cancer cell lines like 4T, LA7, MDA-MB-231, MCF-7 and BT-474.[11,12] It has also been shown to block cell cycle progression, inhibit migration and promote the apoptosis of MDA-MB-231 and BT-474 cells.[13] On the other hand, it has been shown that this drug possesses antiangiogenic effect on human dermal microvascular endothelial cells by inhibition of the migration, proliferation ,tube formation, and expression of *VEGF* both *in vitro* and *in vivo*.[14]

Combination therapies with herbal extract have been proposed to reduce the resistance of several cancerous cells to chemical agents.[15] *Teucrium polium (TP) is* a member of the *Lamaceae* family and has been used for over 2000 years in folk medicine because of its pharmacological properties.[16] This herb consists of more than 300 species and is found in Europe and mainly in the Mediterranean area. Plants of this genus have been used for medicine since ancient Greek times, when they were used for coughs and asthma. *T. polium* has been shown to possess antioxidant, anti-inflammatory, antibacterial, antifungal, antiseptic, antipyretic and hypolipidemic properties.[17]

The anticancer properties of *T. polium* have been shown in some studies on a huge number of cancer cell lines, such as MCF-7 and MDA-MB-231 breast adenocarsinoma,[11,12] bladder carcinoma, epidermoid carcinoma (A431), Skmel-3 Melanoma cell line, Saos-2 osteoblastoma, SW480 colon carcinoma,[18] K562 chronic myelogenous leukemia,[19] REYF-1 glioblastoma multiforme,[20] BT20 human breast ductal carcinoma, PC12 mouse pheochromocytoma and A549 human lung adenocarsinoma cell lines.[21] In addition to the antitumor properties of the crude extract of *T. polium*, different fractions of *T. polium* have also shown promising antitumor activity , namely, the petroleum ether fraction as the most potent fraction that was examined on U87 cells.[22]

A major part of the findings on endothelial cell functions is from *in vitro* experiments with HUVECs line. HUVECs are among the most widely used cells of *in vitro* angiogenesis models. These cells provide a classic model system to study numerous aspects of endothelial function and disease such as normal, abnormal and tumor-associated angiogenesis, oxidative stress, hypoxia and inflammation related pathways in endothelia under normal and pathological conditions.[23] Typical characteristics of *in vitro* angiogenesis assays are proliferation, migration, and the formation of tube-like structures by endothelial cells.[24]

Nitric oxide (NO) is an important signaling factor in many pathological and physiological processes.[25] It is secreted by the endothelium of blood vessels and plays an important role in the angiogenic cascade through the modulation of the activity of angiogenic factors released by tumor cells such as *VEGF*.[26] It has been shown that (NO) is present at higher levels in solid tumors, when compared with normal tissues.[27]

Inhibition of angiogenesis as a new therapeutic option can be considered by following the pivotal role of angiogenesis in tumor growth. It has shown that highly vascular tumors have higher potential of metastasis and poorer prognoses. Since angiogenesis inhibition is an effective antigrowth strategy for treatment of tumor cells, for a causal role of medicinal herbs and the lack of scientific documented evidence regarding antiangiogenic of *T. polium*, attempt has been made to survey the effect of *T. polium* alone and in combination with tranilast on angiogenesis and proliferation of HUVECs. Altogether, the aim of the present study was to investigate possible synergistic antiangiogenic effect of *T. polium in* with tranilast, in with the expectation of creating a more effective anti-tumor treatment strategy.

Materials and Methods

Tranilast was purchased from Sigma-Aldrich, (Mo, USA) and dissolved in dimethyl sulfoxide (DMSO) such thatthe final DMSO concentration in experimental wells did not exceed 0.5% (v/v). Dulbecco's modified Eagle's medium and Ham's F12 (DMEM/F12), fetal bovine serum (FBS), trypsin, and acridine orange (AO) were purchased from Sigma-Aldrich Chemical Co (St. Louis, MO, USA). Gene Matrix Universal RNA Purification Kit was purchased from EURx Ltd. Gdansk (Poland ul). PrimeScriptTM 1st strand cDNA Synthesis Kit and SYBR Premix Ex Taq technology were purchased from Takara (Bio Inc. Japan).

Plant

The areal parts of *T. polium* were collected from Khabr (Kerman, Iran) and identified at the Department of Pharmacognosy, Kerman University of Medical Sciences. A specimen was deposited at the herbarium of the Kerman School of Pharmacy (Voucher number: 28125).

The aerial parts of *T. polium* (200 g) were dried and made into powder. Ethanol extract was provided using maceration method in 80% ethanol for 24 h, followed by evaporation by rotatory evaporator at 50° C. The crude extract was fractionated using petroleum ether by solvent-solvent extraction method. The petroleum ether fraction was concentrated by a rotary evaporator and lyophilized in a freeze dryer. The extract was dissolved in 10μl of DMSO, so that the final concentration of DMSO was adjusted to less than 0.05% in the culture medium.[22]

Cell culture and treatment

(HUVECs) were obtained from the National Cell Bank (Pasteur Institute, Tehran, Iran). The cells were grown in a complete medium consisting of DMEM/F12 medium supplemented with 10% FBS in a humidified atmosphere of 5% CO_2 at 37°C. The cells were treated with 75, 150, 300, 600, and 1200 μM tranilast (base on pilot study) and 25, 50, 100, 200,and 400 μg/ml PE fraction of *T. polium* (base on pilot study*)* for 24, 48 and 72 h. Each treatment was replicated in at least three independent experiments and each was carried out in triplicates.

MTT assay
HUVECs (15×10^3 per well) were plated in 96 well culture plate.The wells were treated with different concentrations of tranilast and *T. polium* in culture medium, and incubated for 24, 48 and 72 h.. The viability of the cells was recorded at an absorbance of 570 nm and the reference wavelength of 630 nm using an ELISA reader. The percentage of cell viability= (Absorbance of treated cell / Absorbance of control cells) × 100, was calculated.[28]

Median effect analysis
Multiple drug effect analysis of Chou and Talaly, based on the median-effect principle, was used to calculate the combined drug effect. This method evaluates the nature of tranilast and *T. polium* interaction (synergistic, additive, or antagonistic). The combination of tranilast and *T. polium* in fixed concentration ratio based on their corresponding IC50 values (302.58 μM for tranilast and 98.7 μg/ml for *T. polium*) in two-fold serial dilutions above and below the IC50 value of agents was done. Combination index (CI) and dose reduction index (DRI) values were calculated using CompuSyn software (ComboSyn, Inc., Paramus, NJ, USA).
The CI values were interpreted as additive ($CI = 1$), synergistic ($CI < 1$) and antagonistic ($CI > 1$). DRI value is the degree to which the concentration of a mean compound can be reduced when used in combination with another compound to maintain an equivalent effect and "Fa" is the fraction of cell death ranging from 0 (no cell killing) to 1 (100% of cell killing). Classical isobolograms were also constructed by plotting drugs concentrations (alone and in combination) that inhibit 50, 75,and 90% viability. In this assay, $CI>1$ is the antagonist effect, $CI = 1$ is the additive effect, and $CI < 1$ is the synergistic effect.[28]

LDH assay
The cells (7×10^4) were cultured in 4 well plates and treated with 1.5 ml medium containing tranilast and *T. polium*. Following 72 h incubation, the supernatant was collected and centrifuged at 250 g for 10 min and lactate dehydrogenase activity was measured following the manufacturer's instructions.[29]

Acridine orange / ethidium bromide (AO/EB) staining
HUVECs were cultured in 24 well plates and incubated for 24 h. The cells were then treated with 300μM tranilast and 100 μg/ml *T. polium* and their combination. The plates were incubated for 72h and were then stained with AO/EB dye mixture. (100 μg/ml of AO and 100 μg/ml of EB in PBS). The cells were observed under a fluorescent microscope.[30]

NO measurement
Griess reaction was used to determine NO using colorimetric detection of nitrite. HUVECs were cultured in 24 well plates and incubated for 24 h. The cells were then treated with 300 μM tranilast, 100 μg/ml *T. polium* and their combination of for 72h. The absorbance was measured using an ELISA reader at 540 and a reference of 630 nm.[31]

Migration assay
In vitro scratch assay was carried out to examine the effect of *T. polium* and/or tranilast on the migratory ability of HUVECs. Cells were cultured in 4-well plates and allowed to form a confluent monolayer. Wounds were made with a plastic tip (1 mm width) and debris was removed by washing with phosphate buffered saline (PBS). The plates were incubated for 72 h and the artificial scratch was then photographed.by an inverted microscope equipped with a digital camera, The length of the wound was then chosen for photograph. After photography, medium containing *T. polium* and/or tranilast were added. Finally, the images were analyzed using TScratch software, Version 1.0 (MathWorks Inc).[32]

Real time RT-PCR
Total RNA was isolated from HUVECs using the GeneMatrix Universal RNA Purification Kit (EURx Ltd. Gdansk Poland ul), according to the manufacturer's instructions. The isolation was performed in three independent replicates for each experiment. Complementary DNA (cDNA) synthesis was carried out using cDNA synthesis kit (PrimeScriptTM 1st strand cDNA Synthesis Kit, Takara) in 20 μl reaction mixture according to the manufacturer's instructions. Real-time PCR was performed using SYBR Premix Ex Taq technology (Takara Bio Inc. Japan) on the Applied Biosystems Real-Time PCR One step System in triplicate. Glyceraldehyde 3-phosphate dehydrogenase (*GAPDH*) was used as an internal control. The primers were designed using the Bio Edit and BLAST program. (http://www.ncbi.nlm.nih.gov) After analyzing the data using One Step Software v3.2, the relative expression level of *BAX* and *BCL-2* genes was calculated using two $^{-\Delta\Delta CT}$ formula. The primers were designed using the program Bio Edit, BLAST searches (http://www.ncbi.nlm.nih.gov) performed to confirm specificity of the selected nucleotide sequences.The sequences of the reverse transcription (RT) primers used were: *BAX* forward: TGTTTGCTGATGGCAACTTC and reverse: GATCAGCTCGGGCACTTTAG; *BCL-2* forward: GGGATGCCTTTGTGGAACTA and reverse: CTCACTTGTGGCCCAGGTAT; *GAPDH* forward: ACTCTGGTAAGTGGATATTGTTC and reverse: GGAAGATGGTGATGGGATTTC.

Statistical analysis
One-way analysis of variance ANOVA test was performed to determine the significance of differences among groups using SPSS statistical software (version 16.0 SPSS Inc.). All data were shown as means ± standard error of mean (SEM) and values of $p<0.05$ were considered significant.

Results

Effects of T. polium, tranilast , and their combination on the viability of HUVECs

The cell viability of HUVECs was decreased from 98.33± 0.88 to 36.66± 0.88, 92.33± 1.76 to 30.33± 0.88 and 73.33± 7.35 to 19.33± 5.20%, respectively, with increase in doses of *T. polium* (25, 50,100.200,and 400 µg/ml), after 24, 48 and 72 h. In addition, incubation of HUVECs by increasing the concentrations of tranilast (75, 150, 300, 600,and 1200 µM) resulted in a decrease in cell viability from 98.66± 0.88 to 47.33± 2.02, 96.33± 0.88 to 37.33± 2.02 and 84.66± 0.88 to 9.66± 0.88 %, respectively after 24, 48 and 72 h incubation (Figure 1).

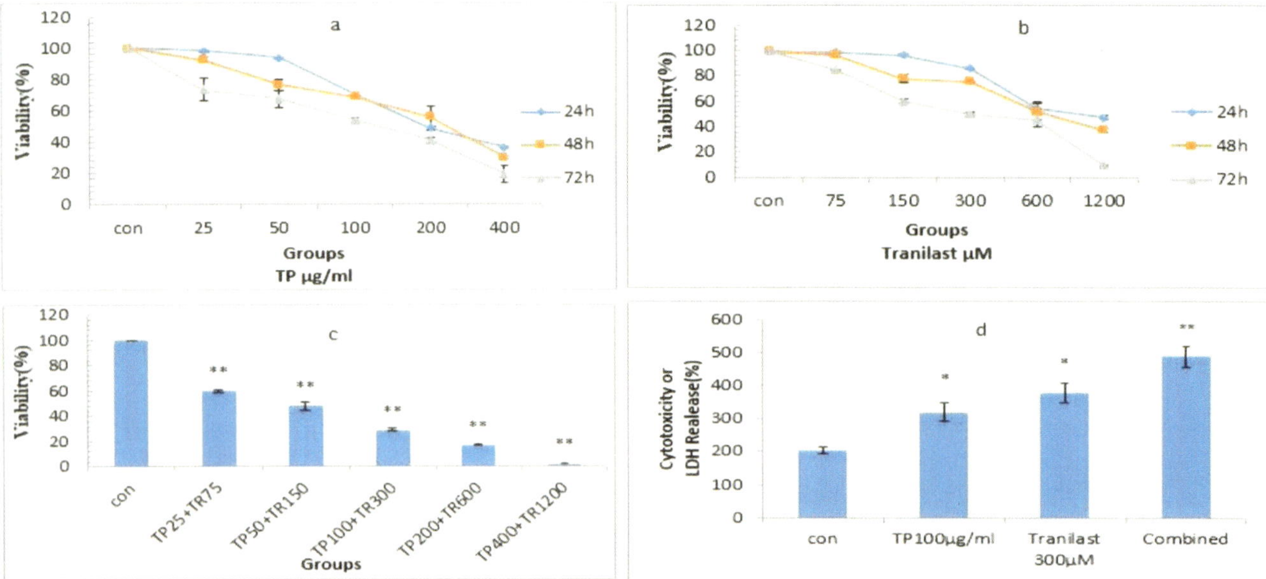

Figure 1. Effects of *T. polium* (a) and tranilast (b) alone and in combination (c) on HUVECs viability and toxicity using MTT and Lactate Dehydrogenase (LDH) assay (d). Cells were treated with *T. polium* and/or tranilast for 24, 48 and 72h and viability was measured by MTT assay. Cells were treated with *TP* and/or Tranilast for 72h and toxicity was measured by LDH assay. Control wells were treated with equivalent amount of medium alone. The values are the mean and SE from triplicated experiments. *TP*: *Teucrium polium* (*P < 0.05; ** P < 0.001 compared with control)

IC50s for *T. polium* and tranilast were about 100 µg/ml and 300 µM, respectively, after 72h, Therefore, 100 µg/ml *T. polium* was used in combination treatment with 300 µM tranilast and cell viability was assessed after 72 h. Combined treatment decreased the cell viability much higher than using either of the agents alone (Figure 1). Combination index (CI plot) , and dose reduction index (DRI), were then calculated.The CI values in all combinations were smaller than one, implying a synergistic effect in all combination tests. The DRI values for both *T. polium* and tranilast were greater than one showing a dose reduction for a given therapeutic effect in both of them (Table 1 and 2).

Table 1. Combination indexa (CI) values for *T.polium* and Tranilast combination

T.Polium(µg/ml)	Tranilast(µM)	CI	Interpretation
25	75	0.71	Synergism
50	150	0.81	Synergism
100	300	0.87	Synergism
200	600	0.92	Synergism
400	1200	0.21	Synergism

Table 2. Dose reduction indexa (DRI) values for *T.polium* and Tranilast combination

Fa	Dose T.polium	Dose Tranilast	DRI T.polium	DRI Tranilast
0.41	68.86	214.5	2.75	2.86
0.55	132.46	341.3	2.64	2.27
0.7	280.2	580.99	2.80	1.93
0.82	608.34	1007.16	3.04	1.67
0.98	9538.88	7102.65	23.84	5.91

Effects of T. polium, tranilast and their combination on LDH activity of HUVECs

Measurement of LDH activity revealed that *T. polium* and/or tranilast significantly increased LDH release after 72 h incubation. Combination of *T. polium* and tranilast significantly increased medium LDH activity ($p<0.001$) more than either *T. polium* or tranilast alone $p<0.05$ (Figure 1).

Effects of T. polium, tranilast and their combination on HUVECs' apoptosis

Apoptosis induction was studied using AO/EB staining in HUVECs treated with *T. polium*, tranilast and their combination after 72 h incubation. As shown in Figure 2A, morphological changes of apoptotic cells include chromatin condensation and cell shrinkage as compared to the control cells. The level of apoptotic HUVECs were 42± 2.30 in 100 μg/ml *T. polium* and 49.3± 3.71% in 300μM tranilast ($p<0.001$). The data showed that HUVECs were more sensitive to combined treatment (81.3± 1.76%) as compared to each drug alone (Figure 2B). By referring to Figure 2A, it was discovered that both early and late apoptotic cells were detected in the presence of 100 μg/ml *TP* and 300-μM tranilast. In the combined treatment, nearly all of the cells were at late apoptotic phase.

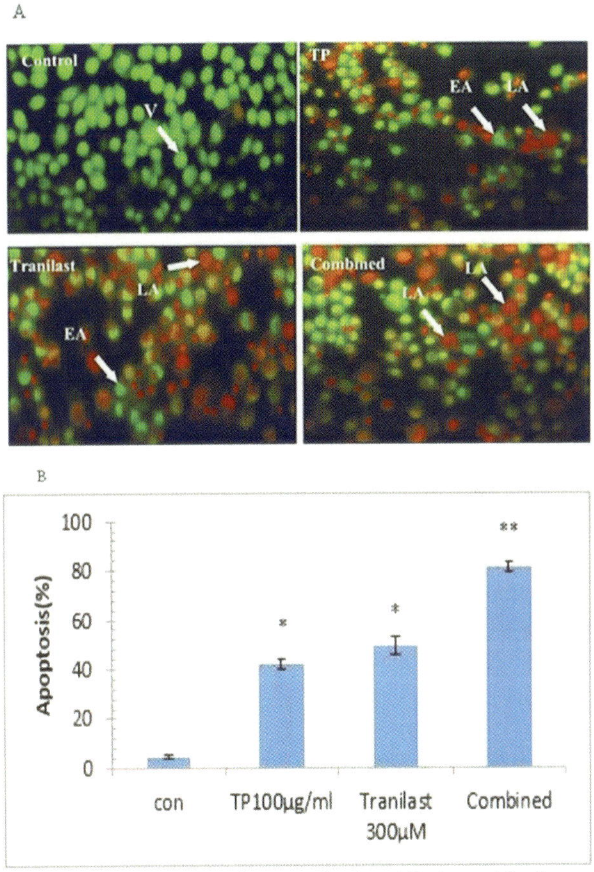

Figure 2. Effects of *T. polium,* tranilast and their combination on apoptosis in HUVECs stained with AO/EB after 72 h. a: Fluorescence Micrographs of cells in control, *T. polium*, tranilast and their combination after 72h. V: viable, EA: early apoptotic, LA: late apoptotic magnification 400x. b: Quantitation of apoptotic HUVEC cells. The values are expressed as mean±S.E. *p<0.05 and **p<0.001. *TP: Teucrium polium*. Con: Control

Effects of T. polium, tranilast and their combination on NO production

The findings of Griess method showed that *T. polium* (P= 0.002) and tranilast (P= 0.01) significantly decreased the NO secretion of HUVECs cells after 72 h compared with the control. Furthermore, *T. polium*/Tranilast combination significantly reduced NO content, the same content for each drug alone (P=0.002) (Figure 3).

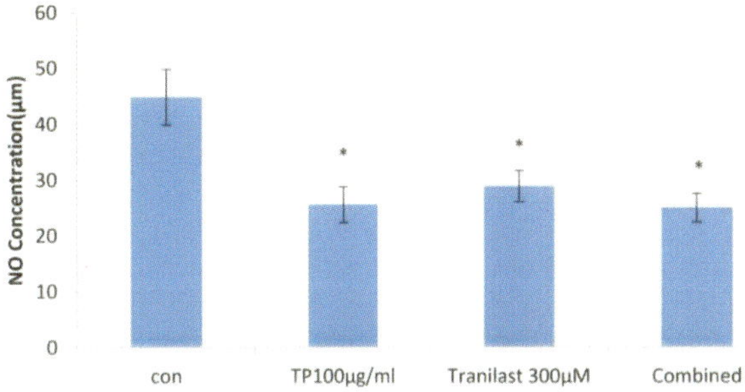

Figure 3. The effects of *T. polium* and/or tranilast on nitric oxide (NO) production in HUVECs. Cells were treated with *T. polium*, tranilast and their combination for 72 h and nitric oxide concentration was measured using Griess assay. Control wells were treated with equivalent amount of medium. The values are mean±SD from triplicated experiments. (*P<0.05 compared to the control). *TP: Teucrium polium*. Con: Control

Effects of T. polium, tranilast and their combination on migration potential of HUVECs'

To evaluate the effects of *TP* and tranilast as a single and/or combined treatment on cell migration, wound healing (scratch) assay in HUVECs was performed. After 72 h treatment, cells in the control group efficiently spread into the wound area to such an extent that the wound boundary was almost indistinguishable, whereas a low number of cells in *TP* or tranilast treated groups crossed the artificial wound boundary. The results clearly showed that *T. polium*(P= 0.00) and tranilast (P=0.00) alone and in combination (P=0.00) significantly decreased the migration of HUVECs (Figure 4).

Effects of T. polium , tranilast and their combination on the expression of BAX and BCL-2

To investigate the mode of action of *T. polium*, tranilast and their combination on cell death, *BAX* and *BCL-2* mRNA expression was evaluated using quantitative real time PCR. *T. polium* , tranilast and their combination increased the expression of *BAX,* a pro-apoptotic molecule, and decreased the expression of *BCL-2*, an anti-apoptotic molecule in HUVECs after 72 h. ($p<0.001$) when compared with the control. As shown in Figure 5, *BAX* / *BCL-2* mRNA ratios were7.7 in *T. polium TP* (P=0.003), 9.3 in tranilast (P= 0.001) and 18 in combined group (P=0.000). Thus, up-regulation of *BAX* and down-regulation of *BCL-2* mRNAs observed in this study may be one of the fundamental mechanisms through which *T. polium* and/or tranilast induces apoptosis in HUVECs.

Discussion

In this study, the synergic effect of *T. polium*, a medicinal plant, and tranilast on HUVECs was studied for the first time. *T. polium* and tranilast alone, and in combination reduced the viability of HUVECs in a dose- and time-dependent manner. Combined treatment significantly increased cytotoxicity with a combination index value between 0.71 and 0.21, showing synergistic effects of *T. polium* and tranilast that were in line with LDH assay.

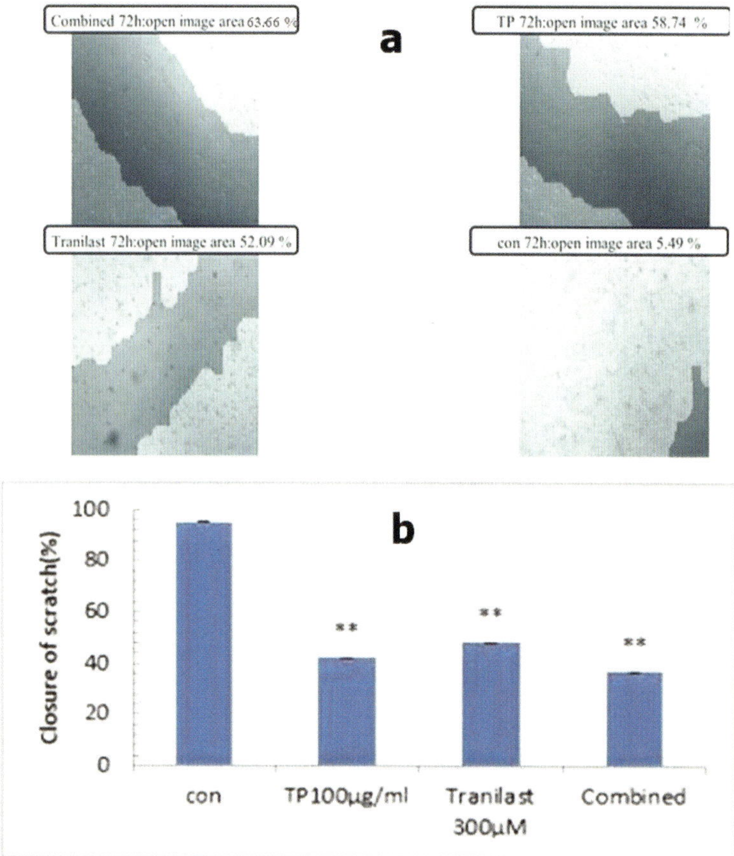

Figure 4. The effects of *T. polium*, tranilast and their combination of them on migration in HUVECs' line. Confluent cells were scratched and then treated with *T. polium*, tranilast and their combination of them for 72 h. Closure of the scratches was photographed (a) and calculated (b) as the percentage of migration. (** p<0.001 vs. control). *TP: Teucrium polium*. Con: Control

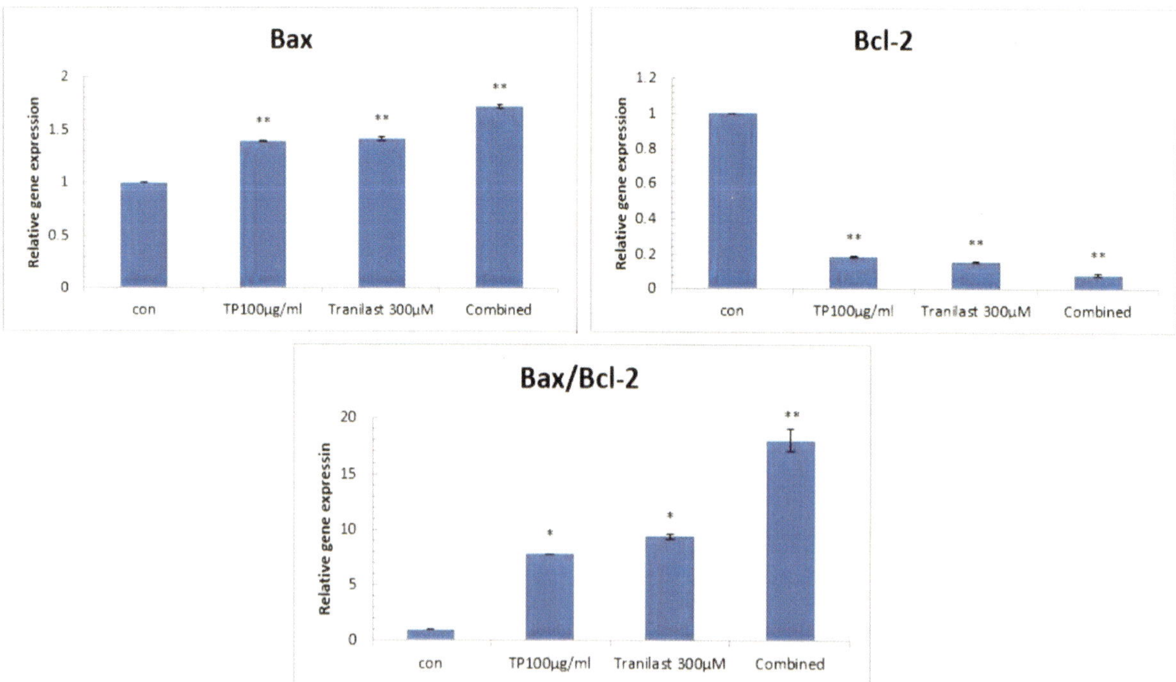

Figure 5. Effects of *TP*, Tranilast and their combination on mRNA expression of *Bax* and *Bcl-2* genes of HUVECs using real-time RT-PCR after 72h. Quantitative RT-PCR was done in HUVECs treated by *TP*, tranilast and combination of them. A significant increase in *BAXx/BCL-2* ratio was observed with combined treatment of TP and Tranilast, respectively, compared to the control. The values are expressed as mean±S.E. *p<0.05 and **p<0.001. *TP: Teucrium polium*. Con: Control

Petroleum ether fraction of *T. polium* has been reported as the most active fraction of *T. polium* on U87 cells.[22] The most anti-proliferative properties of *T. polium* are believed to be related to terpenoids and flavonoids. These compounds in *T. polium* extract are able to influence a variety of cell functions by inhibiting cell proliferation and migration.[19]

Tranilast inhibits the proliferation of human coronary smooth muscle cells (SMCs) in a dose dependent manner. Cell-cycle analysis using flow cytometry showed that tranilast arrests the SMC cell cycle at G1 in growing-phase cells and inhibited the cell-cycle progression from G0:G1 to S phase in G0-arrested cells.[33] To understand the possible mechanisms involved in the antiangiogenic activity of tranilast and *T. polium* combination, the rate of apoptosis in HUVECs was calculated. According to the AO/EB staining results, tranilast and *T. polium* combination significantly induced apoptosis in HUVECs, when compared with the untreated cells and single drug treatments.

The results were consistent with previous study that *T. polium*/vincristine and *T. polium*/vinblastine combinations treatment has induced apoptosis and provoked tumor cell killing in several human cancer cell lines such as MCF7, A431, SW480, Skmel3 and EJ. In agreement with the results, combination of *T. polium* and doxorubicin resulted in a massive apoptosis compared with the effect of individual drugs. Moreover, combinations with *T. polium* extract reduced the cytotoxic effects of known anticancer drugs.[18] Some studies have also shown the ability of tranilast to induce apoptosis in MDA-MB-231 and MCF-7 cell lines. It is the fact that AO/EB staining is a convenient way to diagnose the appearance of dense chromatin, the nuclear fragmentation and the apoptotic bodies in tranilast treated cells.[34]

To elucidate the underlying mechanism involved in the apoptotic properties of tranilast, *T. polium*, and their combination, the expression of apoptosis-related genes have beed evaluated. *BAX* is a proapoptotic *BCL-2* family member that plays an important role in induction of mitochondrial dependent apoptosis. On the other hand, *BCL-2* is an antiapoptotic member that can counteract *BAX* function in initiation of cell death. Modulations of these factors to inhibit or stimulate apoptosis determine the fate of the cells to die or survive.[35]

Some alterations were determined in the expression of *BAX* and *BCL-2* after different treatments. Combination of tranilast and *T. polium* resulted in upregulation of *BAX* and downregulation of *BCL-2*, and an increased ratio *of BAX/BCL2*. The findings of the present study are supported the experiments by Haïdara et al. who reported an increase in *BAX/BCL2* ratio following treatment of MCF-7 and MDA-MB-231 by combination of tranilast and tamoxifen. Flavonoid compounds in *T. polium* also have antiproliferative property that can induce apoptosis via *P53* and other regulators of cell apoptosis.[36] Therefore, cell death induced by *T. polium* extract could be related to *P53* activation and other regulators of cell death and apoptosis.

In mammals including humans, NO is an important cell-signaling molecule involved in many physiological and pathological processes. NO is a mediator of angiogenesis as well.[37] *T. polium* and/ or tranilast in our experiments significantly reduced NO production in HUVECs. Combination of 100 µg/ml *T. polium* and 300-µM tranilast had more profound effect on NO production in HUVECs. It has been reported that tranilast is able to inhibit NO release from N9 microglial cells via suppression of iNOS mRNA expression and iNOS protein accumulation.[38]

The present experiments clearly showed that *in vitro* combination therapy of *T. polium* and tranilast could significantly increase anti-angiogenic properties of these agents in an *in vitro* model of angiogenesis (HUVECs) cells. However, *in vivo* studies on solid tumors in a suitable animal model could highlight the probable potential of *T. polium* /tranilast combination therapy as an antiangiogenic therapy procedure in solid tumors.

Conclusion

These results showed that *T. polium* (*TP*) plus tranilast could be a promising combination therapy for future clinical trials in cancer patients through angiogenesis inhibition. Combination of *T.polium* and tranilast can induce anti-angiogenic effects on HUVECs, which in turn lead to reduced cell viability, increased apoptosis and decreased migration capacity of these cells. Further *in vivo* studies and future clinical trials are proposed to evaluate the efficacy of *T. polium* and tranilast combination therapy for angiogenesis inhibition as a new therapeutic option.

Acknowledgments

This study was part of Ph.D. thesis. The authors appreciate the financial support of this investigation by Kerman and Kermanshah University of Medical Sciences. The authors would like to thank Radan native english edit for editing the manuscript.

Ethical Issues

This experimental *in vitro* study was carried out using HUVECs. This study was approved by ethics committee at Kerman University of Medical Science. Ethical code: IR. KMU.REC.1395.152.

Conflict of Interest

The authors declare that they have no competing interest.

References

1. Scappaticci FA. Mechanisms and future directions for angiogenesis-based cancer therapies. *J Clin Oncol* 2002;20(18):3906-27. doi: 10.1200/JCO.2002.01.033
2. Hanahan D, Folkman J. Patterns and emerging mechanisms of the angiogenic switch during tumorigenesis. *Cell* 1996;86(3):353-64. doi: 10.1016/S0092-8674(00)80108-7

3. Esfandiari N, Khazaei M, Ai J, Nazemian Z, Jolly A, Casper RF. Angiogenesis following three-dimensional culture of isolated human endometrial stromal cells. *Int J Fertil Steril* 2008;2(1):19-22. doi: 10.1016/j.fertnstert.2004.07.157
4. Otrock ZK, Mahfouz RA, Makarem JA, Shamseddine AI. Understanding the biology of angiogenesis: Review of the most important molecular mechanisms. *Blood Cells Mol Dis* 2007;39(2):212-20. doi: 10.1016/j.bcmd.2007.04.001
5. Koda A, Nagai H, Watanabe S, Yanagihara Y, Sakamoto K. Inhibition of hypersensitivity reactions by a new drug, N(3',4'-dimethoxycinnamoyl) anthranilic acid (N-5'). *J Allergy Clin Immunol* 1976;57(5):396-407. doi: 10.1016/0091-6749(76)90054-3
6. Isaji M, Nakajoh M, Naito J. Selective inhibition of collagen accumulation by N-(3,4-dimethoxycinnamoyl)anthranilic acid (N-5') in granulation tissue. *Biochem Pharmacol* 1987;36(4):469-74. doi: 10.1016/0006-2952(87)90353-4
7. Shime H, Kariya M, Orii A, Momma C, Kanamori T, Fukuhara K, et al. Tranilast inhibits the proliferation of uterine leiomyoma cells in vitro through G1 arrest associated with the induction of p21(waf1) and p53. *J Clin Endocrinol Metab* 2002;87(12):5610-7. doi: 10.1210/jc.2002-020444
8. Oshima T, Kurosaka D, Kato K, Kurosaka H, Mashima Y, Tanaka Y, et al. Tranilast inhibits cell proliferation and collagen synthesis by rabbit corneal and Tenon's capsule fibroblasts. *Curr Eye Res* 2000;20(4):283-6. doi: 10.1076/0271-3683(200004)2041-5ft283
9. Izumi K, Mizokami A, Li YQ, Narimoto K, Sugimoto K, Kadono Y, et al. Tranilast inhibits hormone refractory prostate cancer cell proliferation and suppresses transforming growth factor β1-associated osteoblastic changes. *Prostate* 2009;69(11):1222-34. doi: 10.1002/pros.20975
10. Platten M, Wild-Bode C, Wick W, Leitlein J, Dichgans J, Weller M. N-[3,4-dimethoxycinnamoyl]-anthranilic acid (tranilast) inhibits transforming growth factor-β release and reduces migration and invasiveness of human malignant glioma cells. *Int J Cancer* 2001;93(1):53-61. doi: 10.1002/ijc.1289
11. Nie L, Oishi Y, Doi I, Shibata H, Kojima I. Inhibition of proliferation of mcf-7 breast cancer cells by a blocker of ca^{2+}-permeable channel. *Cell Calcium* 1997;22(2):75-82. doi: 10.1016/S0143-4160(97)90107-X
12. Chakrabarti R, Subramaniam V, Abdalla S, Jothy S, Prud'homme GJ. Tranilast inhibits the growth and metastasis of mammary carcinoma. *Anticancer Drugs* 2009;20(5):334-45. doi: 10.1097/CAD.0b013e328327994e
13. Subramaniam V, Ace O, Prud'homme GJ, Jothy S. Tranilast treatment decreases cell growth, migration and inhibits colony formation of human breast cancer cells. *Exp Mol Pathol* 2011;90(1):116-22. doi: 10.1016/j.yexmp.2010.10.012
14. Isaji M, Miyata H, Ajisawa Y, Takehana Y, Yoshimura N. Tranilast inhibits the proliferation, chemotaxis and tube formation of human microvascular endothelial cells in vitro and angiogenesis in vivo. *Br J Pharmacol* 1997;122(6):1061-6. doi: 10.1038/sj.bjp.0701493
15. Nathan M, Scholten R. The complete german commission e monographs: Therapeutic guide to herbal medicines. *Ann Intern Med 1*999;130(5):459. doi: 10.7326/0003-4819-130-5-199903020-00024
16. Simonyan KV, Chavushyan VA. Neuroprotective activity of hydroponic teucrium polium following bilateral ovariectomy. *Metab Brain Dis* 2015;30(3):785-92. doi: 10.1007/s11011-014-9640-2
17. Menichini F, Conforti F, Rigano D, Formisano C, Piozzi F, Senatore F. Phytochemical composition, anti-inflammatory and antitumour activities of four teucrium essential oils from greece. *Food Chem* 2009;115(2):679-86. doi: 10.1016/j.foodchem.2008.12.067
18. Rajabalian S. Methanolic extract of Teucrium polium L. Potentiates the cytotoxic and apoptotic effects of anticancer drugs of vincristine, vinblastine and doxorubicin against a panel of cancerous cell lines. *Exp Oncol* 2008;30(2):133-8.
19. Stankovic MS, Mitrovic TL, Matic IZ, Topuzovic MD, Stamenkovic SM. New Values of Teucrium species: in Vitro Study of Cytotoxic Activities of Secondary Metabolites. *Not Bot Horti Agrobo* 2015;43(1):41-6. doi: 10.15835/nbha4319746
20. Line MC. Evaluation of cytotoxic effect of teuerium polium on a new glioblastoma multiforme cell line (reyf-1) using mtt and soft agar clonogenic assays. *Int J Pharmacol* 2007;3(5):435-7.
21. Nematollahi-Mahani S, Rezazadeh-Kermani M, Mehrabani M, Nakhaee N. Cytotoxic effects of teucrium polium. On some established cell lines. *Pharm Biol* 2007;45(4):295-8. doi: 10.1080/13880200701214904
22. Mahdinia Z, Eftekharvaghefi R, Nabipour F. In vitro inhibition of the growth of glioblastoma by teucrium polium crude extract and fractions. *Int J Phytomed* 2012;4(4):582-8.
23. Nakatsu MN, Sainson RC, Aoto JN, Taylor KL, Aitkenhead M, Perez-del-Pulgar S, et al. Angiogenic sprouting and capillary lumen formation modeled by human umbilical vein endothelial cells (HUVEC) in fibrin gels: The role of fibroblasts and angiopoietin-1. *Microvasc Res* 2003;66(2):102-12.
24. Park EH, Park JY, Yoo HS, Yoo JE, Lee HL. Assessment of the anti-metastatic properties of sanguiin H-6 in HUVECs and MDA-MB-231 human breast cancer cells. *Bioorg Med Chem Lett* 2016;26(14):3291-4. doi: 10.1016/j.bmcl.2016.05.050
25. Mirzaei F, Khazaei M. Role of nitric oxide in biological systems: A systematic review. *J Mazandaran Univ Med Sci* 2017;27(150):192-222.

26. Morbidelli L, Chang CH, Douglas JG, Granger HJ, Ledda F, Ziche M. Nitric oxide mediates mitogenic effect of VEGF on coronary venular endothelium. *Am J Physiol* 1996;270(1):H411-5. doi: 10.1152/ajpheart.1996.270.1.h411
27. Gallo O, Fini-Storchi I, Vergari WA, Masini E, Morbidelli L, Ziche M, et al. Role of nitric oxide in angiogenesis and tumor progression in head and neck cancer. *J Natl Cancer Inst* 1998;90(8):587-96. doi: 10.1093/jnci/90.8.587
28. Pazhouhi M, Sariri R, Rabzia A, Khazaei M. Thymoquinone synergistically potentiates temozolomide cytotoxicity through the inhibition of autophagy in u87mg cell line. *Iran J Basic Med Sci* 2016;19(8):890-8.
29. Pazhouhi M, Sariri R, Khazaei MR, Moradi MT, Khazaei M. Synergistic effect of temozolomide and thymoquinone on human glioblastoma multiforme cell line (U87MG). *J Cancer Res Ther* 2017.
30. Kasibhatla S, Amarante-Mendes GP, Finucane D, Brunner T, Bossy-Wetzel E, Green DR. Acridine orange/ethidium bromide (AO/EB) staining to detect apoptosis. *CSH Protoc* 2006;2006(3). doi: 10.1101/pdb.prot4493
31. Mirzapur P, Rashidi Z, Rezakhani L, Khazaei M. In vitro inhibitory effect of crab shell extract on human umbilical vein endothelial cell. *In Vitro Cell Dev Biol Anim* 2015;51(1):36-41. doi: 10.1007/s11626-014-9810-x
32. Hulkower KI, Herber RL. Cell migration and invasion assays as tools for drug discovery. *Pharmaceutics* 2011;3(1):107-24. doi: 10.3390/pharmaceutics3010107
33. Kusama H, Kikuchi S, Tazawa S, Katsuno K, Baba Y, Zhai YL, et al. Tranilast inhibits the proliferation of human coronary smooth muscle cell through the activation of p21waf1. *Atherosclerosis* 1999;143(2):307-13. doi: 10.1016/S0021-9150(98)00308-6
34. Darakhshan S, Ghanbari A. Tranilast enhances the anti-tumor effects of tamoxifen on human breast cancer cells in vitro. *J Biomed Sci* 2013;20:76. doi: 10.1186/1423-0127-20-76
35. Sharifi S, Barar J, Hejazi MS, Samadi N. Roles of the bcl-2/bax ratio, caspase-8 and 9 in resistance of breast cancer cells to paclitaxel. *Asian Pac J Cancer Prev* 2014;15(20):8617-22. doi: 10.7314/APJCP.2014.15.20.8617
36. Haïdara K, Alachkar A, Al Moustafa AE. Teucrium polium plant extract provokes significant cell death in human lung cancer cells. *Health* 2011;3(6):366-9. doi: 10.4236/health.2011.36062
37. Cooke JP, Losordo DW. Nitric oxide and angiogenesis. *Circulation* 2002;105(18):2133-5. doi: 10.1161/01.CIR.0000014928.45119.73
38. Platten M, Eitel K, Wischhusen J, Dichgans J, Weller M. Involvement of protein kinase Cδ and extracellular signal-regulated kinase-2 in the suppression of microglial inducible nitric oxide synthase expression by N-[3,4-dimethoxycinnamoyl]-anthranilic acid (tranilast). *Biochem Pharmacol* 2003;66(7):1263-70. doi: 10.1016/S0006-2952(03)00449-0

Preparation and Statistical Modeling of Solid Lipid Nanoparticles of Dimethyl Fumarate for Better Management of Multiple Sclerosis

Smriti Ojha[1]*, Babita Kumar[2]

[1] *Vishveshwarya Group of Institutions, Department of Pharmacy, G.B. Nagar, Uttar Pradesh 203207.*
[2] *Sanskar Educational Group, Department of Pharmacy, Ghaziabad, Uttar Pradesh 201302.*

Keywords:
- Box-behnken design
- Dimethyl Fumarate
- Multiple Sclerosis
- Response Surface Method
- Solid lipid nanoparticles
- Polydispersity index

Abstract

Purpose: The objective of this study was to synthesize and statistically optimize dimethyl fumarate (DMF) loaded solid lipid nanoparticles (SLNs) for better management of multiple sclerosis (MS).

Methods: SLNs were formulated by hot emulsion, ultrasonication method and optimized with response surface methodology (RSM). A three factor and three level box-behnken design was used to demonstrate the role of polynomial quadratic equation and contour plots in predicting the effect of independent variables on dependent responses that were particle size and % entrapment efficiency (%EE).

Results: The results were analyzed by analysis of variance (ANOVA) to evaluate the significant differences between the independent variables. The optimized SLNs were characterized and found to have an average particle size of 300 nm, zeta potential value of -34.89 mv and polydispersity index value < 0.3. Entrapment efficiency was found to be 59% and drug loading was 15%. TEM microphotograph revealed spherical shape and no aggregation of nanoparticles. *In-vitro* drug release profile was an indicative of prolonged therapy. *In-vivo* pharmacokinetic data revealed that the relative bioavailability was enhanced in DMF loaded SLNs in Wistar rats.

Conclusion: This study showed that the present formulation with improved characteristics can be a promising formulation with a longer half-life for the better management of MS.

Introduction

MS is a demyelinating, autoimmune disorder and affects central nervous system.[1] MS is a debilitating disease and accompanied by neurological symptoms of varying severity, which leads to accumulation of neurological disabilities over many years.[2] The disease is mediated by a complex interaction of individual's genetics and still unidentified environmental insults. In multiple regions the myelin sheaths deteriorate to scleroses, which are hardened scar or plaques.[3] Dimethyl fumarate (DMF) is a fumarate derivative that is used as a dermatological agent in the treatment of psoriasis and skin disorder.[4]

DMF is recently approved by FDA for the management of relapsing-remitting multiple sclerosis and as per BCS classification it is a class 1 compound.[5,6] In present practice DMF is being prescribed in two strengths of 120 to 240 mg as a delayed release hard gelatin capsule. DMF almost completely absorb from small intestine and is extensively metabolized by esterases before it reaches the systemic circulation. Compromised brain permeability, multiple dosing, poor patient compliance and economic hurdles are the other major challenges in proper utilization of DMF. The elimination half-life of DMF is approximately 1 hour. DMF is associated with the most prevalent side effect of abdominal pain, transient flushing, gastrointestinal irritation, erythema etc.[7] Nanocarriers are an effective platform for a targeted delivery of hydrophilic and lipophilic drugs with increased stability.[8,9] These approaches have some benefits such as increased drug stability, high drug payload, and potential colloidal therapeutic systems able to carry lipophilic or hydrophilic drugs or diagnostics, and no biotoxicity. SLNs are prepared by solid lipids and stabilized by surfactants, while NLCs are also prepared using solid and liquid lipids.[10,11]

Microemulsion based lipid nanoparticle preparation is simple, cost efficient, and also has considerable potential for acting as vehicles of drug delivery by incorporating a wide range of drug molecules.[12] SLNs are a new generation of submicron-sized lipid emulsions where the liquid lipid (oil) has been substituted by a solid lipid. SLNs offer some unique properties such as small size, large surface area, high drug loading and the interaction of phases at the interfaces, and are attractive for their potential to improve performance of pharmaceuticals, neutraceuticals and other materials.[13] The decrease in particle size is connected with a tremendous increase in surface area which is the responsible for the enhanced absorption and improved bioavailability of the drug.

***Corresponding author:** Smriti Ojha, E-mail: smriti.tripathi@vgi.ac.in

They have the potential target for prolonged drug release.[14] The box behnken design is one of the most efficient designs of response surface experimental methodology to study the effect of formulation components on responses for exploring quadratic response surfaces and the second-order polynomial model.[15] The box-behnken model is used to hit the target with reduced variability in experiments that increases the production yield and decreases the amount of waste, and represents opportunities for extensive financial gain.[16]

Materials and Methods

Materials

Components employed in the formulations in this research include stearic acid (m.p. 69.9°C), soy lecithin, tween 80, 1-butanol all are obtained from Chemsworth chemicals,Surat and DMF purchased from Alfa Aesar, a Johnson matthey company. Other chemicals were used only in analytical grade.

Methods

Solubility study of DMF in lipid

The solubility study of DMF in lipid was based on previously described standard procedures.[17,18] An excess amount of DMF was added to the lipids maintained at 70±5 °C were stirred thoroughly and sonicated for maximum solubilization. The solution was sampled at 2, 6, 8, 24, 48 and 72 h to analyze dissolved drug. Approximately 1 ml of the supernatant was transferred into a tared 10 ml volumetric flask and diluted with 7% v/v chloroform in methanol. Samples were further diluted prior to the analysis to allow quantification using the standard curve established. DMF concentrations were subsequently determined by UV-spectrophotometer. Equilibrium solubility was determined as the value when the solubility between two consecutive samples points does not differ practically.

Preparation of solid lipid nanoparticles

Microemulsion method developed by Gasco was used to develop Solid lipid nanoparticles with slight modifications.[19] Solid lipid nanoparticles were prepared by diluting a warm emulsion (o/w) with cold water.[20,21] Accurate quantity of stearic acid (as per the box-behnken design) was weighed and heated to 75°C until the entire lipid melts completely on water bath. To this lipid melt a co-lipid soy lecithin was added. DMF was dissolved in molten lipid mix at 75°C with stirring. Accurate quantity of surfactant (tween 80) was dissolved in distilled water. Temperature of aqueous phase was maintained at 75°C. The lipid phase was added to aqueous phase drop wise. After addition of each drop the aqueous phase was vortexed at 1200 rpm for 5 – 10 minutes and visualized for clarity of solution. If turbidity was observed the sample was sonicated for sufficient time at 75°C to obtain clear solution. The above clear dispersion was poured into distilled water kept at 2-5°C. The ratio of lipid microemulsion to cold water was kept as 1:20.

Box- behnken design for optimization of solid lipid nanoparticles

Design expert10® software version 10.0.6.0 was used to develop and study the influence of three independent parameters namely lipid %w/w, surfactant %w/w and sonication time on two dependent variables namely particle size and drug entrapment efficiency. The independent factors and the dependent variables are listed in the Table 1.

Table 1. Level of variables in Box-behnken design

Independent variables	Low (-1)	Medium (0)	High (+1)
X1- Lipid amount (%g)	20	30	40
X2- Surfactant amount (%g)	2	4	6
X3- Sonication time (min)	1	2	3
Dependent variables		**Constraints**	
R1- Particle size (nm)		Minimum	
R2- %EE		Maximum	

The box-behnken three factors, three levels complete design consisted of 15 experimental runs with 3 central points and were performed in triplicate.

The design of experiment was applied to maximize the efficiency of experiments, to minimize number of experiments and to explore the quadratic response surfaces. The polynomial equation was generated by the experimental design is as follows[22]

$$Y= b_0 + b_1X_1 + b_2X_2 + b_3X_3 + b_{12}X_1X_2 + b_{13}X_1X_3 + b_{23}X_2X_3 + b_{11}X_1^2 + b_{22}X_2^2 + b_{33}X_3^3$$

Where Y is the independent variable, b_0 is the intercept and b_1, b_2, b_3 are regression coefficients which was calculated from the experimental values of independent variables and dependent variables. Analysis of variance (ANOVA) identifies the significant independent factors which may affect the dependent factors and fitness of model.[23] All the batches of solid lipid nanoparticles were evaluated statistically ($p < 0.05$).

Average particle size

The average particle diameter, polydispersity index (PDI) and zeta potential value of the SLNs was determined by Photon correlation spectroscopy (PCS) DelsaNano C (Beckman Coulter Counter, USA) particle size analyser. The samples of SLNs were placed in disposable cuvettes for size and zeta potential measurement. The nanoparticles were dispersed in appropriate volume of HPLC grade water at 25°C, at detection angle of 90° for measuring size and PDI and 120° for zeta potential measurement.

Drug Entrapment Efficiency (% EE)

The % EE was determined as previously reported procedures.[24] DMF loaded SLNs were separated from the solution by ultracentrifugation at12000 rpm for 1 hour. Supernatants recovered from centrifugation were decanted. DMF content in the supernatant was analyzed by a UV-Vis spectrophotometer at 208 nm. The percentage drug entrapment efficiency (%EE) was calculated using the formula give below[25,26]

[% EE= Total amount of DMF added-Free DMF in supernatant/Total amount of DMF added * 100]

In-Vitro Drug release study

In vitro drug release study of the optimized DMF loaded SLNs was carried out using the equilibrium dialysis technique at 37± 1 °C.[26-28] Nanoparticles (equivalent to 1 mg DMF) were suspended in 5 mL of phosphate buffer (pH 7.4) and placed in a dialysis membrane bag. The membrane bag containing DMF loaded nanoparticle suspension was placed in 500 mL PBS and agitated at a speed of 50 rpm. Sink condition was maintained during the experiment and at regular time intervals, 5 mL of the aliquots were collected and replaced with an equal volume of fresh PBS. The collected aliquots were centrifuged at 12000 rpm and the supernatant was analyzed to calculate the cumulative % release of DMF using UV Visible Spectrophotometer at 208 nm.

FT-IR Spectroscopy

In order to evaluate chemical interaction between DMF and lipids spectra of the pure DMF, pure stearic acid and optimized SLN were obtained (by KBr Pellet Method) on FT-IR.[29]

X-ray diffraction

X-ray diffraction (XRD) study was performed to investigate the crystalline structure of SLNs, Stearic acid and the pure DMF.

Electron microscopic Examination

The optimized batch of SLNs was formulated and examined under transmission electron microscope (TEM) to study the morphology and degree of aggregation of prepared nanoparticles.

Stability Studies

Stability evaluation of optimized SLNs suspension was carried out to ascertain its future commercial viability. The SLNs were packed in screw capped amber colored glass bottles and was store at 2-8°C and ambient condition and at (28±4°C) for a period of 90 days. Samples were withdrawn at specified time intervals (1, 30, 60 and 90 days) and evaluated for the average particle size and residual drug content. The results of these parameters before and after the storage are compared and evaluated by means of ANOVA ($p<0.05$).

In-vivo pharmacokinetic study

The oral pharmacokinetic parameters were determined on Wistar rats of both the sex, weighing between 200 to 250 g and 5-6 weeks old. The protocol for animal study was approved by Institutional Animal Ethics Committee (IAEC) and Committee for the Purpose of control and supervision of experiments on animals. The animals were fed with a standard laboratory pellet diet and pure water *adlibitum*. The rats were divided into two groups each consisting of six animals. Group 1 was treated with pure DMF (50 mg/kg) and group 2 was treated with optimized SLNs formulations (equivalent to 3 mg/kg DMF). Blood samples (0.5ml) were collected from retro orbital plexus at predetermined time intervals and kept into heparin solution to prevent clotting. The serum was separated from blood samples by centrifugation. DMF rapidly metabolizes into its active metabolite mono methyl fumarate (MMF), and the content of both were determined using RP-HPLC.[30]

Results

Solubility study

The equilibrium solubility of DMF in Stearic acid was found to be 27 ± 3%w/v. This result predicts that stearic acid is capable to carry high drug load with minimum leakage. Thus stearic acid, a solid lipid could be a good candidate for formulation of SLNs.

Model fitting and experimental design

A total 15 experiments with 3 central points, 3 levels and 3 factors were designed using three independent variables which were % of lipid, % of surfactant and sonication time in order to study their effect on two dependent responses which were average particle size and %EE. The replication of central point gives the result of experimental error.[31,32] The experiments were designed using response surface modeling, box-behnken design with the help of Design Expert 10® software. Except the three independent variables all other parameters were maintained constant. Total 15 formulations as mentioned in Table 2 of SLNs were formulated and analyzed for their response particle size and %EE. Response results of all the variables are listed in the Table 2.

Table 2. Response result of dependent variables

Runs	Factor 1 X1. Lipid % w/w	Factors 2 X2. Surfactant % w/w	Factor 3 X3. Sonication time (min)	Response 1 Particle size (nm)	Response 2 (%) EE
1	0	0	0	298	74
2	0	1	-1	322	88
3	-1	0	1	262	70
4	0	1	1	356	84
5	-1	0	-1	303	82
6	0	0	0	308	74
7	0	0	0	292	74
8	1	0	1	287	66
9	1	-1	0	298	76
10	0	-1	-1	356	75
11	0	-1	1	290	78
12	1	1	0	284	65
13	-1	1	0	300	87
14	-1	-1	0	291	63
15	1	0	-1	314	69

Fitting of model was done by sequential model sum of squares and model summary statistics. It was observed that within linear models, interactive models and quadratic models for particle size and for % EE, the quadratic model was found to be significant with p-value < 0.01.

The polynomial quadratic equation based on the analysis of Design Expert10® was generated by the software and the quantification of the effect of independent variables on responses was done with the help of this equation.

$$Particle\ Size = 299.33 + 3.37 \times A + 3.37 \times B - 12.50 \times c - 5.75 \times AB + 3.50 \times AC + 25.00 \times BC - 22.79 \times A2 + 16.71 \times B2 + 14.96 \times C2$$

$$\%\ EE = 74.00 - 3.25 \times A + 4.00 \times B - 2.00 \times c - 8.75 \times AB + 2.25 \times AC - 1.75 \times BC - 15.37 \times A2 + 4.13 \times B2 + 3.12 \times C2$$

The results were analyzed using ANOVA available in the software and the model was found to be significant with F value of 6.34 for particle size and 12.09 for %EE. The Response surface 3D graphs were constructed using the software. These graphs were used to study the interaction of independent variables on the responses, by keeping one of the variables at constant level. The Graphs obtained for the response particle size and %EE is depicted in the Figure 1.

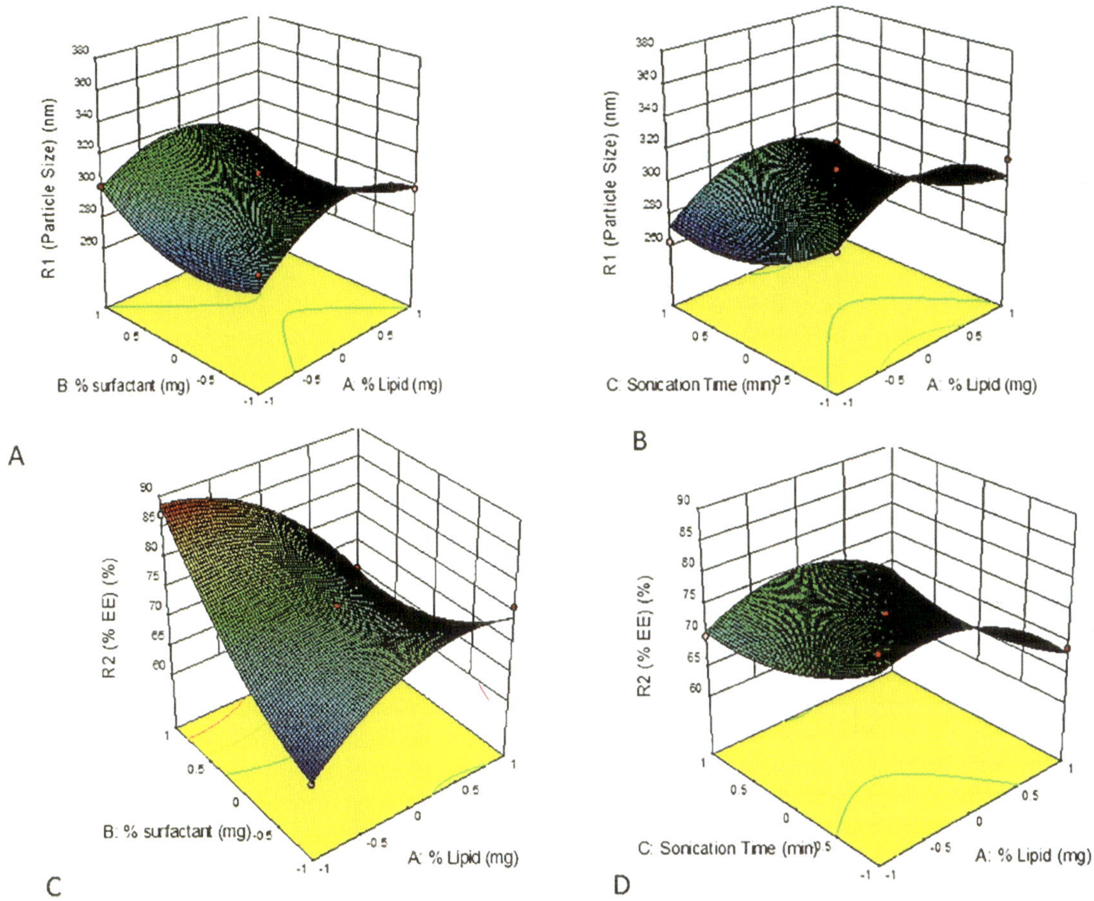

Figure 1. Response surface 3D plot for particle size (R1) and %EE (R2), A. Response surface 3D plot showing the effect of % lipid and % surfactant on R1, B- Response surface 3D plot showing the effect of % lipid and sonication time on R1, C. Response surface 3D plot showing the effect of % lipid and % surfactant on R2, D. Response surface 3D plot showing effect of sonication time and % lipid on R2.

Numerical optimization

Numerical optimization of SLNs was done by Design Expert10 ® software and the response variables were optimized using RSM, box-behnken modeling. The optimized formulation was then prepared with 30% w/w stearic acid, 15% w/w surfactant and 4 min sonication time with desirability 0.87. The optimized batch of SLNs was further evaluated for average particle size, Zeta potential, PDI, % EE and % cumulative drug release. The observed responses of variables were compared with predicted responses and the calculated % error was found significant with values less than 0.05%.

Size analysis and surface morphology

TEM microphotograph of optimized batch of SLN was obtained and shown in the Figure 2. The image revealed that the nanoparticles are of spherical shape and their average particle diameter was in the range of 300 nm. The average particle diameter as obtained by the Zetasizer instrument is 298 ± 4 nm (Figure 2), which also confirms the TEM result of particle size.

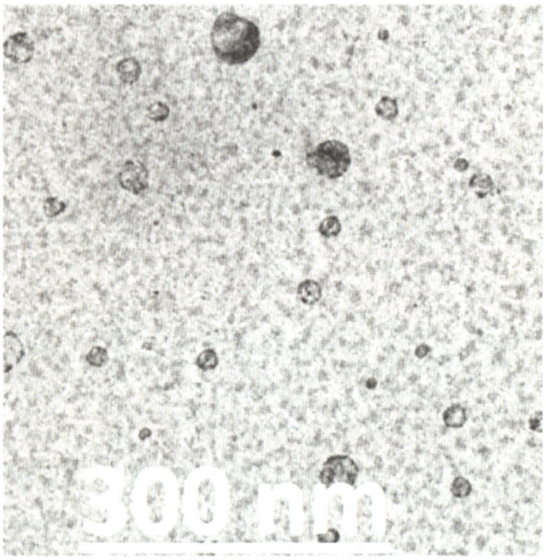

Figure 2. Transmission Electron Photomicrograph of optimized SLNs.

Zeta potential is the difference in the potential between the surface of tightly bound layer and the electro neutral region of the solution.[33] The value of zeta potential of optimized SLNs was found to be -34.89 mv.

IR spectroscopy and drug interaction

IR spectroscopy method was used to study the drug–lipid interactions. IR spectroscopy of DMF shows all the characteristic peaks of functional groups present in the DMF. The absence of chemical interactions between drug and excipients were confirmed by the characteristic peaks of functional groups in the IR spectra of DMF, stearic acid and SLNs (Figure 3). The characteristic peaks of DMF were observed at 3428, 3022, 1719, 1445, 1297, 1164, 998, 889, 778 and 521 cm^{-1}; for stearic acid 2900, 1450, 1467, 1385, 1395 cm^{-1}. The characteristic peaks of DMF were also observed with IR spectra of SLNs which were at 3400, 2918, 2850, 1129, 1099 and 948cm^{-1}. Similarly, the characteristic peaks of stearic acid were also observed at 2955 and 726 cm^{-1} in SLNs IR spectra.

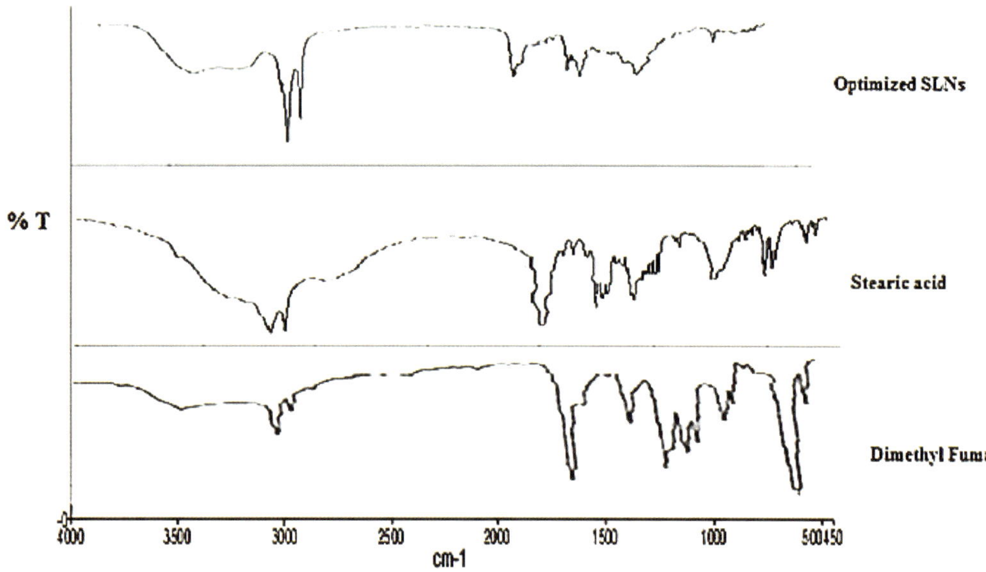

Figure 3. Overlay FT-IR spectra of DMF, stearic acid and optimized SLNs

XRD analysis

XRD studies were performed to indicate the reduction of the crystallinity of DMF in SLNs. The XRD of DMF, Stearic acid and optimized formulation were obtained (Figure 4). The diffraction spectrum of pure DMF and pure Stearic acid showed that the drug and the lipid were crystalline in nature. DMF presented many characteristic peaks observed in range 17.485, 20.013, 20.577and 30.47 at various 2θ values. The diffractograms of SA exhibit sharp peaks at 2h scattered angles of 7.07, 20.60, 21.71, and 24.05, indicating the lipid crystalline nature. Compared with the pure lipid, the peak intensities of SLN are much weaker, XRD pattern of SLNs showed that it is less crystalline and indicating amorphous nature of drug.

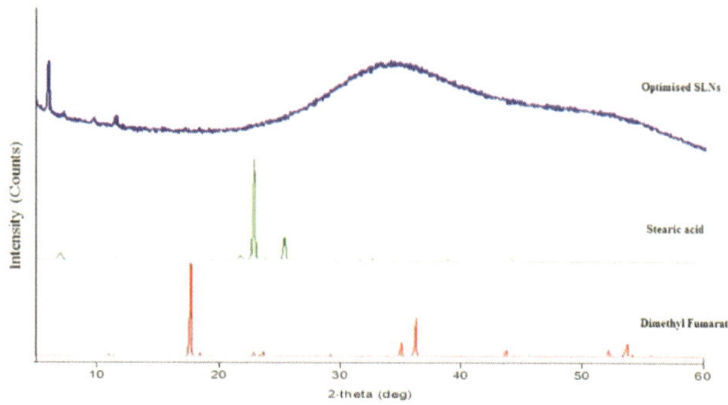

Figure 4. Overlay diffractograms of DMF, stearic acid and optimized SLNs

In-vitro drug release

In-vitro release profile of optimized SLNs was shown in the Figure 5. The cumulative percent drug release of DMF was 70.46±1.17% and 71.79±0.79 in 0.1 N HCl and 7.4

pH PBS respectively over a period of 24h. The percentage drug release of DMF was 52.24±0.85% in 0.1 N HCl and 54.55±0.45% in 7.4 PBS respectively after 2 h. Different kinetic models for *in-vitro* cumulative % drug release such as zero order (cumulative amount of drug released vs. time), first order (log cumulative % of drug remaining vs. time), Higuchi model (cumulative percentage of drug released vs. square root of time), korsmeyer-peppas model (log% cumulative release Vs. log time) and Hixson Crowell model (% drug remained Vs. time) were applied to study the drug release kinetics from the optimized formulations. Korsmeyer-peppas model was found to be the best-fit model with a highest R^2 value of 0.903 in 0.1N HCl and 0.925 in 7.4 PBS.

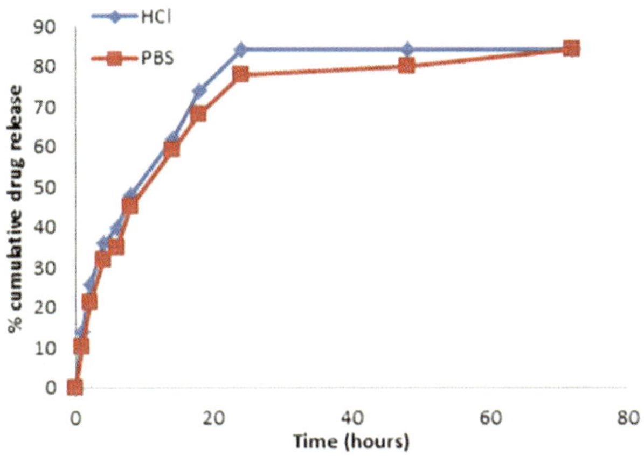

Figure 5. *In-vitro* cumulative % drug release profile of DMF from optimized SLNs.

Stability study

The samples were analyzed for average particle size, % drug retained after 1 day, 30 days, 60 days and 90 days. Average particle size was found to be increased about 15 nm with storage at 28°C for 90 days, which was higher than the SLNs stored at 2-4°C. The result of % drug retained was found to be stable on storage for a period of 90 days.

***In-vivo* pharmacokinetic study**

The oral pharmacokinetic profile of pure DMF and DMF loaded SLNs is tabulated in Table 3. The pharmacokinetic parameters of pure DMF were compared with DMF loaded SLNs. In comparison with the pure DMF the values of C_{max}, T_{max}, and AUC were found to be increased with DMF loaded SLNs, which indicates the fast onset of action and long absorption phase of the present formulation. The half-life was also higher in SLNs formulation.

Table 3. Pharmacokinetic parameters

Parameters (unit)	DMF	DMF loaded SLNs
C_{max}(ng.ml^{-1})	1054.51	1323.85
T_{max}(h)	1.58	3.45
K_E (h^{-1})	0.187	0.165
K_a (h^{-1})	1.28	6.53
$t_{1/2}$ (h)	3.5	5.8
$[AUC]_0^\infty$ (ng.ml^{-1}.h)	7398.84	18543.78
$[AUMC]_0^\infty$ (ng.ml^{-1}.h^2)	94249.66	369762.97
MRT (h)	12.74	19.94

Discussion

15 SLN formulations were prepared as per RSM box-behnken design by the method hot emulsification and ultrasonication. The model was fitted with help of software and quadratic model was found to be best fit model among all with predicted R^2 value of 0.9853 and PRESS value of 9674 for particle size and R^2 value of 0.9561 and PRESS value of 592 for %EE. The main focus of the design is to obtain maximum R^2 value and minimum PRESS value. The value of $F< 0.05$ indicates that the model terms are significant. A good correlation was observed between predicted and observed values with a higher value of R^2.

Factors with positive values in the above quadratic equation indicated that the response increases with increase in factor value and negative value indicates an inverse relationship.[34,35]

It was clear by the graph that on increasing the amount of lipid the size of SLN also increases, which results into and increased surface tension.[36] The decrease in average particle size was associated with an increased percentage of surfactant. This phenomenon is probably due to the hydrophobic interactions between the lipid and surfactant. It has been reported that the size of SLNs decreases as the ratio of phospholipids to stearic acid increases.[37] Drug %EE increases as lipid percentage increases due to the high drug dissolution in an increased and molten lipid amount. Higher surfactant concentration resulted in lower entrapment efficiency, as this would increase the partitioning of drug from internal phase to external phase. This increased partitioning might result from increased solubility of drug in the external phase.[38]

The results of numerical optimization were used to formulate the optimized SLNs and evaluated for its particle size and % EE. Further analysis and statistical modeling revealed that the predicted responses are very close to the actual response results. A low value of prediction error validates the method and quadratic model.

Zeta potential measure is important to predict the long term kinetic stability of formulations as well as to understand the state of the surface morphology of the nanoparticles. This parameter is not only responsible for the stability of colloidal dispersions but it provides an indication of the degree of repulsion between particles with identical charge in the dispersion.[39]

Nanoparticles are considered to be kinetically stable with a zeta potential value higher than +25 mv or lower than -25 mv. Zeta potential analysis revealed that the optimized batch was stable with a zeta potential value of -34 mv. Negative value of zeta potential may be an indication of presence of fatty acid in SLNs preparation which provides rigid hydrophobic interactions. Higher zeta potential (either positive or negative) require higher energy for bringing two particles in contact with each other i.e. it possess high energy barrier in between the particles.[40]

TEM microphotograph of optimized batch of SLNs was obtained. TEM image clearly shows that the nanoparticles were spherical in shape with smooth surface morphology. The TEM study also revealed that the average particle size of SLNs were 300 nm. No particle aggregation was visible in the TEM microphotograph. As reported in various literatures it can be concluded that the lower size assures better brain delivery of the formulation which could be a good candidate for the treatment of MS.[41,42]

The XRD results seem to indicate that SA in SLNs was partially recrystallized or less ordered. These changes are because of the presence of a mixture of polymorphs in the nanoparticles and the method of obtaining the SLNs. It can also be seen that in the diffractograms of SLNs, the crystalline peaks of DMF is absent which could be because of conversion of crystalline DMF to amorphous DMF.

In-vitro release kinetics was fitted with various dissolution models and on the basis of correlation coefficient (R^2) value the best fit model was selected. Korsmeyer-peppas model showed a highest R^2 value of 0.903 in 0.1 N HCl and 0.925 in PBS with 7.4 pH indicated that release kinetics follows a diffusion coupled with lipoidal matrix relaxation. All the formulations exhibited an initial burst release followed by a controlled drug release for a period of 500 minutes. The initial burst release can be explained by the surface adsorption of DMF which is a main characteristic of nano and microparticles. Controlled release profile was observed which is mainly due to the diffusion of drug from inner lipid matrix.

The accelerated stability study data reveals that the prepared SLNs are stable and retains its property on storage. Further result showed a higher stability at low temperature conditions hence the prepared SLNs need to be stored at 5°C or low temperature to get a better shelf life.

The oral pharmacokinetic results confirmed that the bioavailability of DMF loaded SLNs was much higher as compared to free DMF which may be because of low particle size in SLNs. The increase in C_{max} and AUC values of SLNs indicates that the present optimized formulation may be helpful to reduce the dose of DMF. The relative bioavailability results of also confirmed that the present formulation may have an improved therapeutic activity and to reduce the dose of DMF. T_{max} value is delayed which can be explained by a sustained release rate profile of SLNs. MRT and half-life was also found to be increased which may be helpful to reduce the frequency of dosing and to reduce the side effects.

Conclusion

DMF loaded SLN were successfully prepared by the method hot emulsion ultrasonication and optimized by three level three factors box-behnken design through RSM. The effect of all the three independent variables was studied and they are found to affect the dependent responses significantly. Observed response values were found to be in a linear correlation with predicted response values with a low predicted error result which also validates the quadratic model. The optimized formulation was prepared and characterized for particle size, % EE, zeta Potential and PDI. TEM image of the optimized SLN reveals a spherical shape and no aggregation of particles. FTIR study showed that the present SLNs formulation is free from any kind of drug interactions and the DMF original functional groups were present in the formulation also. The results of in-vitro study showed that the % cumulative drug release is 82% and approximately 40% of the drug was released in the first 180 minutes. Stability study was performed till 90 days and the results showed that the formulation is able to maintain its original property with insignificant changes. The results of the present study demonstrated that DMF loaded controlled release SLNs could be a promising candidate for the better management of the multiple sclerosis disease. Future in vivo study should be conducted to evaluate the effectiveness of the formulation in the management of the disease.

Acknowledgments

The authors would like to thank the Vishveshwarya Group of Institution, G. B. Nagar for its support. The authors also extend this acknowledgment to CDRI, Lucknow for providing TEM images and FTIR spectra and IIT BHU, Varanasi for providing XRD diffractograms and results of zeta sizing.

Ethical Issues

The study was approved by the Institutional Animal Ethical Committee and their guidelines were followed throughout the study.

Conflict of Interest

All the authors declared that there is no conflict of interest.

References

1. Noseworthy JH, Lucchinetti C, Rodriguez M, Weinshenker BG. Multiple sclerosis. *N Engl J Med* 2000;343(13):938-52. doi: 10.1056/nejm200009283431307
2. Compston A, Coles A. Multiple sclerosis. *Lancet* 2008;372(9648):1502-17. doi: 10.1016/s0140-6736(08)61620-7
3. Gerard JT, Bruan HD. Principle of Anatomy and Pathophysiology. 11th ed. New York: Wiky International; 2014.
4. Mrowietz U, Christophers E, Altmeyer P. Treatment of psoriasis with fumaric acid esters: Results of a prospective multicentre study. German multicentre study. *Br J Dermatol* 1998;138(3):456-60.
5. Vargas DL, Tyor WR. Update on disease-modifying therapies for multiple sclerosis. *J Investig Med* 2017;65(5):883-91. doi: 10.1136/jim-2016-000339
6. Bomprezzi R. Dimethyl fumarate in the treatment of relapsing-remitting multiple sclerosis: An overview. *Ther Adv Neurol Disord* 2015;8(1):20-30. doi: 10.1177/1756285614564152

7. Linker RA, Gold R. Dimethyl fumarate for treatment of multiple sclerosis: Mechanism of action, effectiveness, and side effects. *Curr Neurol Neurosci Rep* 2013;13(11):394. doi: 10.1007/s11910-013-0394-8
8. Vyas SP, Khar RK. Targetted and controlled drug delivery, Novel carrier systems. Delhi: CBS publishers and distributers; 2007.
9. Jourghanian P, Ghaffari S, Ardjmand M, Haghighat S, Mohammadnejad M. Sustained release curcumin loaded solid lipid nanoparticles. *Adv Pharm Bull* 2016;6(1):17-21. doi: 10.15171/apb.2016.004
10. Bennewitz MF, Saltzman WM. Nanotechnology for delivery of drugs to the brain for epilepsy. *Neurotherapeutics* 2009;6(2):323-36. doi: 10.1016/j.nurt.2009.01.018
11. Wissing SA, Kayser O, Muller RH. Solid lipid nanoparticles for parenteral drug delivery. *Adv Drug Deliv Rev* 2004;56(9):1257-72. doi: 10.1016/j.addr.2003.12.002
12. Lawrence MJ, Rees GD. Microemulsion-based media as novel drug delivery systems. *Adv Drug Deliv Rev* 2000;45(1):89-121.
13. Cavalli R, Caputo O, Gasco MR. Solid lipospheres of doxorubicin and idarubicin. *Int J Pharm* 1993;89(1):R9–R12. doi: 10.1016/0378-5173(93)90313-5
14. Attama AA, Schicke BC, Muller-Goymann CC. Further characterization of theobroma oil-beeswax admixtures as lipid matrices for improved drug delivery systems. *Eur J Pharm Biopharm* 2006;64(3):294-306. doi: 10.1016/j.ejpb.2006.06.010
15. Motwani SK, Chopra S, Talegaonkar S, Kohli K, Ahmad FJ, Khar RK. Chitosan-sodium alginate nanoparticles as submicroscopic reservoirs for ocular delivery: Formulation, optimisation and in vitro characterisation. *Eur J Pharm Biopharm* 2008;68(3):513-25. doi: 10.1016/j.ejpb.2007.09.009
16. Hosny KM. Alendronate sodium as enteric coated solid lipid nanoparticles; preparation, optimization, and in vivo evaluation to enhance its oral bioavailability. *PLoS One* 2016;11(5):e0154926. doi: 10.1371/journal.pone.0154926
17. Sacchetti M, Nejati E. Prediction of drug solubility in lipid mixtures from the individual ingredients. *AAPS PharmSciTech* 2012;13(4):1103-9. doi: 10.1208/s12249-012-9830-3
18. Kossena GA, Boyd BJ, Porter CJ, Charman WN. Separation and characterization of the colloidal phases produced on digestion of common formulation lipids and assessment of their impact on the apparent solubility of selected poorly water-soluble drugs. *J Pharm Sci* 2003;92(3):634-48. doi: 10.1002/jps.10329
19. Muthu MS, Rawat MK, Mishra A, Singh S. PLGA nanoparticle formulations of risperidone: Preparation and neuropharmacological evaluation. *Nanomedicine* 2009;5(3):323-33. doi: 10.1016/j.nano.2008.12.003
20. Seju U, Kumar A, Sawant KK. Development and evaluation of olanzapine-loaded PLGA nanoparticles for nose-to-brain delivery: In vitro and in vivo studies. *Acta Biomater* 2011;7(12):4169-76. doi: 10.1016/j.actbio.2011.07.025
21. Gasco MR. Inventor solid lipid microspheres having a narrow size distribution and method for producing them. Europ. Patent, EP0526666A1. 2002.
22. Ojha S, Kumar B. Formulation and optimization of chitosan nanoparticles of dimethyl fumarate using box-behnken design. *Int J App Pharm* 2016;8(4):10-7. doi: 10.22159/ijap.2016v8i4.13450
23. Vieira AC, Chaves LL, Pinheiro M, Ferreira D, Sarmento B, Reis S. Design and statistical modeling of mannose-decorated dapsone-containing nanoparticles as a strategy of targeting intestinal M-cells. *Int J Nanomedicine* 2016;11:2601-17. doi: 10.2147/ijn.s104908
24. Esposito E, Ravani L, Mariani P, Huang N, Boldrini P, Drechsler M, et al. Effect of nanostructured lipid vehicles on percutaneous absorption of curcumin. *Eur J Pharm Biopharm* 2014;86(2):121-32. doi: 10.1016/j.ejpb.2013.12.011
25. Hemant KJ, Archana AG. Stability indicating RP-HPLC assay method for estimation of dimethyl fumarate in bulk and capsules. *Int J Appl Pharm* 2017;9(5):121-7. doi: 10.22159/ijap.2017v9i5.20944.
26. Luo Y, Chen D, Ren L, Zhao X, Qin J. Solid lipid nanoparticles for enhancing vinpocetine's oral bioavailability. *J Control Release* 2006;114(1):53-9. doi: 10.1016/j.jconrel.2006.05.010
27. Huang G, Zhang N, Bi X, Dou M. Solid lipid nanoparticles of temozolomide: Potential reduction of cardial and nephric toxicity. *Int J Pharm* 2008;355(1-2):314-20. doi: 10.1016/j.ijpharm.2007.12.013
28. Chaves LL, Vieira AC, Ferreira D, Sarmento B, Reis S. Rational and precise development of amorphous polymeric systems with dapsone by response surface methodology. *Int J Biol Macromol* 2015;81:662-71. doi: 10.1016/j.ijbiomac.2015.08.009
29. Bhalekar MR, Pokharkar V, Madgulkar A, Patil N, Patil N. Preparation and evaluation of miconazole nitrate-loaded solid lipid nanoparticles for topical delivery. *AAPS PharmSciTech* 2009;10(1):289-96. doi: 10.1208/s12249-009-9199-0
30. Gennari O, Montesano D, Salzano A, Albrizio S, Grumetto L. Determination of dimethyl fumarate in desiccant and antimould sachets by reversed-phase liquid chromatography. *Biomed Chromatogr* 2011;25(12):1315-8. doi: 10.1002/bmc.1602
31. Gunday Tureli N, Tureli AE, Schneider M. Optimization of ciprofloxacin complex loaded plga nanoparticles for pulmonary treatment of cystic fibrosis infections: Design of experiments approach.

Int J Pharm 2016;515(1-2):343-51. doi: 10.1016/j.ijpharm.2016.10.025

32. Rahman Z, Zidan AS, Habib MJ, Khan MA. Understanding the quality of protein loaded plga nanoparticles variability by plackett-burman design. *Int J Pharm* 2010;389(1-2):186-94. doi: 10.1016/j.ijpharm.2009.12.040
33. Xu Z, Chen L, Gu W, Gao Y, Lin L, Zhang Z, et al. The performance of docetaxel-loaded solid lipid nanoparticles targeted to hepatocellular carcinoma. *Biomaterials* 2009;30(2):226-32. doi: 10.1016/j.biomaterials.2008.09.014
34. Gannu R, Yamsani VV, Yamsani SK, Palem CR, Yamsani MR. Optimization of hydrogels for transdermal delivery of lisinopril by box-behnken statistical design. *AAPS PharmSciTech* 2009;10(2):505-14. doi: 10.1208/s12249-009-9230-5
35. Chopra S, Patil GV, Motwani SK. Release modulating hydrophilic matrix systems of losartan potassium: Optimization of formulation using statistical experimental design. *Eur J Pharm Biopharm* 2007;66(1):73-82. doi: 10.1016/j.ejpb.2006.09.001
36. Tanvir S, Qiao L. Surface tension of nanofluid-type fuels containing suspended nanomaterials. *Nanoscale Res Lett* 2012;7(1):226. doi: 10.1186/1556-276x-7-226
37. Mao S, Wang P, Bi D. Investigations on 5-fluorouracil solid lipid nanoparticles (SLN) prepared by hot homogenization. *Pharmazie* 2005;60(4):273-7.
38. Yang Q, Owusu-Ababio G. Biodegradable progesterone microsphere delivery system for osteoporosis therapy. *Drug Dev Ind Pharm* 2000;26(1):61-70.
39. Ma S, Chen F, Ye X, Dong Y, Xue Y, Xu H, et al. Intravenous microemulsion of docetaxel containing an anti-tumor synergistic ingredient (brucea javanica oil): Formulation and pharmacokinetics. *Int J Nanomedicine* 2013;8:4045-52. doi: 10.2147/ijn.s47956
40. Olivier JC, Huertas R, Lee HJ, Calon F, Pardridge WM. Synthesis of pegylated immunonanoparticles. *Pharm Res* 2002;19(8):1137-43.
41. Lockman PR, Koziara JM, Mumper RJ, Allen DD. Nanoparticle surface charges alter blood-brain barrier integrity and permeability. *J Drug Target* 2004;12(9-10):635-41. doi: 10.1080/10611860400015936
42. Ojha S, Kumar B. A review on nanotechnology based innovations in diagnosis and treatment of multiple sclerosis. *J Cell Immunother* 2018;1-9. doi: 10.1016/j.jocit.2017.12.001

Combination of Vildagliptin and Ischemic Postconditioning in Diabetic Hearts as a Working Strategy to Reduce Myocardial Reperfusion Injury by Restoring Mitochondrial Function and Autophagic Activity

Goltaj Bayrami[1], Alireza Alihemmati[1], Pouran Karimi[2], Aniseh Javadi[3,4], Rana Keyhanmanesh[1,5], Mustafa Mohammadi[1], Milad Zadi-Heydarabad[4], Reza Badalzadeh[1,5,6]*

[1] *Drug Applied Research Center, Tabriz University of Medical Sciences, Tabriz, Iran.*
[2] *Neurosciences Research Center, Tabriz University of Medical Sciences, Tabriz, Iran.*
[3] *Cardiovascular Research Center, Tabriz University of Medical Sciences, Tabriz, Iran.*
[4] *Student Research Committee, Tabriz University of Medical Sciences, Tabriz, Iran.*
[5] *Department of Physiology, Faculty of Medicine, Tabriz University of Medical Sciences, Tabriz, Iran.*
[6] *Molecular Medicine Research Center, Tabriz University of Medical Sciences, Tabriz, Iran.*

Keywords:
- Ischemic postconditioning
- Diabetes
- Reperfusion injury
- Autophagy
- Mitochondrial function

Abstract

Purpose: Diabetic hearts are resistant to cardioprotection by ischemic-postconditioning (IPostC). Protection of diabetic hearts and finding related interfering mechanisms would have clinical benefits. This study investigated the combination effects of vildagliptin (Vilda) and IPostC on cardioprotection and the levels of autophagy and mitochondrial function following myocardial ischemia/reperfusion (I/R) injury in type-II diabetic rats.

Methods: Diabetes was established by high fat diet/low dose of streptozotocin and lasted for 12 weeks. The diabetic rats received Vilda (6 mg/kg/day, orally) for one month before I/R. Myocardial regional ischemia was induced through the ligation of left coronary artery, and IPostC was applied immediately at the onset of reperfusion. The infarct size was assessed by a computerised planimetry and left ventricles samples were harvested for cardiac mitochondrial function studies (ROS production, membrane potential and staining) and western blotting was used for determination of autophagy markers.

Results: None of Vilda or IPostC but combination of them could significantly reduce the infarct size of diabetic hearts, comparing to control ($P<0.001$). IPostC could not significantly affect p62 expression level in diabetic hearts, but pre-treatment with Vilda alone ($p<0.05$) and in combination with IPostC ($p<0.01$) more significantly decreased p62 expression in comparison with corresponding control group. The expression of LC3B-II and LC3BII/LC3BI as well as mitochondrial ROS production were decreased significantly in treatment groups ($p<0.001$). Mitochondrial membrane depolarization was significantly higher and mitochondrial density was lower in untreated diabetic I/R hearts than treated groups ($p<0.001$). IPostC in combination with vildagliptin prevented the mitochondrial membrane depolarization and increased the mitochondrial content more potent than IPostC alone in diabetic hearts.

Conclusion: Combination of vildagliptin and IPostC in diabetic hearts was a well-working strategy to reduce myocardial I/R damages by restoring mitochondrial membrane potential and ROS production and modulating the autophagic activity in I/R hearts.

Introduction

Myocardial ischemia/repefusion (I/R) injury is defined as the reversible or irreversible cardiomyocyte damages following reperfusion therapy, leading to excessive reactive oxygen species (ROS) generation, inflammatory reactions, mitochondrial dysfunction and subsequently cell death.[1] Diabetes mellitus is a main cardiovascular comorbidity which exacerbates myocardial function following myocardial I/R injuries and reduces the efficiency of cardioprotective interventions.[2,3] Diabetic heart is accompanied with the development of cardiac dysfunction, myocardial hypertrophy, myocardial interstitial fibrosis, increased apoptosis, mitochondrial dysfunction, dysregulated autophagy and upregulation of oxidative stress and pro-inflammatory mediators.[4,5] The prevalence of type-II diabetes is rapidly increasing world-wide and insulin resistance is a critical metabolic abnormality among these diabetic patients, resulting in hyperglycemia, hyperinsulinemia, pancreatic β-islet cell dysfunction in advanced stages of diabetes and lack of insulin effects in the periphery.[4,6]

***Corresponding author:** Reza Badalzadeh, Email: badalzadehr@tbzmed.ac.ir

Autophagy is a bulk degradation of long-live protein, oxidized proteins and dysfunctional organelles inside the cells. Both protective or negative roles of autophagy have been reported in experimental settings of I/R injury and diabetes, depending on the type and duration of the stress conditions in different organs.[7,8] Thus, whether the alternations in autophagy are beneficial or detrimental under I/R injury remains controversial and needs more investigations, particularly in diabetes. It is evident that modification of the excessive autophagic response via various means would be associated with the restoration of myocardial functions during I/R insults.

Ischemic postconditioning (IPostC) is a clinically applicable cardioprotective intervention in which some short alternative cycles of ischemia and reperfusion is applied immediately at the early minutes of reperfusion.[5,9] It is a mechanical strategy with significant cardioprotection in non-diabetic (healthy) animal experiments. Recent evidence showed that autophagy can be regulated by postconditioning during reperfusion.[9,10] In addition, numerous studies showed that the diabetes abrogates cardioprotective effects of IPostC following myocardial reperfusion injury, due to the numerous less-known underlying mechanisms, including dysfunctions in cell survival signaling pathways.[11,12] Using an adjuvant therapy to increase the potency of IPostC in diabetic myocardium may be one of the promising strategies to restore the diabetes-induced loss of cardioprotection.[13]

Vildagliptin (as a potent dipeptidyl peptidase 4 (DPP-4) inhibitor) acts as an enhancer of glucagon-like peptide 1 (GLP-1) hormone, having multiple beneficial effects besides reducing hyperglycaemia, such as increasing glucose-stimulated insulin release,[14] improving mitochondrial function,[15] and anti-inflammatory[16] and antioxidative[17] effects. Also, it has been reported to exert positive cardiovascular effects in both preclinical and clinical studies under healthy or diabetic circumstances.[15,18] In our previous work, we showed that pre-treatment of diabetic rats with vildagliptin could improve the failure of IPostC on the recovery of myocardial hemodynamic function after ischemic event and this effect was associated somewhat with anti-oxidative and anti-inflammatory properties.[19] There is less or no information about the effect of vildagliptin on autophagy and mitochondrial function in normal condition or in type-II diabetic myocardium following I/R injury.[20,21] Due to the positive therapeutic potentials of vildagliptin in cardiovascular medicine, in this experiment we have combined vildagliptin and IPostC to investigate their cardioprotective effects by focusing on autophagy and mitochondrial function in (chronic) type-II diabetic hearts with regional I/R injury.

Materials and Methods

Animals

The 8-week-old male Wistar rats (200-250g) were used in this study. The rats were housed in animal room with free access to food and water and maintained at 22±2°C on a 12 h light/dark cycle. They were under strict surveillance until the end of the study. All steps of the experiment were carried out in line with the Guide for the Care and Use of Laboratory Animals published by the US National Institutes of Health (NIH publication No 85-23, revised 1996) and officially accepted by the Ethical Commission of Tabriz University of Medical Sciences.

Induction of type-II diabetes

Type-II diabetes with insulin resistance was induced by the method of high-fat diet-fed and low-dose streptozotocin, according to the previous reports.[22] The diabetic period was lasted for 12 weeks for simulation of chronic diabetes. After a week of acclimatization, diabetic rats were fed for 6 weeks *ad libitum* with a high-fat diet, containing 35% normal pellet, 30% lard, 4% sucrose, 24% casein, 1% cholesterol, 0.3% DL-Methionine (62% calories from fat, and total caloric value was about 4.6 kcal/g). Non-diabetic healthy rats were fed with normal diet. At the end of 6th week, the diabetic rats were then administered with a low dose of streptozotocin (35 mg/kg in citrate buffer, pH 4, i.p.) after 8 hours fasting. Blood samples were obtained 72 hours after STZ injection for confirmation of diabetes. Rats with blood glucose levels higher than 250 mg/dl were enrolled to the further study.

Experimental Preparation and Protocols

The animals were randomly divided into five diabetic and two non-diabetic subgroups, n=5-6/each. Diabetic (D) groups included: D-Sham, D-Control, D-IPostC (diabetic hearts of rats received IPostC), D-Vilda (diabetic rats received vildagiliptin) and D-Vilda-IPostC (diabetic rats received vildagiliptin and then their hearts received IPostC). Non-diabetic healthy (H) animals were divided into H-Sham and H-Control subgroups. Rats in D-Vilda and D-Vilda-IPostC groups were treated with vildagliptin (6 mg/kg/day) through feeding gavage in the last 5 weeks.[15,19]

Myocardial I/R modeling

At the end of treatment, all hearts of animals were isolated as mentioned previously.[23,24] Briefly, before the anesthetization of rats with the intra-peritoneal injection of ketamine (60 mg/kg) and xylasine (10 mg/kg), they were heparinized (500 IU) to avoid blood clotting during surgery. Then, the hearts of animals were rapidly isolated and mounted on a constant-pressure (80 mmHg) mode of Langendorff perfusion apparatus (ML176-V, AD Instruments, Australia) and perfused with a Krebs–Henseleit solution containing (in mM/l): NaCl 118; KCl 4.7; $CaCl_2$ 2.5; $MgSO_4$ 1.2; $NaHCO_3$ 25; KH_2PO_4 1.2; glucose 11.1. The perfusion solution was gassed with a mixture of 95% O2, 5% CO2 at 37°C and pH 7.4. For measurement of interventricular pressure changes, a water-filled latex balloon was inserted into the left ventricle and the signals were delivered to the related transducer through a connecting pressure catheter. In all experimental groups, a 5-10 mmHg of left ventricular end-diastolic pressure was produced by adjusting the balloon volume. Following stabilization on Langendorff perfusion system, the isolated hearts were assigned to receive one of these protocols:

- H-Sham: the hearts were subjected to 105 min full perfusion only.
- H-Control: the hearts were subjected to 35 min ischemia + 60 min reperfusion.
- D-Sham: the hearts were subjected to 105 min full perfusion only.
- D-Control: the hearts were subjected to 35 min ischemia + 60 min reperfusion.
- D-IPostC: the hearts were subjected to 35 min ischemia + 6 cycles of 10s ischemia /10s reperfusion immediately at the onset of 60 min reperfusion.[25]
- D-Vilda: the hearts of vildagliptin-receiving rats were subjected to 35 min ischemia + 60 min reperfusion
- D-Vilda-IPostC: the hearts of vildagliptin-receiving rats were subjected to 35 min ischemia + 6 cycles of 10s ischemia /10s reperfusion immediately at the onset of 60 min reperfusion.

Regional ischemia (for 35 minutes) was induced by tightening a 5-0 silk suture around the left anterior descending (LAD) coronary artery, close to its origin. The snare was then removed and the hearts received reperfusion for 60 minutes. At the end of reperfusion, the left ventricle of each heart was isolated from whole heart and then the ischemic zone were harvested and divided in half, one part were paraffinized for mitochondrial staining method and the other part frozen in liquid nitrogen and stored at -70°C until use.

HOMA1-IR index measurement for confirmation of type-II diabetes and insulin resistance

Fasting blood glucose level was measured with a glucometer device (elegance CT-X12, Convergent Technologies, Germany) and fasting plasma insulin levels were determined using a rat-specific insulin ELISA kit (Cayman chem., Ann Arbor, MI, USA) according to the manufacturer's instructions. Insulin resistance was identified with the homeostasis model assessment of insulin resistance (HOMA1-IR) index, using the following formula: fasting blood glucose (mmol/l) × fasting insulin (μu/l)/22.5.[26]

Infarct size evaluation

In a separate grouping of animals, the infarct sizes were measured as described previously.[23] At the end of reperfusion, the LAD coronary artery was occluded again and the hearts were perfused with 2 ml Evans blue dye (0.25%). Then, 2 mm slices were prepared from the hearts and immersed in 2,3,5-triphenylte-trazolium chloride (TTC, 1%) in phosphate buffer solution (pH 7.4). A computerized planimetry and ImageJ software were employed to determine the Left ventricular, risk zones and infarcted areas, by an investigator blinded to the animal grouping. The infarct sizes were reported as a percentage of the left ventricular risk zones.

Preparation of tissue homogenates

At the end of each Langendorff experiment, the left ventricles were separated and the ischemic zones were sampled and cut into pieces in lysis buffer containing (mM/ml) 1 KH2PO4, 1 KCL, 50 Tris–HCl pH 7.4, 1 EDTA, 1 NaF, 1 Na3VO4, and 1% triton 100X and protease inhibitor cocktail (Sigma-Aldrich, USA) and then homogenized with a Dounce glass tissue homogenizer (Sigma, Germany) in ice-cold. The homogenate was underwent centrifugation at 10,000 RCF for 10 min at 4°C. The obtained supernatants were quickly frozen at -70°C.[23] The Bradford method was used for detection of the amount of proteins in supernatants.[27]

Western blotting

The western blotting was performed as described previously.[20] Briefly, protein of the samples were separated in 12% SDS-gels, and then transferred to PVDF membranes at an hour for all gels. Subsequently, the blocking of membranes were done in 5% skim milk buffer containing 0.1% Tween-20 for 1.5 h and then probed with primary antibodies against microtubule-associated proteins 1A/1B light chain 3B (LC3B) (1:1000, Cell Signaling), P62/SQSTM1 (1:500, Santa Cruz) and β-actin (1:500, Cell Signaling) overnight at 4°C on a shaker incubator. After 4×5 min washing with Tris buffer saline containing 0.1% Tween-20, HRP-conjugated secondary antibody (1:7000, Cell Signaling) was added on the membranes. After for an hour incubation on shaker, the membranes were bathed in wash buffer and washed at least 3×5 min. Then, the membranes were incubated with the enhanced chemiluminescence (ECL, Amersham) reagents in dark room. This step was followed by the exposing of the membrane to an X-ray film and visualization of the chemiluminescence of the binding by means of a visualizing machine. The intensity of the bands was calculated using Image J software (IJ 1.46r version, NIH, USA) and normalized to each sample based on the intensity of β-actin as internal control.

Mitochondrial function studies

Isolation of cardiac mitochondria

For mitochondrial studies, at the end of reperfusion time of each isolated heart, the area at risk (AAR) of left ventricle was rapidly harvested for mitochondria isolation. All operations were performed on ice at 4°C, freshly. Myocardial AAR (40 mg) was minced with a scissor and homogenized in isolation buffer containing 70 mmol/L sucrose, 210 mmol/L mannitol, and 1 mmol/L EDTA in 50 mmol/L Tris/HCl, pH 7.4 (approx.1 mL buffer/15 mg tissue) by pre-cooled 2.0-ml Dounce Homogenizer. After centrifugation of the homogenates at 1300*g* for 3 minutes, the supernatant was centrifuged again at 10000*g* for 10 minutes. The mitochondrial pellet was obtained and suspended in 100 μl storage buffer containing 70 mmol/L sucrose and 210 mmol/L mannitol in 50 mmol/L Tris/HCl, pH 7.4

and was used freshly within 4 hours. Protein content was assayed by the bicinchoninic acid method with BSA as a standard.[28]

Cardiac mitochondrial ROS production

For mitochondrial ROS production study, the mitochondrial pellets were incubated with 2 μM dichlorofluorescin diacetate (DCFDA) dye at room temperature for 30 minutes. DCFDA, a fluorogenic dye, measures hydroxyl, peroxyl and other ROS activity within the cell and its organelles. After diffusion into organelle, DCFDA is oxidized by ROS into a highly fluorescent compound, 2', 7'-dichlorofluorescein (DCF). DCF fluorescence was detected by a fluorometric method with the excitation and emission wavelengths of 480 nm and 530 nm, respectively. An increase in the fluorescent intensity indicated an increased mitochondrial ROS production.[29]

Cardiac mitochondrial membrane potential changes

Cardiac mitochondrial membrane potential changes were determined using the 5,5',6,6'-tetrachloro-1,1',3,3'-tetraethylbenzimidazolylcarbocyanine iodide (JC-1) by an isolated mitochondrial staining kit according to the manufacturer's protocol (Sigma, Germany). In brief, 5 μg isolated mitochondria were diluted in 100 μl assay buffer containing 0.2 μg/ml JC-1 and incubated in the dark at room temperature for 10-20 min. JC-1 aggregates (red fluorescent, in healthy cells) were exited at 525 nm wavelength and detected at 590 nm emission wavelength, and JC-1 monomers (green fluorescent, in unhealthy cells) were exited at 485 nm wavelength and detected at 530 nm emission wavelength. Fluorescent intensity was recorded using spectrofluorometer (FP-750). A decrease in the red/green fluorescent intensity ratio is a representative of depolarization of mitochondrial membrane.[30]

Cain's method for staining mitochondria

The ischemic zone of left ventricular sections from mid-myocardial parts were deparaffinized and placed in hot aniline acid-fuschin solution for about 10 min and incubated in 0.1% sodium carbonate solution until pale pink. Following a quick rinse in 1% hydrochloric acid, sections were rinsed in distilled water, and then counterstained in methyl blue. Sections were again rinsed in water, dipped in 1% HCl, rinsed once more in water, and then dehydrated in graded alcohols and cleared in Xylol and infiltrated in paraffin. Sections were imaged using Olympus Bx40 microscope (Olympus Japan),[31] then evaluated according to Table 1. All processes of histological evaluations were done in a blind and random manner.

Statistical analysis

All values were expressed as means ± SEM. Comparison between groups were analysed through *one-way ANOVA* followed by *Tukey* post hoc or Student's t-tests as appropriate, using SPSS v16. A $p<0.05$ was considered statistically significant.

Table 1. Grading system for evaluation of mitochondrial density in cardiac cells.

Scoring	Intensity of Staining	Percentage Score
1	weak staining	< 25% positive
2	moderate staining	25% - 50% positive
3	strong staining	> 50% positive

Results

FBS* and *HOMA1-IR index analysis

Analysis of variance showed that the diabetic rats had a significantly higher blood glucose, plasma insulin and HOMA1-IR index ($p<0.001$, for all) comparing to those of non-diabetic control group. Pre-treatment of diabetic rats with vildagliptin significantly reduced hyperglycaemia ($p<0.001$) and increased plasma insulin level ($p<0.001$) and decreased HOMA1-IR index ($p<0.05$) comparing to the diabetic group (Table 2).

Table 2. Fasting blood sugar (FBS), plasma level of insulin and HOMA-IR test at the end of treatment protocol.

Groups	Non-Diabetic	Diabetic	Diabetic+Vilda
FBS (mmol/l)	5.28±0.18	28.60±0.50***	20.06±0.25$^{***,+++}$
Insulin (μu/ml)	4.64± 0.27	7.33±0.14***	9.52±0.20$^{***,+++}$
HOMA1-IR	1.08±0.05	9.31±0.18***	8.23±0.50$^{***,+}$

The data were expressed as mean ± SEM. n=10 for each group. Vilda: vildagliptin; HOMA1-IR: homeostasis model assessment-estimated insulin resistance. $^{***}p<0.001$ as compared with non-diabetic group and $^{++}p<0.01$ and $^{+++}p<0.001$ as compared with diabetic group.

Myocardial Infarct size

Induction of I/R injury through occluding of LAD provided similar risk zones in both control and diabetic hearts and this indicates no difference in the degree of ischemic stimulus in all groups. Instead, I/R injury led to induction of 42±2% infarct size in control hearts vs. 38±2% in diabetic hearts. Neither IPostC nor vildagliptin significantly reduced the infarct size in diabetic rats (17.02% and 21.73% lower than those of D-Control group, respectively). However, combined administration of IPostC with vildagliptin had a greater and more significant infarct sparing effect (up to 48.18% reduction) as compared with diabetic control group ($P<0.001$) (Figure 1).

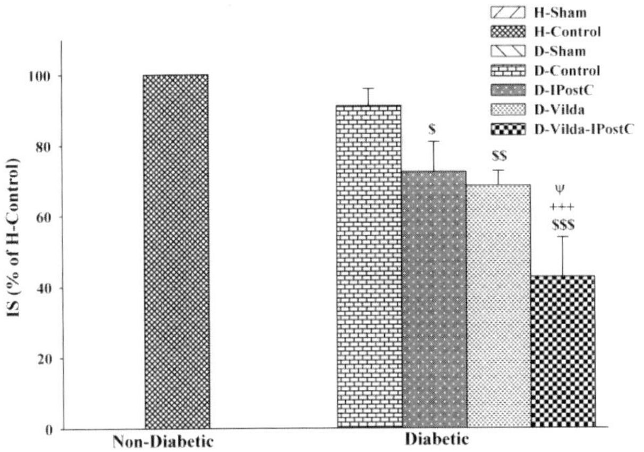

Figure 1. The changes of infarct sizes (IS) in experimental groups. IS was evaluated by evan's blue and triphenyltetrazolium chloride staining method, in non-diabetic and diabetic hearts subjected to 35 min regional ischemia and 60 min reperfusion. The data were expressed as mean±SEM. n=5-6 for each group. H: healthy; D: diabetic; IPostC: ischemic postconditioning; Vilda: vildagliptin. $^{\$}p<0.05$, $^{\$}p<0.01$ and $^{\$}p<0.001$ as compared to H-control; $^{+++}p<0.001$ as compared to D-Control group; $^{\Psi}p<0.05$ as compared to D-Vilda and D-IPostC groups.

Detection of autophagy and autophagic flux

To determine the autophagic changes, western blotting were performed for the autophagic markers, proteins LC3B-II and p62 (a selective substrate of autophagy) in area at risk of left ventricle in all groups. LC3B-II expression correlates with the increased levels of autophagic vesicles. P62 is subjected to the autophagic degradation at the lysosome, so autophagic flux is indicated by a reduction in the level of this proteins. The results revealed that in H-Control group the expression of p62 as well as expression of LC3BII and the ratio of LC3BII/LC3BI were increased to some extent as compared with those of H-Sham group, but there was no significant difference between them (Figure 2-A and B). It seems that autophagy tends to be unregulated very slightly with I/R injury in healthy hearts. In diabetic hearts, the expression of p62 and LC3B-II and the ratio were significantly increased in D-Sham group as compared with H-Sham healthy group (p<0.001) (Figure 2-A and B). These results showed that in this chronic model of type-II diabetes after 12 weeks, the autophagy was unregulated but the autophagic flux was more likely impaired at the late process of lysosomal degradation, as indicated indirectly by the lack of reduction of p62 level in diabetic hearts.

As shown in Figure 2, autophagic activity in D-Control group was significantly increased as compared with D-Sham group (p<0.01 for p62, and p<0.001 for both LC3B-II and the ratio).

Treatment of diabetic hearts decreased the expression of p62, so that this reduction was statistically significant in groups D-Vilda (p<0.05) and D-Vilda-IPostC (p<0.01) in comparison with D-Control group (Figure 2-A). IPostC alone could not significantly influence the levels of p62 expression in diabetic hearts, but the combination of IPostC with vildagliptin pre-treatment modulated the p62 levels significantly as compared with IPostC group (p < 0.05). In addition, the expression of LC3B-II and the ratio of LC3BII/LC3BI were decreased significantly in all treatments groups as compared with D-Control group (p<0.001 for all). While, the expression of LC3B-I was similar among all groups. These results showed that in treated diabetic hearts subjected to I/R injury, autophagy were decreased as compared with diabetic I/R heart with no treatments. It seems that addition of vildagliptin to IPostC administration increased the potency of IPostC to reduce the expressions of p62 and LC3-II proteins expression, and vildagilptin restored the autophagy flux in diabetic I/R hearts receiving IPostC.

Mitochondrial function

Cardiac mitochondrial ROS production

The level of cardiac mitochondrial ROS production in isolated mitochondria from area at risk of myocardium was expressed as fluorescence intensity of DCF, indicating the levels of ROS production. Figure 3-A showed that the levels of ROS production between groups were statistically significant (p<0.001). ROS production level in control hearts was higher than sham hearts, but this was statistically significant only in D-Contol group compared to D-Sham group (p<0.001). ROS production levels were significantly reduced in D-IpostC, D-Vilda and D-Vilda-IPostC groups in comparison with those of D-Control group (p<0.001, for all). In addition, the level of ROS production in vildagliptin-treated diabetic hearts was higher than D-IPostC hearts (Figure 3-A).

Cardiac mitochondrial membrane potential changes

Changes of cardiac mitochondrial membrane potential were expressed as red/green fluorescent intensity ratio of JC-1 staining in isolated mitochondria from area at risk of the myocardium (Figure 3-B). The greater red/green ratios correlate with normal membrane potentials (lack of unwanted depolarization). The ratio was significantly lower in control groups versus sham groups in non-diabetic and diabetic hearts (p<0.001/both), indicating the decreased or collapsed membrane potentials (more depolarization) in these I/R hearts. Mitochondrial membrane depolarization was significantly higher in D-Control than other treated-diabetic groups (p<0.001); thus, IPostC alone, vildagliptin alone and combination of vildagliptin with IPostC prevented the further depolarization of mitochondrial membrane potential. In addition, the ratio of red/green fluorescent intensity in combination treatment was significantly higher than those of IPostC alone group (p<0.001), indicating the increased efficiency of IPostC on mitochondrial functional preservation, when combined with vildagliptin pre-treatment (Figure 3-B).

Mitochondrial density

To test whether mitochondrial content and density was affected in area at risk of left ventricle, the myocardial sections from all groups were subjected to histological analysis using Cain's Method to specifically visualize the mitochondria. Increased intensity of staining indicates to increased mitochondrial density in Cain's method. As indicated by histological images in Figure 4 and intensity scoring in Figure 5, the mitochondrial density was significantly lowered in H-Control group versus H-Sham group and so in D-Control group versus D-Sham group (p<0.001 for both). In addition, mitochondrial density was significantly increased in vildagliptin-treated diabetic groups as compared with D-Control group (p<0.01, and p<0.001, respectively). However, higher mitochondrial densities were seen in hearts treated with combination of vildagliptin and IPostC compared to IPostC and D-Control hearts (p<0.01) (Figure 5).

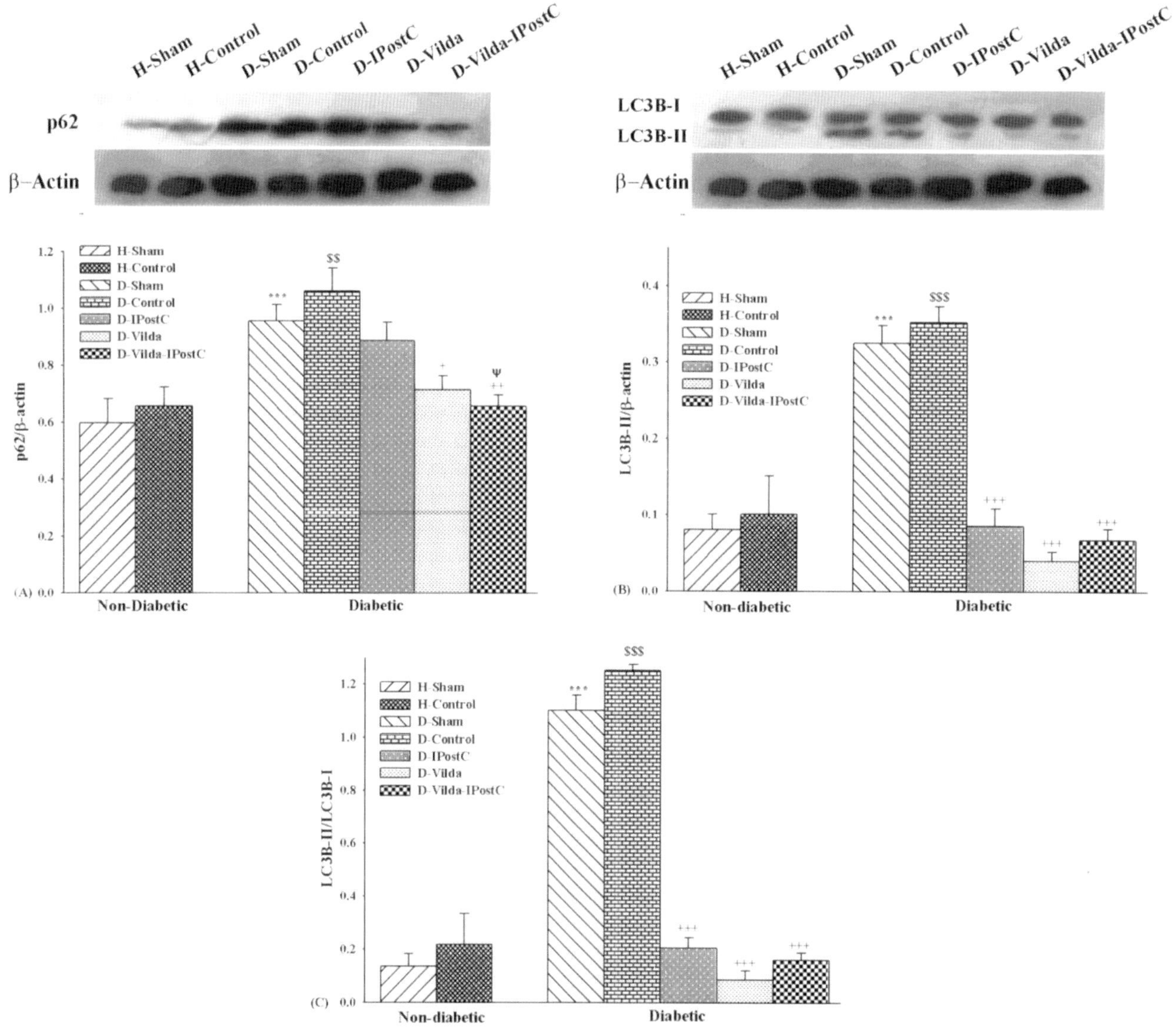

Figure 2. Changes of autophagy markers in experimental groups. The data were expressed as mean ±SEM. n=5 for each group. **A)** Changes of p62 protein expression; **B)** Changes of LC3B-II protein expression; and **C)** Changes of the ratio of LC3BII/LC3BI. H: healthy; D: diabetic; IPostC: ischemic-postconditioning; Vilda: vildagliptin. Levels of β-actin protein were used as the loading control. $^{\$\$}$p<0.01 and $^{\$\$\$}$p<0.001 as compared with H-Control group; $^{+}$p<0.05, $^{++}$p<0.01 and $^{+++}$p<0.001 as compared with D-Control group; $^{\Psi\Psi}$p<0.001 as compared with D-IPostC group.

Discussion

This experimental study showed that pretreatment of type-II diabetic rats with vildagliptin significantly restored the positive effects of IPostC on cardioprotection, autophagic flux and mitochondrial function following reperfusion injury, characterized by improved myocardial infarction, decreased autophagic markers LC3B-II and p62, reduced mitochondrial ROS generation, decreased mitochondrial membrane depolarization and increased mitochondrial number and density. Type-II diabetic patients with insulin resistance are characterized by hyperglycemia, hyperlipidemia, hyperinsulinemia, glucose intolerance and insulin resistance.[6] In this study, the diabetic rats demonstrated glucose intolerance at the end of 7th week and high FBS, hyperinsulinemia and increased HOMA1-IR at the end of 12th week, confirming that the animals were suffered with type-II diabetes and insulin-resistance. Oxidative stress, impaired mitochondrial function, apoptotic and autophagic stresses are common in the pathophysiology of diseases like diabetes and I/R injury.[4,32]

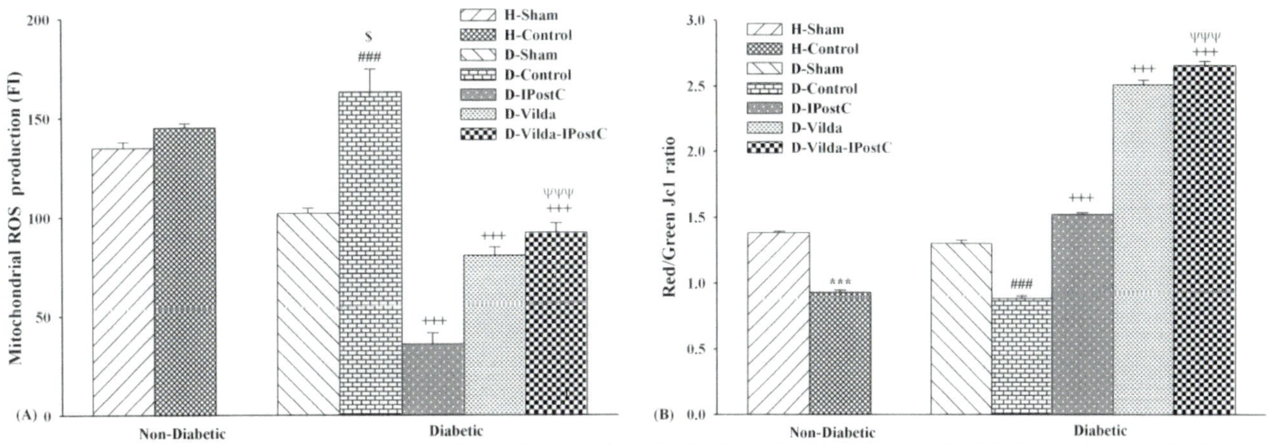

Figure 3. Mitochondrial functional studies. A) Cardiac mitochondrial ROS production assessed by DCFH-DA dye; and **B)** Cardiac mitochondrial membrane potential changes assessed by JC-1 dye. The data were expressed as mean ± SEM. n=6 for each group. H: Healthy; D: diabetic; IPostC: ischemic postconditioning; Vilda: vildagliptin. $^{***}p<0.001$ as compared with H-Sham group; $^{\#\#\#}p<0.001$ as compared with D-Sham group; $^{\$}p<0.05$ as compared with H-Control group; $^{+++}p<0.001$ as compared with D-Control group; $^{\Psi\Psi\Psi}p<0.001$ as compared with D-IPostC group.

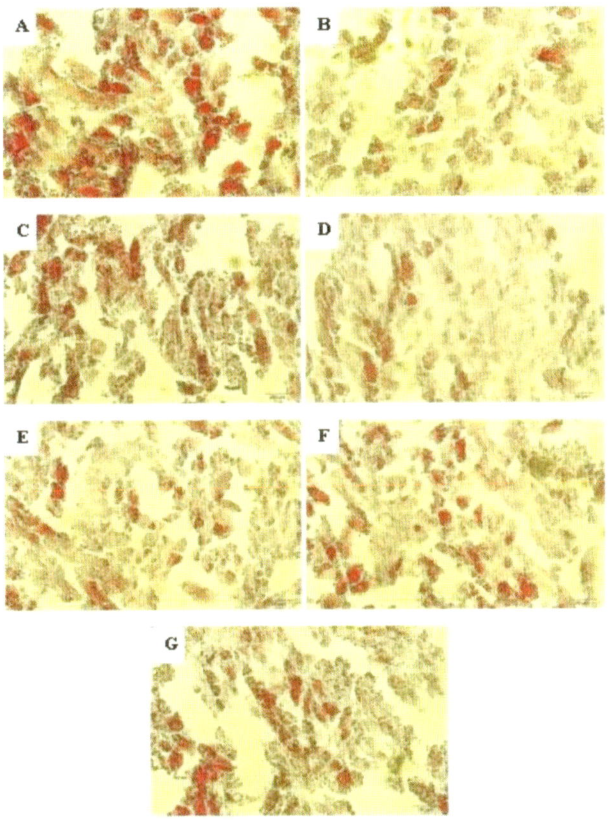

Figure 4. Photomicrographs of mitochondrial density in cardiomyocytes of experimental groups. Area at risk of left ventricle sections stained using Cain's method for mitochondrial density. Scale bar: 20 µm. A) H-Sham; B) H-Control; C) D-Sham; D) D-Control; E) D-IPostC; F) D-Vilda; G) D-Vilda-IPostC groups.

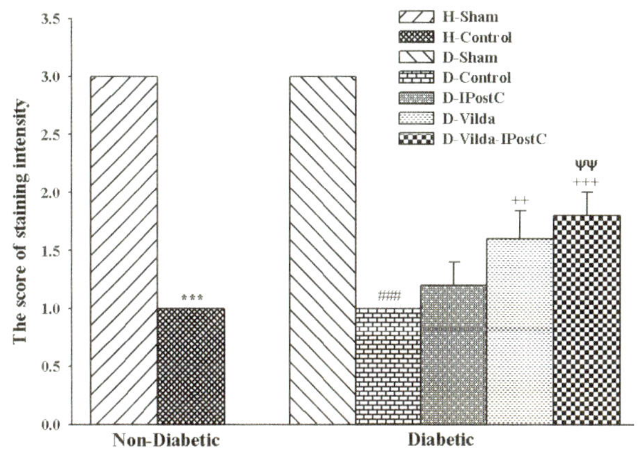

Figure 5. The scoring of staining intensity for determining mitochondrial densities by Cain's method. The data were expressed as mean ± SEM. n=5 for each group. H: Healthy; D: diabetic; IPostC: ischemic postconditioning; Vilda: vildagliptin. $^{***}p<0.001$ as compared with H-Sham group; $^{\#\#\#}p<0.001$ as compared with D-Sham group; $^{++}$ $p<0.001$, $^{+++}p<0.001$ as compared with D-Control group; $^{\Psi\Psi}$ $p<0.01$ as compared with D-IPostC group.

In type-II diabetes, increased plasma lipid profile leads to increased free fatty acid (FA) levels, because of inability of insulin to suppress the hormone sensitive lipase in the adipose tissue and the secretion of very low-density lipoproteins in the liver. In this condition, myocardial metabolism is switched to FA uptake and oxidation.[33] Therefore, diabetic heart is subjected to excessive oxidative stress, inflammation and lipotoxiciy that contribute to insulin resistance, functional impairment of the mitochondria, cardiomyocyte hypertrophy, apoptosis and dysregulation of autophagic activity.[34] Vildagilptin, as an enhancer of GLP1 hormone, increased plasma levels of insulin, decreased glucose intolerance and HOMA1-IR, so increased insulin sensitivity in our type-II diabetic rats. Some parts of these effects of vildagliptin can come back to its improving effects on the diabetes-induced alterations in plasma lipid profile.[19] At the time of reperfusion in diabetic hearts, various intracellular alterations switch the source of energy requirements to more fatty acid metabolism, inducing rapid opening of mitochondrial permeability transition pore (mPTPs) and decreasing mitochondrial membrane potential. These changes, in turn, cause overproduction of ROS by dysfunctional mitochondria, thus a defective cycle develops and leads to irreversible cellular injury triggered by necrosis, apoptosis and autophagy process.[1,35,36]

At basal level, autophagy has physiological function in the heart by restoring normal energy and cellular homeostasis and bioenergetics. However, the shift of autophagy to lower or higher than physiological levels may give rise to cell death, by accumulation of toxic molecules and damaged organelles or by degrading many essential proteins and organelles, respectively.[7,37] The role of autophagy in cardiac complications of diabetes is not well elucidated. Some studies demonstrated that during myocardial I/R injury the autophagic activity is enhanced to the detrimental level.[37] There is also a controversy that whether modulating autophagy is protective or harmful for myocardial I/R injury.[7] Recent experimental studies show that myocardial I/R injury and high fat diet lead to the upregulation of autophagy and impairment of autophagosome clearance.[38,39] It has been demonstrated that autophagy flux in the heart under diabetes is impaired as shown indirectly by up-regulation of LC3B-II and p62 protein level[36,37] or inhibited as shown by down-regulation of LC3B-II and up-regulation of p62.[38] In our study, myocardial I/R injury led to the elevation of the expression of both proteins LC3B-II and p62 in diabetic hearts. Although the autophagic flux was not directly examined in the present study due to some limitations, related results of this experiment are consistent with previous studies, indicating the impairment of autophagy flux in diabetic and I/R hearts as compared with non-diabetic ones.

Mitochondrial ROS generation and resultant autophagosome accumulation are associated with further ROS overproduction and mitochondrial permeabilization, leading to cell death by apoptosis.[36] Restoration of autophagosome clearance through adjusting the autophagic flux to an appropriate levels is thought to maintain cellular homeostasis and cell survival; this restoration was beneficial for the heart, by reducing cell apoptosis, oxidative stress and mitochondrial dysfunction in diabetic mice.[36,38] Similarly, application of vildagliptin with or without IPostC reduced the expression levels of LC3B-II and p62, accompanying with improved mitochondrial function and cardioprotection. Even though IPostC alone reduced mitochondrial ROS generation considerably, this effect was not associated with a significant reduction in infarct size by this strategy. This may possibly because the other arms of protection process (e.g. restoration of p62 levels and autophagosome clearance) are not affected by IPostC during diabetes. This finding likely indicates that reduction of mitochondrial ROS by itself could not responsible for cardioprotection and there should be an effective co-activation or coordination of multiple protective mechanisms. However, further study could overcome our limitation in evaluation of the reliance of this hypothesis.

Beside its hypoglycemic effect, vildagliptin decreased mitochondrial ROS production and mitochondrial depolarization, increased mitochondrial counts and improved the indications of autophagy flux accompanied with significant cardioprotection in diabetic hearts with I/R injury. It is demonstrated that vildagliptin has various important effects including decreasing lipid profile,[40] and anti-oxidative,[41] anti-inflammatory,[42] and anti-apoptotic[43] features in type-II diabetes, which they can contribute partly to observed cardioprotective actions. Because of these benefits of vildagliptin, the myocardial salvaging effects and cardio–cerebrovascular safety of this DPP-4 inhibitor has been reported in animals and patients with type-II diabetes.[44] In rats with isoproterenol-induced myocardial infarction (MI) and in non-diabetic obese rats with myocardial I/R injury, vildagliptin have reduced infarct size and recovered cardiac function through mitochondrial protection, and anti-oxidative and anti-apoptotic properties.[15,45] In addition, in the OLETF, a rat model of type-II diabetes, vildagliptin reduced diabetes-induced post-MI acute mortality possibly by restoring the autophagic response through attenuation of Bcl-2-Beclin-1 interaction.[46]

Previous studies have shown that IPostC could not restore diabetic heart function and infarct size following I/R injury.[13,47] Our studies proposed that IPostC could act more effectively if it was accompanied with a pharmacological agent.[13] As mentioned for diabetes, there is no conclusive and unequivocal evidence about the exact effects of postconditioning on the autophagic activity following myocardial I/R injury. In some studies, for example, postconditioning with sevoflurane,[10] and IPostC[9,48] promote autophagic activity via inhibiting the phosphorylation of mTOR during early reperfusion in non-diabetic hearts. In contrast, other studies have shown that cardioprotective effect of IPostC was associated with the inhibition of autophagic activity by the regulation of beclin-1 and AMPK/mTOR signaling pathway[49] or by preventing apoptotic and autophagic cell death in cardiomyocytes culture.[50] Our present results were in accord with the latter, as we found IPostC alone or in combination with vildagliptin tended to reduce the levels of autophagic markers, LC3B-II and p62, in diabetic hearts. These diverse results may be related mostly to the designs of the basic and pre-clinical studies. IPostC is conducted with different algorithms, resulting in dissimilar effects in diabetic or healthy hearts. The important variables possibly leading to these differences are the variability in activation levels of cell survival pathways and mediators, and presence or absence of end effectors (e.g. normal mitochondrial function) in diabetic or healthy hearts, and intrinsic characteristics of the tissues as well as the methodological discrepancies.[51] On the other hand, we observed that the mitochondrial and autophagy variables were affected constantly by combination of IPostC with vildagliptin and these effects were associated with full and greater cardioprotection rather than individual treatments. It seems that vildagliptin potentiates the cardioprotective influences of IPostC on diabetic myocardium. Due to the interfering effects of diabetes-induced changes with cardioprotection, it is plausible that the potency of IPostC may be reduced during diabetes. However, concomitant application of vildagliptin can normalize some abnormal metabolic and cellular changes of diabetes and thus increase the effectiveness of IPostC in this scenario, not in all but in most aspects of protective ways.

Conclusion

Combination of vildagliptin and IPostC in type-II diabetic hearts was a well-working strategy to reduce myocardial I/R damages by restoring mitochondrial membrane potential and mitochondrial function and modulating the autophagic activity in risk zones of I/R hearts. However, additional studies are necessary to elucidate the contribution of signaling pathways in the regulatory effects of Vildagliptin/IPostC on autophagy and mitochondrial biogenesis and function, especially in the models of *in vivo* I/R injury.

Acknowledgments

This work was supported in part by a grant from the National Elite Foundation of the Islamic Republic of Iran, and a grant from Drug Applied Research Centre, Tabriz University of Medical Sciences, Tabriz-Iran. The authors declare that they have no conflict of interest with respect to the research, authorship, and/or publication of this article.

Ethical Issues

All steps of the experiment were carried out in line with the Guide for the Care and Use of Laboratory Animals published by the US National Institutes of Health (NIH publication No 85-23, revised 1996) and approved by the Ethical Commission of Tabriz University of Medical Sciences (ethical number: 5.4.10696).

Conflict of Interest

The authors declare no conflict of interests.

References

1. Yellon DM, Hausenloy DJ. Myocardial Reperfusion Injury. *N Engl J Med* 2007;357(11):1121-35. doi: 10.1056/NEJMra071667
2. Luciani N, Nasso G, Gaudino M, Abbate A, Glieca F, Alessandrini F, et al. Coronary artery bypass grafting in type II diabetic patients: a comparison between insulin-dependent and non-insulin-dependent patients at short- and mid-term follow-up. *Ann Thorac* Surg 2003;76(4):1149-54. doi: 10.1016/S0003-4975(03)00838-5
3. Szabó Z, Håkanson E, Svedjeholm R. Early postoperative outcome and medium-term survival in 540 diabetic and 2239 nondiabetic patients undergoing coronary artery bypass grafting. *Ann Thorac Surg* 2002;74(3):712-9. doi: 10.1016/S0003-4975(02)03778-5
4. Huynh K, Bernardo BC, McMullen JR, Ritchie RH. Diabetic cardiomyopathy: mechanisms and new treatment strategies targeting antioxidant signaling pathways. *Pharmacol Ther* 2014;142(3):375-415. doi: 10.1016/j.pharmthera.2014.01.003
5. Badalzadeh R, Mokhtari B, Yavari R. Contribution of apoptosis in myocardial reperfusion injury and loss of cardioprotection in diabetes mellitus. *J Physiol Sci* 2015;65(3):201-15. doi: 10.1007/s12576-015-0365-8
6. Yang ZH, Peng XD. Insulin resistance and heart injury in rats with insulin resistance or type 2 diabetes mellitus. *Acta Cardiol* 2010;65(3):329-35. doi: 10.2143/AC.65.3.2050350
7. Matsui Y, Takagi H, Qu X, Abdellatif M, Sakoda H, Asano T, et al. Distinct roles of autophagy in the heart during ischemia and reperfusion: Roles of amp-activated protein kinase and beclin 1 in mediating autophagy. *Circ Res* 2007;100(6):914-22. doi: 10.1161/01.RES.0000261924.76669.36
8. Zou MH, Xie Z. Regulation of interplay between autophagy and apoptosis in the diabetic heart: new role of AMPK. *Autophagy* 2013;9(4):624-5. doi: 10.4161/auto.23577
9. Wei C, Li H, Han L, Zhang L, Yang X. Activation of autophagy in ischemic postconditioning contributes to cardioprotective effects against ischemia/reperfusion injury in rat hearts. *J Cardiovasc Pharmacol* 2013;61(5):416-22. doi: 10.1097/FJC.0b013e318287d501
10. Zhang YL, Yao YT, Fang NX, Zhou CH, Gong JS, Li LH. Restoration of autophagic flux in myocardial tissues is required for cardioprotection of sevoflurane postconditioning in rats. *Acta Pharmacol Sin* 2014;35(6):758-69. doi: 10.1038/aps.2014.20
11. Badalzadeh R, Azimi A, Alihemmati A, Yousefi B. Chronic type-I diabetes could not impede the anti-inflammatory and anti-apoptotic effects of combined postconditioning with ischemia and cyclosporine A in myocardial reperfusion injury. *J Physiol Biochem* 2017;73(1):111-20. doi: 10.1007/s13105-016-0530-4
12. Ferdinandy P, Hausenloy DJ, Heusch G, Baxter GF, Schulz R. Interaction of Risk Factors, Comorbidities, and Comedications with Ischemia/Reperfusion Injury and Cardioprotection by Preconditioning, Postconditioning, and Remote Conditioning. *Pharmacol Rev* 2014;66(4):1142-74. doi: 10.1124/pr.113.008300

13. Badalzadeh R, Mohammadi M, Najafi M, Ahmadiasl N, Farajnia S, Ebrahimi H. The additive effects of ischemic postconditioning and cyclosporine-A on nitric oxide activity and functions of diabetic myocardium injured by ischemia/reperfusion. *J Cardiovasc Pharmacol Ther* 2012;17(2):181-9. doi: 10.1177/1074248411416118
14. Burkey BF, Li X, Bolognese L, Balkan B, Mone M, Russell M, et al. Acute and chronic effects of the incretin enhancer vildagliptin in insulin-resistant rats. *J Pharmacol* Exp *Ther* 2005;315(2):688-95. doi: 10.1124/jpet.105.087064
15. Apaijai N, Pintana H, Chattipakorn SC, Chattipakorn N. Effects of vildagliptin versus sitagliptin, on cardiac function, heart rate variability and mitochondrial function in obese insulin-resistant rats. *Br J Pharmacol* 2013;169(5):1048-57. doi: 10.1111/bph.12176
16. Akarte AS, Srinivasan BP, Gandhi S, Sole S. Chronic DPP-IV inhibition with PKF-275-055 attenuates inflammation and improves gene expressions responsible for insulin secretion in streptozotocin induced diabetic rats. *Eur J Pharm Sci* 2012;47(2):456-63. doi: 10.1016/j.ejps.2012.07.003
17. Hamamoto S, Kanda Y, Shimoda M, Tatsumi F, Kohara K, Tawaramoto K, et al. Vildagliptin preserves the mass and function of pancreatic β cells via the developmental regulation and suppression of oxidative and endoplasmic reticulum stress in a mouse model of diabetes. *Diabetes Obes Metab* 2013;15(2):153-63. doi: 10.1111/dom.12005
18. Yin M, Sillјé HH, Meissner M, van Gilst WH, de Boer RA. Early and late effects of the DPP-4 inhibitor vildagliptin in a rat model of post-myocardial infarction heart failure. *Cardiovasc Diabetol* 2011;10:85. doi: 10.1186/1475-2840-10-85
19. Bayrami G, Karimi P, Agha-Hosseini F, Feyzizadeh S, Badalzadeh R. Effect of Ischemic postconditioning on Myocardial Function and Infarct Size Following Reperfusion Injury in Diabetic Rats Pretreated with Vildagliptin. *J Cardiovasc Pharmacol Ther* 2018;23(2):174-83. doi: 10.1177/1074248417729881
20. Badalzadeh R, Mohammadi M, Yousefi B, Farajnia S, Najafi M, Mohammadi S. Involvement of glycogen synthase kinase-3beta and oxidation status in the loss of cardioprotection by postconditioning in chronic diabetic male rats. *Adv Pharm Bull* 2015;5(3):321-7. doi: 10.15171/apb.2015.045
21. Jang JH, Baerts L, Waumans Y, De Meester I, Yamada Y, Limani P, et al. Suppression of lung metastases by the CD26/DPP4 inhibitor Vildagliptin in mice. *Clin Exp Metastasis* 2015;32(7):677-87. doi: 10.1007/s10585-015-9736-z
22. Srinivasan K, Viswanad B, Asrat L, Kaul CL, Ramarao P. Combination of high-fat diet-fed and low-dose streptozotocin-treated rat: a model for type 2 diabetes and pharmacological screening. *Pharmacol Res* 2005;52(4):313-20. doi: 10.1016/j.phrs.2005.05.004
23. Mokhtari B, Badalzadeh R, Alihemmati A, Mohammadi M. Phosphorylation of GSK-3β and reduction of apoptosis as targets of troxerutin effect on reperfusion injury of diabetic myocardium. *Eur J Pharmacol* 2015;765:316-21. doi: 10.1016/j.ejphar.2015.08.056
24. Badalzadeh R, Norouzzadeh A, Mohammadi M, Asgari A, Khoshbaten A. Cardiac responsiveness to beta-adrenergics in rats with lead-induced hypertension. *Biol Med* 2009;1(4):75-81.
25. Wu N, Zhang X, Guan Y, Shu W, Jia P, Jia D. Hypercholesterolemia abrogates the cardioprotection of ischemic postconditioning in isolated rat heart: roles of glycogen synthase kinase-3β and the mitochondrial permeability transition pore. *Cell Biochem Biophys* 2014;69(1):123-30. doi: 10.1007/s12013-013-9778-2
26. Geloneze B, Vasques AC, Stabe CF, Pareja JC, Rosado LE, Queiroz EC, et al. HOMA1-IR and HOMA2-IR indexes in identifying insulin resistance and metabolic syndrome: Brazilian Metabolic Syndrome Study (BRAMS). *Arq Bras Endocrinol Metabol* 2009;53(2):281-7. doi: 10.1590/S0004-27302009000200020
27. Bradford MM. A rapid and sensitive method for the quantitation of microgram quantities of protein utilizing the principle of protein-dye binding. *Anal Biochem* 1976;72(1-2):248-54. doi: 10.1016/0003-2697(76)90527-3
28. Gomez L, Paillard M, Thibault H, Derumeaux G, Ovize M. Inhibition of GSK3β by postconditioning is required to prevent opening of the mitochondrial permeability transition pore during reperfusion. *Circulation* 2008;117(21):2761-8. doi: 10.1161/CIRCULATIONAHA.107.755066
29. Thummasorn S, Kumfu S, Chattipakorn S, Chattipakorn N. Granulocyte-colony stimulating factor attenuates mitochondrial dysfunction induced by oxidative stress in cardiac mitochondria. *Mitochondrion* 2011;11(3):457-66. doi: 10.1016/j.mito.2011.01.008
30. Forini F, Kusmic C, Nicolini G, Mariani L, Zucchi R, Matteucci M, et al. Triiodothyronine prevents cardiac ischemia/reperfusion mitochondrial impairment and cell loss by regulating miR30a/p53 axis. *Endocrinology* 2014;155(11):4581-90. doi: 10.1210/en.2014-1106
31. Corum DG, Tsichlis PN, Muise-Helmericks RC. AKT3 controls mitochondrial biogenesis and autophagy via regulation of the major nuclear export protein CRM-1. *FASEB J* 2014;28(1):395-407. doi: 10.1096/fj.13-235382
32. Schrauwen P, Hesselink MK. Oxidative Capacity, Lipotoxicity, and Mitochondrial Damage in Type 2 Diabetes. *Diabetes* 2004;53(6):1412-7. doi: 10.2337/diabetes.53.6.1412
33. Boden G. Role of fatty acids in the pathogenesis of insulin resistance and NIDDM. *Diabetes* 1997;46(1):3-10. doi: 10.2337/diab.46.1.3

34. Hsu HC, Chen CY, Lee BC, Chen MF. High-fat diet induces cardiomyocyte apoptosis via the inhibition of autophagy. *Eur J Nutr* 2016;55(7):2245-54. doi: 10.1007/s00394-015-1034-7
35. Badalzadeh R, Yousefi B, Tajaddini A, Ahmadian N. Diosgenin-induced protection against myocardial ischaemia-reperfusion injury is mediated by mitochondrial KATP channels in a rat model. *Perfusion* 2015;30(7):565-71. doi: 10.1177/0267659114566064
36. Gottlieb RA, Mentzer Jr RM. Autophagy during cardiac stress: joys and frustrations of autophagy. *Annu Rev Physiol* 2010;72:45-59. doi: 10.1146/annurev-physiol-021909-135757
37. Munasinghe PE, Katare R. Maladaptive autophagy in diabetic heart disease. *Int J Clin Exp Physiol* 2016;3(4):155-65. doi: 10.4103/2348-8832.196893
38. Xie J, Cui K, Hao H, Zhang Y, Lin H, Chen Z, et al. Acute hyperglycemia suppresses left ventricular diastolic function and inhibits autophagic flux in mice under prohypertrophic stimulation. *Cardiovasc Diabetol* 2016;15(1):136. doi: 10.1186/s12933-016-0452-z
39. Sciarretta S, Boppana VS, Umapathi M, Frati G, Sadoshima J. Boosting autophagy in the diabetic heart: a translational perspective. *Cardiovasc Diagn Ther* 2015;5(5):394-402. doi: 10.3978/j.issn.2223-3652.2015.07.02
40. Matikainen N, Mänttäri S, Schweizer A, Ulvestad A, Mills D, Dunning BE, et al. Vildagliptin therapy reduces postprandial intestinal triglyceride-rich lipoprotein particles in patients with type 2 diabetes. *Diabetologia* 2006;49(9):2049-57. doi: 10.1007/s00125-006-0340-2
41. de Lima Ávila D, de Araújo GR, Silva M, de Amorim Miranda PH, Diniz MF, Pedrosa ML, et al. Vildagliptin ameliorates oxidative stress and pancreatic beta cell destruction in type 1 diabetic rats. *Arch Med Res* 2013;44(3):194-202. doi: 10.1016/j.arcmed.2013.03.004
42. Rizzo MR, Barbieri M, Marfella R, Paolisso G. Reduction of oxidative stress and inflammation by blunting daily acute glucose fluctuations in patients with type 2 diabetes: Role of dipeptidyl peptidase-IV inhibition. *Diabetes care* 2012;35(10):2076-82. doi: 10.2337/dc12-0199
43. Wu YJ, Guo X, Li CJ, Li DQ, Zhang J, Yang Y, et al. Dipeptidyl peptidase-4 inhibitor, vildagliptin, inhibits pancreatic beta cell apoptosis in association with its effects suppressing endoplasmic reticulum stress in db/db mice. *Metabolism* 2015;64(2):226-35. doi: 10.1016/j.metabol.2014.08.006
44. Schweizer A, Dejager S, Foley JE, Couturier A, Ligueros-Saylan M, Kothny W. Assessing the cardio-cerebrovascular safety of vildagliptin: meta-analysis of adjudicated events from a large Phase III type 2 diabetes population. *Diabetes Obes Metab* 2010;12(6):485-94. doi: 10.1111/j.1463-1326.2010.01215.x
45. Bingyan G, Yongjun L. GW25-e4168 Dipeptidyl peptidase (DPP) -4 inhibitor exhibits anti-apoptosis effects in isoproterenol-induced myocardial infarcted rats by inhibiting oxidative stress. *J* Am *Coll Cardiol* 2014;64(16):C43. doi: 10.1016/j.jacc.2014.06.206
46. Murase H, Kuno A, Miki T, Tanno M, Yano T, Kouzu H, et al. Inhibition of DPP-4 reduces acute mortality after myocardial infarction with restoration of autophagic response in type 2 diabetic rats. *Cardiovasc Diabetol* 2015;14:103. doi: 10.1186/s12933-015-0264-6
47. Bouhidel O, Pons S, Souktani R, Zini R, Berdeaux A, Ghaleh B. Myocardial ischemic postconditioning against ischemia-reperfusion is impaired in ob/ob mice. *Am J Physiol Heart Circ Physiol* 2008;295(4):H1580-6. doi: 10.1152/ajpheart.00379.2008
48. Hao M, Zhu S, Hu L, Zhu H, Wu X, Li Q. Myocardial Ischemic Postconditioning Promotes Autophagy against Ischemia Reperfusion Injury via the Activation of the nNOS/AMPK/mTOR Pathway. *Int J Mol Sci* 2017;18(3):614. doi: 10.3390/ijms18030614
49. Guo L, Xu JM, Mo XY. Ischemic postconditioning regulates cardiomyocyte autophagic activity following ischemia/reperfusion injury. *Mol Med Rep* 2015;12(1):1169-76. doi: 10.3892/mmr.2015.3533
50. Dosenko VE, Nagibin VS, Tumanovskaya LV, Moibenko AA, Vaage J. Postconditioning prevents apoptotic necrotic and autophagic cardiomyocyte cell death in culture. *Fiziol Zh* 2005;51(3):12-7.
51. Feyzizadeh S, Badalzadeh R. Application of ischemic postconditioning's algorithms in tissues protection: response to methodological gaps in preclinical and clinical studies. *J Cell Mol Med* 2017;21(10):2257-67. doi: 10.1111/jcmm.13159

The Eeffect of Metformin Combined with Calcium-Vitamin D3 Against Diet-Induced Nonalcoholic Fatty Liver Disease

Sara Shojaei Zarghani[1], Samin Abbaszadeh[2], Mohammad Alizadeh[3], Maryam Rameshrad[4], Alireza Garjani[4], Hamid Soraya[2]*

[1] *Student Research Committee, Urmia University of Medical Sciences, Urmia, Iran.*

[2] *Cellular and Molecular Research Center, Department of Pharmacology, Faculty of Pharmacy, Urmia University of Medical Sciences, Urmia, Iran.*

[3] *Department of Nutrition, Food and Beverages Safety Research Center, Faculty of Medicine, Urmia University of Medical Sciences, Urmia, Iran.*

[4] *Department of Pharmacology and Toxicology, Faculty of Pharmacy, Tabriz University of Medical Sciences, Tabriz, Iran.*

Keywords:

- AMP-activated protein kinase
- Calcium
- Metformin
- Nonalcoholic fatty liver disease
- Vitamin D_3

Abstract

Purpose: Metformin is one of the most popular drugs tested against nonalcoholic fatty liver disease (NAFLD). The present study aimed to investigate whether calcium-vitamin D_3 cosupplementation will intensify the effect of metformin on the prevention of high-fat, high-fructose (HFFr) diet-induced hepatic steatosis.

Methods: Male wistar rats (210±16 g) were assigned into the following seven groups: a Control group to receive a standard chow and six HFFr-fed groups to receive diets containing either normal (0.5% calcium and 1000 IU/kg vitamin D_3) or high amount of calcium and vitamin D_3 (2.4% calcium and 10000 IU/kg vitamin D_3) (CaD), in combination with gastric gavage administration of either saline or 25 or 200 mg/kg body weight/day metformin. After 60 days, rats were assessed with respect to their anthropometric, metabolic and hepatic parameters, as well as their hepatic AMP-activated protein kinase (AMPK) phosphorylation.

Results: Metformin and CaD, either alone or in combination, caused a significant reduction in HFFr diet-induced high serum aspartate aminotransferase (AST), hepatic steatosis and lipid accumulation without effect on insulin resistance and AMPK phosphorylation. In addition, slightly (and non-significantly) better effects of the combination in ameliorating steatosis and hepatic cholesterol content were observed.

Conclusion: Taken together, our results suggest that metformin and CaD could protect against the onset of HFFr diet-induced NAFLD in an insulin and AMPK-independent manner, without any marked additional benefits of their combination.

Introduction

Nonalcoholic fatty liver disease (NAFLD) has become the most common form of chronic liver disease in the world, which is characterized by abnormal triglyceride accumulation in hepatocytes, not due to excess alcohol consumption or other causes of secondary hepatic steatosis.[1,2] A growing body of evidence suggests a bidirectional relationship between NAFLD and components of metabolic syndrome,[3,4] although insulin resistance may still play an important role in the pathogenesis of NAFLD.[5] It is believed that insulin resistance and adiposity are associated with an imbalance between delivery and export of free fatty acid to the liver.[1,5] Therefore, it is not surprising that several studies have investigated the efficacy of natural or pharmacological insulin sensitizers on the prevention and management of NAFLD.

Among pharmacological insulin sensitizers, metformin has acquired a fundamental role in the management of many disorders associated with insulin resistance. Metformin is believed to exert its anti-diabetic effects through inhibition of mitochondrial respiratory chain complex I,[6,7] resulting in a fall in the ATP/AMP ratio and activation of AMP-activated protein kinase (AMPK), a master kinase regulating cellular energy homeostasis.[8] The activation of AMPK in the liver could both induce catabolic pathways, such as β-oxidation of fatty acids, and suppress anabolic pathways like lipogenesis, thus potentially leading to reduced hepatic steatosis.[8,9] As some studies have shown that metformin could protect against the development of steatosis in animal models,[10,11] however human studies are controversial.[12]

There is now some evidence that vitamin D could be a natural insulin sensitizer, especially in combination with calcium.[13,14] Dietary calcium or $VitD_3$ (cholecalciferol) intake, as well as calcitriol administration have been shown to prevent adiposity, insulin resistance[14,15] and hepatic fatty changes[16,17] and to be related to AMPK activation in different tissues in animal models.[18,19] On the

***Corresponding author:** Hamid Soraya, Email: soraya.h@umsu.ac.ir other hand, Shalata *et al.*[20] reported that vitamin D could intensify the effects of sitaglibtin/metformin drugs on treatment of steatosis and on decreasing hepatic triglyceride and malondialdehyde (MDA) content. So the hypothesis that combined calcium and vitamin D_3 supplementation augments the protective effects of metformin on the onset of diet-induced steatosis was tested in the present study, and the role of AMPK signaling in mediating observed effects was also determined.

Materials and Methods

Animals and diets

Male Wistar rats (210±16 g) were housed at a room temperature of 22±2°C under a 12-h light–dark cycle. The rats were acclimated to the new conditions for one week before receiving their experimental diets. Then, rats were randomly assigned to two groups to feed on either a standard chow (Control, n=6) or high-fat, high-fructose (HFFr) diet (n=42) for a period of 60 days. Rats had continuous access either to plain tap water or to water containing 20% fructose solution, respectively. The HFFr-fed rats were nourished ad libitum with a normal calcium (0.5%) and $VitD_3$ (1000 IU/kg) diet or a high calcium (2.4%) and $VitD_3$ (10000 IU/kg) diet (CaD). These rats were also randomized to receive, by gastric gavage, *either* 1 ml of saline alone (S) or 25 or 200 mg/kg body weight metformin, once a day. The standard chow contained recommended levels of calcium (0.5%) and $VitD_3$ (1000 IU/kg).[21] The highest amount of vitamin D_3 (10000 IU/kg diet) was selected as the optimal level of vitamin D_3 intake without any adverse effect on rats.[22] Details of Control and HFFr diets are provided in Table 1. The HFFr diet used has been shown to induce NAFLD, previously.[23] Throughout the experiment, daily feed intake and weekly body weight measurements were taken to monitor the health of the rats. This study was conducted in accordance with the Guide for the Care and Use of Laboratory Animals of Urmia University of Medical Sciences. In addition, all animal protocols were approved by the Ethics Committee of Urmia Medical Sciences University.

Table 1. Macronutrient composition and energy contents of the control and high fat high fructose (HFFr) diets

-	Constituent	Control	HFFr
Macronutrients (% by weight)	**Carbohydrate**	52.8	47.9
	Starch	52.8	30.4
	Fructose	0	17.5
	Fat	5	27.8
	Soybean oil	5	2.8
	Hydrogenated oil	0	5
	Sheep tallow	0	20
	Protein	20	11.5
Macronutrients (% Kcal)	**Carbohydrate**	59.7	37.3
	Fat	14.5	53
	Protein	25.8	9.7
	Energy (Kcal/g)	3.1	4.72

Evaluation of animal and organ weights

At the end of the 60th day of the diet, the animals were anesthetized by an *ip* injection of a mixture of ketamin (60 mg/kg) and xylazin (10 mg/kg). Then, after blood sampling, the livers and visceral fat from both epididymal and perirenal areas were rapidly excised and weighed. Next, the livers were stored at -80 for further analysis.

Serum analysis

At the end of the treatment period and after a 16 h fast with free access to water, blood samples were collected via portal vein from anaesthetized animals. Blood samples were centrifuged and serum was frozen at -80°C for subsequent analysis. Serum fasting glucose, alanine aminotransferase (ALT), aspartate aminotransferase (AST), triglycerides, total and high-density lipoprotein (HDL) cholesterol concentrations were determined by an enzymatic method using individual commercial kits (Pars azmun, Tehran, Iran) and an automatic biochemical analyzer (BT 4500, Biotechnica, Italy). Non-HDL-C was calculated as total cholesterol minus HDL-C. Serum insulin (Bioassay Technology Laboratory, China) and complement C1q/tumor necrosis factor-α related protein-3 (CTRP3) (zellBio, Germany) levels were quantified with ELISA kits. In addition, we used the homeostasis model assessment of insulin resistance (HOMA-IR) method to estimate insulin resistance as [Fasting insulin×Fasting glucose/405].

Hepatic lipid quantitation and lipid peroxidation

The hepatic lipids were extracted according to the method described by Folch *et al.*[24] Hepatic triglyceride and cholesterol content was quantified using commercially colorimetric assay kits (Pars azmun, Iran). Results were given as mg triglyceride or cholesterol per gram liver. Hepatic malondialdehyde (MDA), a product of lipid peroxidation, was also measured to evaluate the degree of oxidative stress, as described by Yousefi *et al.*[25]

Histological examination

Immediately after removal, fragments of liver tissues were fixed in a solution of 10% buffered formaldehyde. Sections of the formalin-fixed and paraffin-embedded tissues were stained with hematoxylin and eosin to semi-quantitatively assess the fatty degeneration using the NAFLD activity score (NAS). The histological features were numerically scored according to the percentage of distributions and blinded regarding treatment groups. Scores for steatosis (score 0 to 3), lobular inflammation (score 0 to 3), and ballooning (score 0 to 2), were also summed to produce the NAS, thus they ranged from 0 to 8.

Western blot analysis

Powdered liver tissue, was homogenized (10% w/v) in homogenization buffer containing 50 mM Tris-Hcl, 150 mM Nacl, 5mM Sodium Pyrophosphate (NaPPi), 50mM NaF, 1mM EDTA, 1mM dithiothreitol (DTT), 0.1%SDS (w/v), 1% TXT-100 (v/v), and protease inhibitor cocktail. Tissue homogenates were centrifuged at 1000g for 10 min at 4 °C and supernatants were stored in 50 µl aliquots at -80 °C for further analysis. Bradford Protein Assay kit was used to evaluate the protein content of the supernatant. SDS-polyacrylamide gel electrophoresis, followed by transfer to nitrocellulose membranes was performed using 50 µg of homogenate protein. Then membranes were blocked in 5% non-fat milk in Tris-buffered saline Tween-20 and incubated overnight with rabbit antibodies against phospho-AMPK (p-AMPKThr172) and AMPK (1:1000 dilution - Cell Signaling Technology Inc., Danvers, Massachusetts, USA) in 5 % BSA (wt/vol). After extensive washing, the membranes were incubated with a peroxidase-conjugated goat anti-rabbit secondary antibody (1:5000 dilution, Cell Signaling Technology Inc. Danvers, Massachusetts, USA) in 5% skim milk (wt/vol). After washing, antibodies were visualized using the BM Chemiluminescence kit (Roche; Germany). Densitometric analyses of immunoblots were performed using Image J software (National Institute of Health, Bethesda, Maryland).[26]

Statistical analysis

All data are presented as mean ± standard error (SE). Data were tested by one-way analysis of variance (ANOVA, SPSS19). When ANOVA results were significant ($p<0.05$), the post hoc Tukey test was also applied to find where differences existed.

Results and Discussion

Body and Tissue Weights

The initial body weight of rats was similar (*p-value*=0.19). At the end of the experimental period, the HFFr+S rats had a near doubling of visceral fat weight compared to the Control group (6.9±1.1 g vs. 3.4±0.4 g, *p-value*=0.009), while it was slightly and non-significantly lower in the other groups, especially in the rats gavaged with the high dose of metformin (200 mg/kg/day). After 60 days, no significant differences were found between the groups regarding final body weight and liver/body weight percentage (Table 2). It means that the excess energy intake of HFFr rats have led to a greater adiposity, but not to a higher body weight.

Table 2. Body and tissue weight-related measurements

-	Control	HFFr+S	+Met25	+CaD+Met25	+Met200	+CaD+Met200	+CaD+S
Initial Body Weight (g)	213.3±6.5	218.7±6.8	208±5.6	203±3.9	201.6±6	203±5.4	221.1±9
Final Body Weight (g)	288.3±13.6	278.8±11.1	243.7±9.4	255.1±7	238.7±9.5	244.5±13.1	262.3±6.5
Liver/ body weight (%)	3.02±0.05	2.9±0.05	3±0.07	3.1±0.09	3.1±.1	3.1±0.09	2.9±0.1
Visceral fat weight (g)	3.4±0.4	6.9±1.1*	5.5±0.6	5.1±0.3	4.6±0.5	4.7±0.3	5.1±0.5
Visceral fat/body weight (%)	1.1±0.13	2.4±0.3*	2.3±0.2	2.01±0.14	1.91±0.14	2.02±0.14	1.94±0.2

HFFr: High-Fat, High-Fructose diet, S: Saline, +Met25: HFFr+25 mg/kg body weight metformin, +Met200: HFFr+200 mg/kg body weight metformin, +CaD: HFFr+2.4% Calcium plus 10000 IU/kg vitamin D_3. Data are mean ± SE. n = 6–7 in each group. (*) $P<0.05$ versus the Control group. (one way ANOVA, Tukey post hoc test).

Serum Biochemistry

Compared to the Control rats, the HFFr+S rats displayed a non-significant increase in glucose levels and HOMA-IR scores and a decrease in insulin levels. The CaD+S rats had also greater glucose and lower insulin levels compared to the metformin-gavaged rats (not significantly in some cases), although no meaningful differences were observed in HOMA-IR between the groups (*p-value*=0.34).

Vitamin D and calcium have been linked to the improvement of insulin sensitivity, activation of the Ca^{2+}-mediated apoptotic pathway in adipose tissues,[14] inhibition of lipogenesis and promotion of lipid oxidation.[17,27] The beneficial effects of metformin are also thought to be through some mechanisms, including activation of AMPK,[28] and increasing insulin receptor activation, glucose uptake[29] and leptin sensitivity in liver.[30] In the present study, we tested the hypothesis that whether or not CaD augments the ameliorating effects of metformin on insulin resistance, as the major pathogenic factor of NAFLD. Surprisingly, to the contrary of our hypothesis, neither metformin nor CaD did not alter the increased levels of HOMA-IR induced by HFFr diet, so exerted their protective effects independent of insulin action. The inability of metformin therapy to reduce indexes of insulin resistance has been reported in both humans[31,32] and animal studies,[10,33] that in part may be due to the unaltered insulin signaling within skeletal muscle and whole-body, and gluconeogenesis after metformin treatment.[31,34] In this line, Linden *et al.*[35,36] reported that metformin (300 mg/kg/day) lowered adiposity, hemoglobin A1c levels, hepatic triglycerides and markers of hepatic de novo lipogenesis in diabetic Otsuka Long-Evans Tokushima Fatty (OLETF) rats, which were not accompanied by an improvement in the both fasting and postchallenge glycemic control and in the increased serum levels of triglyceride and free fatty acids. Indeed, there are some other studies which have found no effect exerted by either dietary calcium and/or vitamin D on glucose intolerance.[37-41]

In this study, HFFr diet, calcium-vitamin D_3 supplementation and oral gavage administration of metformin did not alter the serum concentrations of triglycerides, total cholesterol and Non-HDL-C (*p-*

value>0.05). The rats in the CaD+S group exhibited clearly higher levels of serum HDL-C compared to the groups receiving recommended levels of calcium and vitamin D_3. Moreover, the levels of serum CTRP3 was significantly higher in the +Met200 group compared to the other groups (except the +CaD+Met200 group). There was no effect of HFFr diet and no additive effect of metformin and CaD on serum HDL-C and CTRP3 (Table 3).

Table 3. Serum Biochemical Parameters

-	Control	HFFr+S	+Met25	+CaD+Met25	+Met200	+CaD+Met200	+CaD+S
Triglycerides (mg/dl)	49.3±3.8	41.2±4.1	35.1±2.7	48.5±2.9	44.2±5.2	45.8±6.2	38±6.8
Cholesterol (mg/dl)	63±4.7	59.6±1	66±3.8	64.2±4.5	56.1±4.1	62.6±2.3	65.8±3.8
HDL-C (mg/dl)	20±0.9	20.3±0.4^{a}	22.1±1.1^{a,c}	23.3±0.7^{a,b}	22.2±1.4^{a,c}	26±0.8^{b,c}	26.6±0.8^{b}
Non-HDL-C (mg/dl)	41.7±4.2	39.6±1.4	43.8±3.1	44.1±3.3	33.8±3.6	36.6±2.1	39.1±4.6
Glucose (mg/dl)	114±8.3	170.5±9^{a,b}	135±16.2^{a}	152.8±19.9^{a,b}	167.2±20.7^{a,b}	154.5±14.9^{a,b}	216.8±5.8^{b}
Insulin (mg/dl)	13.01±0.9	12.4±0.3^{a,b}	13.4±0.7^{a}	13.2±0.5^{a}	12.1±0.8^{a,b}	14.4±0.4^{a}	10.38±0.5^{b}
HOMA-IR	3.8±0.4	5.2±0.3	4.9±0.4	5.4±0.8	4.9±0.6	5.5±0.6	5.3±0.2
CTRP3 (ng/ml)	128.4±18.1	127.6±22.3^{a}	131.8±10^{a}	140.3±16.1^{a}	235.6±12.9^{b}	168.2±21.4^{a,b}	98.1±16.6^{a}

HFFr: High-Fat, High-Fructose diet, S: Saline, +Met25: HFFr+25 mg/kg body weight metformin, +Met200: HFFr+200 mg/kg body weight metformin, +CaD: HFFr+2.4% Calcium plus 10000 IU/kg vitamin D_3, HDL-C: High-density lipoprotein cholesterol, HOMA-IR: Homeostatic model assessment of insulin resistance, CTRP3: Complement C1q/tumor necrosis factor-α related protein-3. Data are mean ± SE. n = 6–7 in each group. (*) P<0.05 versus the Control group. Values with different letters are significantly different (P<0.05) (one way ANOVA, Tukey post hoc test).

CTRP3 (also known as cartonectin, cartducin, CORS-26) is a novel adipokine and a member of CTRP superfamily, which has been shown to reduce glucose levels, hepatic steatosis and gluconeogenesis, by its regulatory effects on lipid and glucose metabolism.[42,43] Moreover recent studies have suggested that some beneficial effects of CTRP3 could be mediated through AMPK signaling.[44-46] The reduced levels of circulating and tissue expression of CTRP3 are reported in both human and rodent models of obesity and diabetes.[43,47-49] Nonetheless, choi *et al.*[50] reported an elevated circulating CTRP-3 concentrations in diabetic compared to non-diabetic adults and in the another study no difference was found between patients with and without metabolic syndrome.[51] In the present study, although neither the HFFr diet nor CaD supplementation did not alter the circulating levels of this adipokine, metformin administration at a dose of 200 mg/kg led to the highest levels of CTRP3, but not the most improvement in AMPK activation and steatosis. This was, in part, in accordance with findings *of* Tan and coworkers[52] who for the first time investigated the effects of metformin therapy on CTRP3 levels. They demonstrated lower serum and omental adipose tissue CTRP3 in women with PCOS, which was increased after 6 months of metformin therapy.

Moreover, in the present study, the HFFr+S rats showed higher levels of serum ALT and AST compared to the Control group (131.9±17.6 IU/l vs. 65.2±8.1 IU/l, *p-value*= 0.02 and 239.8±27.9 IU/l vs. 171.5±12 IU/l, *p-value*=0.12, respectively). CaD supplementation and oral gavage of metformin significantly prevented the increase in the serum concentration of AST, although ALT levels reduced non-significantly, without any differences between groups. (Figure 1).

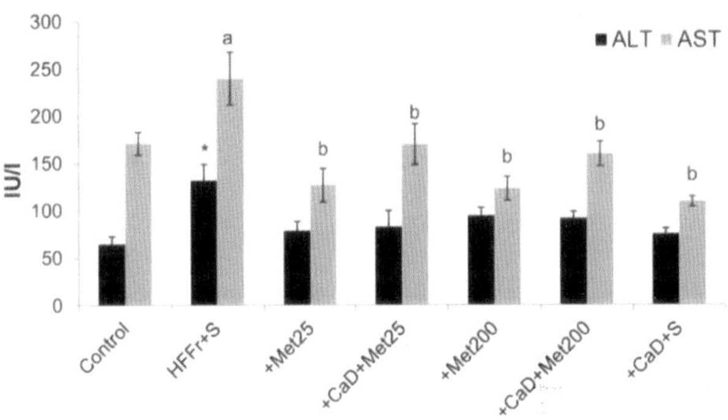

Figure 1. Effect of experimental diets on liver enzymes. HFFr: High-Fat, High-Fructose diet, S: Saline, +Met25: HFFr+25 mg/kg body weight metformin, +Met200: HFFr+200 mg/kg body weight metformin, +CaD: HFFr+2.4% Calcium plus 10000 IU/kg vitamin D_3, ALT: Alanine aminotransferase, AST: Aspartate aminotransferase. Data are mean ± SE. n = 6–7 in each group. (*) P<0.05 versus the Control group. Values with different letters are significantly different (P<0.05) (one way ANOVA, Tukey post hoc test).

Hepatic lipid content and lipid peroxidation

The HFFr+S rats exhibited the expected increases in the hepatic fat deposition (hepatic triglyceride, 5.75±0.59 mg/g tissue weight vs. 1.83±0.25 mg/g tissue weight, *p-value*< 0.001 and hepatic cholesterol 1.2±0.13 mg/g tissue weight vs. 0.88±0.06 mg/g tissue weight, *p-value*=0.04, respectively), while it was significantly attenuated in the other groups. There was no marked differences in the hepatic triglyceride and cholesterol content between CaD-supplemented and/or metformin-gavaged groups.

HFFr diet did not increase the lipid peroxidation in livers, which was determined by measurement of hepatic MDA contents, although the concentration of hepatic MDA was significantly decreased in the +Met200 group compared to the HFFr+S group (Figure 2).

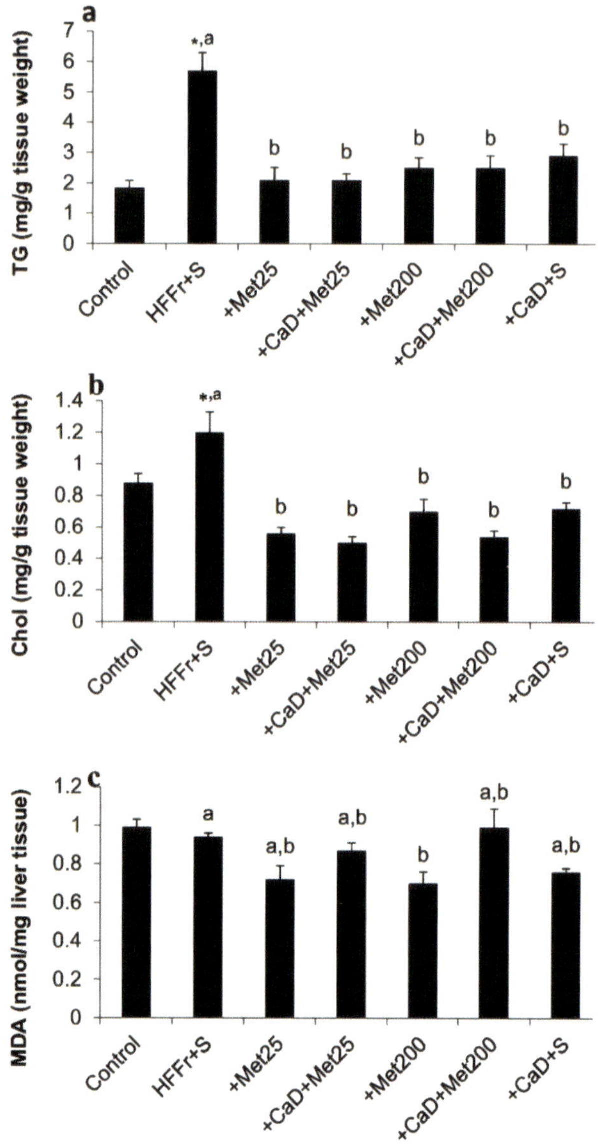

Figure 2. Effect of experimental diets on hepatic lipid content and malondialdehyde. **a** hepatic TG, **b** hepatic Chol, **c** hepatic MDA content. HFFr: High-Fat, High-Fructose diet, S: Saline, +Met25: HFFr+25 mg/kg body weight metformin, +Met200: HFFr+200 mg/kg body weight metformin, +CaD: HFFr+2.4% Calcium plus 10000 IU/kg vitamin D_3, TG: Triglyceride, Chol: Cholesterol, MDA: Malondialdehyde. Data are mean ± SE. n = 6–7 in each group. (*) P<0.05 versus the Control group. Values with different letters are significantly different (P<0.05) (one way ANOVA, Tukey post hoc test).

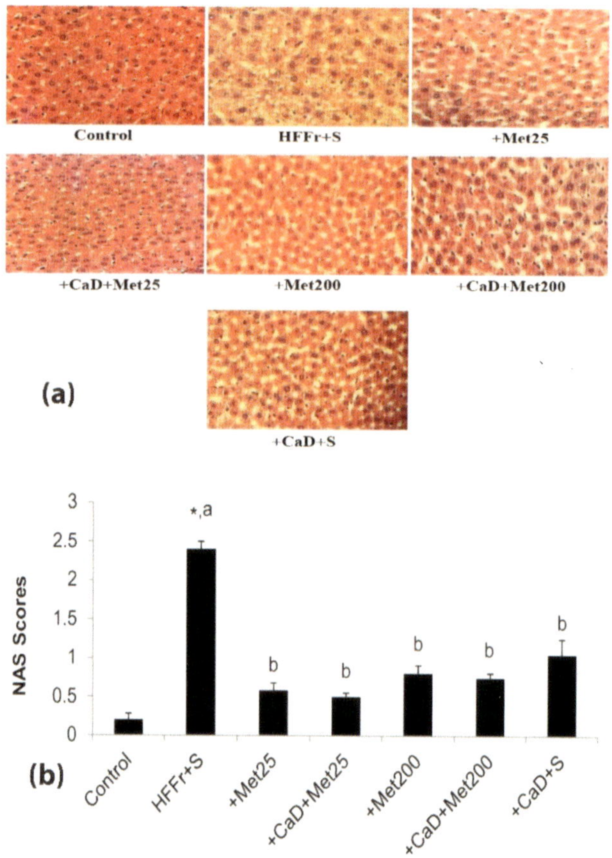

Figure 3. a: Histopathological assessment after haematoxylin–eosin staining of liver sections. Sections from liver tissues of the HFFr+S rats showed hepatic steatosis and only slightly ballooning degeneration. Other five groups, especially the metformin-gavaged groups, showed lower fat accumulation (magnification×400). **b**: The NAFLD activity score (NAS) was determined based on histopathological analysis (steatosis, inflammation and ballooning). HFFr: High-Fat, High-Fructose diet, S: Saline, +Met25: HFFr+25 mg/kg body weight metformin, +Met200: HFFr+200 mg/kg body weight metformin, +CaD: HFFr+2.4% Calcium plus 10000 IU/kg vitamin D_3. Data are mean ± SE. n = 6–7 in each group. (*) P<0.05 versus the Control group. Values with different letters are significantly different (P<0.05) (one way ANOVA, Tukey post hoc test).

Liver Histology

The livers from HFFr+S rats displayed evidence of fatty liver, with macro and microvesicular steatosis. Although steatosis and NAS scores were significantly attenuated in the other five groups, especially in the metformin groups, compared to that in the HFFr+S group, in accordance with the hepatic triglyceride content. The hepatic histological examination of liver fragments showed no sign of inflammation, and only slightly ballooning degeneration, as is shown in Figure 3.

Excessive fat accumulation in hepatocytes is the earliest and the most common manifestation of NAFLD.[53] In the present study, although liver weight did not differ between groups, serum markers of liver function, hepatic lipid content and steatosis scores were raised in the HFFr+S rats and similarly attenuated in the treated groups in an *insulin*-independent manner. However, metformin, especially in the dose of 25 mg/kg/day, showed slightly more favorable effects on steatosis and hepatic lipid content. Our present results demonstrated that using the combination of metformin and CaD, was no more effective than each of them alone on the different parameters studied. Although they slightly intensified the hepatoprotective effects of each other on HFFr diet-induced steatosis and hepatic cholesterol accumulation, but not on the increased serum liver enzymes levels and hepatic lipid peroxidation. These results are consistent with the findings of some earlier studies which have demonstrated the protective effects of each of metformin,[10,11] calcium[16] or 1,25 $(OH)_2$ vitamin

D_3,[17] separately, and CaD[54] against the development of steatosis in animal models.

Calcium-vitamin D has been shown to increase the effects of metformin therapy on symptoms of women with polycystic ovary syndrome (PCOS).[55,56] Nevertheless, according to the best of our knowledge, no report exists on the effect of combined calcium-vitamin D and metformin on the development of diet-induced NAFLD. Shalata *et al*. reported that vitamin D could intensify the effects of sitaglibtin/metformin drugs on treatment of steatosis.[20] Moreover, a very recent study demonstrated the synergistic protective effects of vitamin D (6 ng/kg SC) and metformin (100 mg/kg) on the improvement of some metabolic and structural abnormalities and, hepatic steatosis induced by 8 weeks of high fat diet feeding in wistar rats.[57] In this study no possible mechanism was mentioned for the observed synergistic effects, except a speculation of the involvement of AMPK.

Western blot analysis

There was no statistical difference between the seven groups with respect to the hepatic phosphorylation of AMPK (p-value>0.05) (Figure 4).

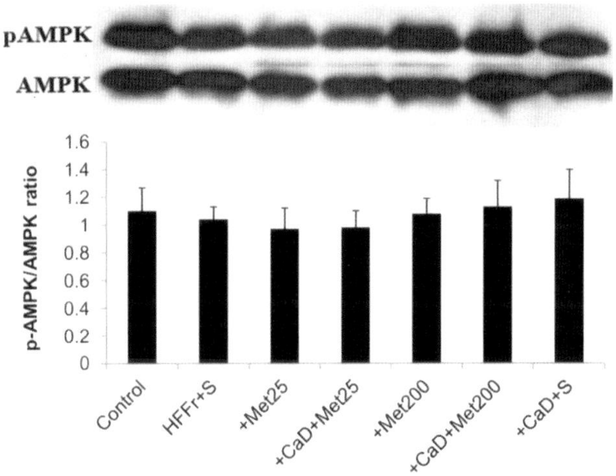

Figure 4. Western blotting analysis of AMPK and p-AMPK expression in the livers of experimental rats. Image shows demonstrative bands of the analyzed proteins in the livers. Bars represent the ratio of phosphorylated AMPKα to total AMPKα. HFFr: High-Fat, High-Fructose diet, S: Saline, +Met25: HFFr+25 mg/kg body weight metformin, +Met200: HFFr+200 mg/kg body weight metformin, +CaD: HFFr+2.4% Calcium plus 10000 IU/kg vitamin D3, *AMPK: AMP-activated protein kinase.* Data are mean ± SE. n = 6–7 in each group. There were no significant differences between groups (P>0.05).

The suggested key role of AMPK in mechanism of metformin action prompted us to examine the involvement of AMPK in the observed findings. Here, we demonstrated that the phosphorylation of AMPK was not affected by neither HFFr diet nor different doses of metformin and/or calcium-vitamin D_3. These findings are discordant from a large body of literature, which suggests that a high-fat diet exposure could decrease hepatic p-AMPK and metformin and calcitriol are activators of this intracellular energy sensor.[19,44,58,59] In contrast, and in agreement with our findings, Foretz *et al.*[60] reported that mice lacking hepatic AMPK exhibited normal blood glucose levels and gluconeogenic gene expression compared to those in wild-type mice. The maintenance of the antidiabetic effects of metformin in these animals as well as the reduction of intracellular ATP content clearly revealed that metformin suppressed gluconeogenesis independently of the liver-kinase B1 (LKB1)/AMPK pathway and via lowering hepatic energy status. This finding has been subsequently confirmed by other investigators,[35,36,61] who disclosed the AMPK-independent effects of metformin in the management of type 2 diabetes and NAFLD, and suggested that metformin could ameliorate hepatic steatosis through silent mating type information regulation 2 homolog1 (SIRT1) -mediated effects on the autophagy machinery. In this study, we did not assess inflammatory pathways and fatty acid metabolism-related gene expressions, which could provide a direction for future research.

Conclusion

In conclusion, our results suggest that both metformin and calcium-vitamin D_3 provide similar hepatoprotective effects in an insulin and AMPK-independent manner, with slightly additional protective benefits of their combination on the steatosis scores and hepatic cholesterol content. *Ultimately,* the increased CTRP3 levels after metformin administration was also observed in the present study.

Acknowledgments

The authors would like to express their gratitude towards Dr. Amir Abbas Farshid and Dr. Ali Asghar Tehrani for conducting the pathological assessments. The authors would also like to thank the Pharma chemie, Arya and Daana Pharmaceutical Companies and Beyza 21 Feed Mill Company. Financially, this study was supported by Urmia University of Medical Sciences.

Ethical Issues

This study was conducted in accordance with the guide for care and use of laboratory animals approved by the Animal Ethical Committee of Urmia University of Medical Sciences.

Conflict of Interest

The authors declare that they have no conflict of interest.

References

1. Smith BW, Adams LA. Non-alcoholic fatty liver disease. *Crit Rev Cl Lab Sci* 2011;48(3):97-113. doi: 10.3109/10408363.2011.596521
2. Chalasani N, Younossi Z, Lavine JE, Diehl AM, Brunt EM, Cusi K, et al. The diagnosis and management of non-alcoholic fatty liver disease: Practice guideline by the american association for the study of liver diseases, american college of gastroenterology, and the american gastroenterological association. *Am J Gastroenterol* 2012;107(6):811-26. doi: 10.1038/ajg.2012.128

3. Wainwright P, Byrne CD. Bidirectional relationships and disconnects between nafld and features of the metabolic syndrome. *Int J Mol Sci* 2016;17(3):367. doi: 10.3390/ijms17030367
4. Ballestri S, Zona S, Targher G, Romagnoli D, Baldelli E, Nascimbeni F, et al. Nonalcoholic fatty liver disease is associated with an almost twofold increased risk of incident type 2 diabetes and metabolic syndrome. Evidence from a systematic review and meta-analysis. *J Gastroenterol Hepatol* 2016;31(5):936-44. doi: 10.1111/jgh.13264
5. Berlanga A, Guiu-Jurado E, Porras JA, Auguet T. Molecular pathways in non-alcoholic fatty liver disease. *Clin Exp Gastroenterol* 2014;7:221-39. doi: 10.2147/CEG.S62831
6. El-Mir MY, Nogueira V, Fontaine E, Averet N, Rigoulet M, Leverve X. Dimethylbiguanide inhibits cell respiration via an indirect effect targeted on the respiratory chain complex i. *J Biol Chem* 2000;275(1):223-8.
7. Owen MR, Doran E, Halestrap AP. Evidence that metformin exerts its anti-diabetic effects through inhibition of complex 1 of the mitochondrial respiratory chain. *Biochem J* 2000;348 Pt 3:607-14.
8. Zhou G, Myers R, Li Y, Chen Y, Shen X, Fenyk-Melody J, et al. Role of amp-activated protein kinase in mechanism of metformin action. *J Clin Invest* 2001;108(8):1167-74. doi: 10.1172/JCI13505
9. Browning JD, Horton JD. Molecular mediators of hepatic steatosis and liver injury. *J Clin Invest* 2004;114(2):147-52. doi: 10.1172/jci22422
10. Kita Y, Takamura T, Misu H, Ota T, Kurita S, Takeshita Y, et al. Metformin prevents and reverses inflammation in a non-diabetic mouse model of nonalcoholic steatohepatitis. *PLoS One* 2012;7(9):e43056. doi: 10.1371/journal.pone.0043056
11. Spruss A, Kanuri G, Stahl C, Bischoff SC, Bergheim I. Metformin protects against the development of fructose-induced steatosis in mice: Role of the intestinal barrier function. *Lab Invest* 2012;92(7):1020-32. doi: 10.1038/labinvest.2012.75
12. Tang W, Xu Q, Hong T, Tong G, Feng W, Shen S, et al. Comparative efficacy of anti-diabetic agents on nonalcoholic fatty liver disease in patients with type 2 diabetes mellitus: A systematic review and meta-analysis of randomized and non-randomized studies. *Diabetes Metab Res Rev* 2016;32(2):200-16. doi: 10.1002/dmrr.2713
13. Pittas AG, Lau J, Hu FB, Dawson-Hughes B. The role of vitamin d and calcium in type 2 diabetes. A systematic review and meta-analysis. *J Clin Endocrinol Metab* 2007;92(6):2017-29. doi: 10.1210/jc.2007-0298
14. Sergeev IN, Song Q. High vitamin d and calcium intakes reduce diet-induced obesity in mice by increasing adipose tissue apoptosis. *Mol Nutr Food Res* 2014;58(6):1342-8. doi: 10.1002/mnfr.201300503
15. Nobre JL, Lisboa PC, Santos-Silva AP, Lima NS, Manhaes AC, Nogueira-Neto JF, et al. Calcium supplementation reverts central adiposity, leptin, and insulin resistance in adult offspring programed by neonatal nicotine exposure. *J Endocrinol* 2011;210(3):349-59. doi: 10.1530/joe-11-0172
16. Hidayat M, Prahastuti S, Tiono H, Dianawati D. Effect of calcium against weight gain and improved histopathologic fatty liver on male wistar rats that fed high fat food. *Obes Res Clin Pract* 2013;7:15-6. doi: 10.1016/j.orcp.2013.08.051
17. Yin Y, Yu Z, Xia M, Luo X, Lu X, Ling W. Vitamin d attenuates high fat diet-induced hepatic steatosis in rats by modulating lipid metabolism. *Eur J Clin Invest* 2012;42(11):1189-96. doi: 10.1111/j.1365-2362.2012.02706.x
18. He YH, Li ST, Wang YY, Wang G, He Y, Liao XL, et al. Postweaning low-calcium diet promotes later-life obesity induced by a high-fat diet. *J Nutr Biochem* 2012;23(10):1238-44. doi: 10.1016/j.jnutbio.2011.07.004
19. Gao L, Cao JT, Liang Y, Zhao YC, Lin XH, Li XC, et al. Calcitriol attenuates cardiac remodeling and dysfunction in a murine model of polycystic ovary syndrome. *Endocrine* 2016;52(2):363-73. doi: 10.1007/s12020-015-0797-1
20. Shalata A, Vintfield Y, Krichevsky L, Svzalb S, Grosovski M, Djibre A, et al. The effect of vitamin d and sitaglibtin/metformin combination on hepatic fat and triglyceride content in mo-1 mice with fatty liver disease. *J Hepatol* 2013;58(1):S531.
21. National Research Council. Nutrient requirements of laboratory animals, 4th ed. Washington, D.C: The National Academy Press; 1995.
22. Fleet JC, Gliniak C. Modeling human vitamin D status in experimental rodents. *FASEB J* 2007;21(6): A1110-A1110.
23. Shojaei Zarghani S, Soraya H, Zarei L, Alizadeh M. Comparison of three different diet-induced non alcoholic fatty liver disease protocols in rats: A pilot study. *Pharm Sci* 2015;22(1): 9-15. doi: 10.15171/PS.2016.03
24. Folch J, Lees M, Sloane Stanley GH. A simple method for the isolation and purification of total lipides from animal tissues. *J Biol Chem* 1957;226(1):497-509.
25. Yousefi K, Soraya H, Fathiazad F, Khorrami A, Hamedeyazdan S, Maleki-Dizaji N, et al. Cardioprotective effect of methanolic extract of marrubium vulgare l. On isoproterenol-induced acute myocardial infarction in rats. *Indian J Exp Biol* 2013;51(8):653-60.
26. Soraya H, Farajnia S, Khani S, Rameshrad M, Khorrami A, Banani A, et al. Short-term treatment with metformin suppresses toll like receptors (tlrs) activity in isoproterenol-induced myocardial infarction in rat: Are ampk and tlrs connected? *Int Immunopharmacol* 2012;14(4):785-91. doi: 10.1016/j.intimp.2012.10.014

27. Sun C, Wang L, Yan J, Liu S. Calcium ameliorates obesity induced by high-fat diet and its potential correlation with p38 mapk pathway. *Mol Biol Rep* 2012;39(2):1755-63. doi: 10.1007/s11033-011-0916-x
28. Kim YD, Park KG, Lee YS, Park YY, Kim DK, Nedumaran B, et al. Metformin inhibits hepatic gluconeogenesis through amp-activated protein kinase-dependent regulation of the orphan nuclear receptor shp. *Diabetes* 2008;57(2):306-14. doi: 10.2337/db07-0381
29. Gunton JE, Delhanty PJ, Takahashi S, Baxter RC. Metformin rapidly increases insulin receptor activation in human liver and signals preferentially through insulin-receptor substrate-2. *J Clin Endocrinol Metab* 2003;88(3):1323-32. doi: 10.1210/jc.2002-021394
30. Tang X, Li J, Xiang W, Cui Y, Xie B, Wang X, et al. Metformin increases hepatic leptin receptor and decreases steatosis in mice. *J Endocrinol* 2016;230(2):227-37. doi: 10.1530/joe-16-0142
31. Karlsson HK, Hallsten K, Bjornholm M, Tsuchida H, Chibalin AV, Virtanen KA, et al. Effects of metformin and rosiglitazone treatment on insulin signaling and glucose uptake in patients with newly diagnosed type 2 diabetes: A randomized controlled study. *Diabetes* 2005;54(5):1459-67.
32. Haukeland JW, Konopski Z, Eggesbo HB, von Volkmann HL, Raschpichler G, Bjoro K, et al. Metformin in patients with non-alcoholic fatty liver disease: A randomized, controlled trial. *Scand J Gastroenterol* 2009;44(7):853-60. doi: 10.1080/00365520902845268
33. Eskens BJM, Vink H, VanTeeffelen JWGE. Improvement of insulin reistance in diet-induced obese mice by sulodexide, an endothelial glycocalyx mimetic. *J Endocrinol Diabetes Obes* 2014;2:1027
34. Basu R, Shah P, Basu A, Norby B, Dicke B, Chandramouli V, et al. Comparison of the effects of pioglitazone and metformin on hepatic and extra-hepatic insulin action in people with type 2 diabetes. *Diabetes* 2008;57(1):24-31. doi: 10.2337/db07-0827
35. Linden MA, Lopez KT, Fletcher JA, Morris EM, Meers GM, Siddique S, et al. Combining metformin therapy with caloric restriction for the management of type 2 diabetes and nonalcoholic fatty liver disease in obese rats. *Appl Physiol Nutr Metab* 2015;40(10):1038-47. doi: 10.1139/apnm-2015-0236
36. Linden MA, Fletcher JA, Morris EM, Meers GM, Kearney ML, Crissey JM, et al. Combining metformin and aerobic exercise training in the treatment of type 2 diabetes and nafld in oletf rats. *Am J Physiol Endocrinol Metab* 2014;306(3):E300-10. doi: 10.1152/ajpendo.00427.2013
37. Alkharfy KM, Al-Daghri NM, Yakout SM, Hussain T, Mohammed AK, Krishnaswamy S. Influence of vitamin d treatment on transcriptional regulation of insulin-sensitive genes. *Metab Syndr Relat Disord* 2013;11(4):283-8. doi: 10.1089/met.2012.0068
38. de Wit NJ, Bosch-Vermeulen H, Oosterink E, Muller M, van der Meer R. Supplementary dietary calcium stimulates faecal fat and bile acid excretion, but does not protect against obesity and insulin resistance in c57bl/6j mice. *Br J Nutr* 2011;105(7):1005-11. doi: 10.1017/s0007114510004654
39. Gagnon C, Daly RM, Carpentier A, Lu ZX, Shore-Lorenti C, Sikaris K, et al. Effects of combined calcium and vitamin d supplementation on insulin secretion, insulin sensitivity and beta-cell function in multi-ethnic vitamin d-deficient adults at risk for type 2 diabetes: A pilot randomized, placebo-controlled trial. *PLoS One* 2014;9(10):e109607. doi: 10.1371/journal.pone.0109607
40. Geldenhuys S, Hart PH, Endersby R, Jacoby P, Feelisch M, Weller RB, et al. Ultraviolet radiation suppresses obesity and symptoms of metabolic syndrome independently of vitamin d in mice fed a high-fat diet. *Diabetes* 2014;63(11):3759-69. doi: 10.2337/db13-1675
41. Ryu OH, Chung W, Lee S, Hong KS, Choi MG, Yoo HJ. The effect of high-dose vitamin d supplementation on insulin resistance and arterial stiffness in patients with type 2 diabetes. *Korean J Intern Med* 2014;29(5):620-9. doi: 10.3904/kjim.2014.29.5.620
42. Peterson JM, Seldin MM, Wei Z, Aja S, Wong GW. Ctrp3 attenuates diet-induced hepatic steatosis by regulating triglyceride metabolism. *Am J Physiol Gastrointest Liver Physiol* 2013;305(3):G214-24. doi: 10.1152/ajpgi.00102.2013
43. Peterson JM, Wei Z, Wong GW. C1q/tnf-related protein-3 (ctrp3), a novel adipokine that regulates hepatic glucose output. *J Biol Chem* 2010;285(51):39691-701. doi: 10.1074/jbc.M110.180695
44. Woo SL, Xu H, Li H, Zhao Y, Hu X, Zhao J, et al. Metformin ameliorates hepatic steatosis and inflammation without altering adipose phenotype in diet-induced obesity. *PLoS One* 2014;9(3):e91111. doi: 10.1371/journal.pone.0091111
45. Wang S, Zhou Y, Yang B, Li L, Yu S, Chen Y, et al. C1q/tumor necrosis factor-related protein-3 attenuates brain injury after intracerebral hemorrhage via ampk-dependent pathway in rat. *Front Cell Neurosci* 2016;10:237. doi: 10.3389/fncel.2016.00237
46. Zhang CL, Feng H, Li L, Wang JY, Wu D, Hao YT, et al. Globular ctrp3 promotes mitochondrial biogenesis in cardiomyocytes through ampk/pgc-1alpha pathway. *Biochim Biophys Acta* 2017;1861(1 Pt A):3085-94. doi: 10.1016/j.bbagen.2016.10.022
47. Ban B, Bai B, Zhang M, Hu J, Ramanjaneya M, Tan BK, et al. Low serum cartonectin/ctrp3 concentrations in newly diagnosed type 2 diabetes mellitus: In vivo regulation of cartonectin by glucose. *PLoS One* 2014;9(11):e112931. doi: 10.1371/journal.pone.0112931

48. Wolf RM, Steele KE, Peterson LA, Magnuson TH, Schweitzer MA, Wong GW. Lower circulating c1q/tnf-related protein-3 (ctrp3) levels are associated with obesity: A cross-sectional study. *PLoS One* 2015;10(7):e0133955. doi: 10.1371/journal.pone.0133955
49. Li X, Jiang L, Yang M, Wu YW, Sun SX, Sun JZ. Expression of ctrp3, a novel adipokine, in rats at different pathogenic stages of type 2 diabetes mellitus and the impacts of glp-1 receptor agonist on it. *J Diabetes Res* 2014;2014:398518. doi: 10.1155/2014/398518
50. Choi KM, Hwang SY, Hong HC, Yang SJ, Choi HY, Yoo HJ, et al. C1q/tnf-related protein-3 (ctrp-3) and pigment epithelium-derived factor (pedf) concentrations in patients with type 2 diabetes and metabolic syndrome. *Diabetes* 2012;61(11):2932-6. doi: 10.2337/db12-0217
51. Yoo HJ, Hwang SY, Hong HC, Choi HY, Yang SJ, Choi DS, et al. Implication of progranulin and c1q/tnf-related protein-3 (ctrp3) on inflammation and atherosclerosis in subjects with or without metabolic syndrome. *PLoS One* 2013;8(2):e55744. doi: 10.1371/journal.pone.0055744
52. Tan BK, Chen J, Hu J, Amar O, Mattu HS, Adya R, et al. Metformin increases the novel adipokine cartonectin/ctrp3 in women with polycystic ovary syndrome. *J Clin Endocrinol Metab* 2013;98(12):E1891-900. doi: 10.1210/jc.2013-2227
53. Than NN, Newsome PN. A concise review of non-alcoholic fatty liver disease. *Atherosclerosis* 2015;239(1):192-202. doi: 10.1016/j.atherosclerosis.2015.01.001.
54. Shojaei Zarghani S, Soraya H, Alizadeh M. Calcium and vitamin d3 combinations improve fatty liver disease through ampk-independent mechanisms. *Eur J Nutr* 2016. doi: 10.1007/s00394-016-1360-4
55. Rashidi B, Haghollahi F, Shariat M, Zayerii F. The effects of calcium-vitamin d and metformin on polycystic ovary syndrome: A pilot study. *Taiwan J Obstet Gynecol* 2009;48(2):142-7. doi: 10.1016/s1028-4559(09)60275-8
56. Tehrani HG, Mostajeran F, Shahsavari S. The effect of calcium and vitamin d supplementation on menstrual cycle, body mass index and hyperandrogenism state of women with poly cystic ovarian syndrome. *J Res Med Sci* 2014;19(9):875-80.
57. Mostafa DK, Nasra RA, Zahran N, Ghoneim MT. Pleiotropic protective effects of vitamin d against high fat diet-induced metabolic syndrome in rats: One for all. *Eur J Pharmacol* 2016;792:38-47. doi: 10.1016/j.ejphar.2016.10.031.
58. Yogalakshmi B, Bhuvaneswari S, Sreeja S, Anuradha CV. Grape seed proanthocyanidins and metformin act by different mechanisms to promote insulin signaling in rats fed high calorie diet. *J Cell Commun Signal* 2014;8(1):13-22. doi: 10.1007/s12079-013-0210-x
59. Liu Y, Wan Q, Guan Q, Gao L, Zhao J. High-fat diet feeding impairs both the expression and activity of ampka in rats' skeletal muscle. *Biochem Biophys Res Commun* 2006;339(2):701-7. doi: 10.1016/j.bbrc.2005.11.068
60. Foretz M, Hebrard S, Leclerc J, Zarrinpashneh E, Soty M, Mithieux G, et al. Metformin inhibits hepatic gluconeogenesis in mice independently of the lkb1/ampk pathway via a decrease in hepatic energy state. *J Clin Invest* 2010;120(7):2355-69. doi: 10.1172/jci40671
61. Song YM, Lee YH, Kim JW, Ham DS, Kang ES, Cha BS, et al. Metformin alleviates hepatosteatosis by restoring sirt1-mediated autophagy induction via an amp-activated protein kinase-independent pathway. *Autophagy* 2015;11(1):46-59. doi: 10.4161/15548627.2014.984271

Nanotechnology in Wound Healing; Semisolid Dosage Forms Containing Curcumin-Ampicillin Solid Lipid Nanoparticles, *in-Vitro*, *Ex-Vivo* and *in-Vivo* Characteristics

Solmaz Ghaffari[1,2]*, Faezeh Alihosseini[1], Seyed Mahdi Rezayat Sorkhabadi[1,3,4], Sepideh Arbabi Bidgoli[1,5], Seyyedeh Elaheh Mousavi[6], Setareh Haghighat[7], Ahoo Afshar Nasab[1], Nooshin Kianvash[2]

[1] *Pharmaceutical Sciences Research Center, Pharmaceutical Sciences Branch, Islamic Azad University (IAUPS), Tehran, Iran.*
[2] *Young Researchers and Elite Club, Pharmaceutical Sciences Branch, Islamic Azad University (IAUPS), Tehran, Iran.*
[3] *Department of Medical Nanotechnology, School of Advanced Sciences and Technology in Medicine, Tehran University of Medical Sciences (TUMS), Tehran, Iran.*
[4] *Department of Pharmacology and Toxicology, Pharmaceutical Sciences Branch, Islamic Azad University, (IAUPS), Tehran, Iran.*
[5] *Department of Toxicology, Pharmaceutical Sciences Branch, Islamic Azad University (IAUPS), Tehran, Iran.*
[6] *Department of Pharmacology, School of Medicine, Tehran University of Medical Sciences, Tehran, Iran.*
[7] *Department of Microbiology, Faculty of Advanced Sciences and Technology, Pharmaceutical Sciences Branch, Islamic Azad University (IAUPS), Tehran, Iran.*

Keywords:
- Wound healing
- Solid Lipid Nanoparticles
- *In-vivo*
- Semi solids

Abstract

Purpose: Wound healing is a natural biologic process, but the duration of it may take too long. Trying to shorten this process is one of the challenges for scientists. Many technologies were applied to achieve this goal as well as nanotechnology. In this study semi solid formulations containing curcumin and ampicillin solid lipid nanoparticles (SLNs) were prepared to evaluate as burn wound healing agent.

Methods: Curcumin as an anti-inflammatory and anti-bacterial agent and ampicillin as an antibiotic were applied. *In-vitro* and *in-vivo* evaluations were carried out. Particle size, loading efficiency, release profile, morphology and anti-bacterial efficacy of desired nanoparticles were evaluated at first. Then the remaining of the antibacterial effect in semi solid preparations was studied. Animal studies for both toxicology using rabbits and skin burn model using rats were designed. Pathology studies after applying of formulations was done too.

Results: Desired nanoparticles were spherical in shape and particle size in range of 112-121 nm, with low zeta potential. For increasing stability of particles they were freeze dried using cryoprotectant. Lyophilized particles show no significant size enlargement. Results showed that both ointment and gel preparations have reasonable anti-bacterial effects, both of them cause increasing in the rate of wound healing in comparison with placebos and control groups and none of the formulations showed acute toxicity.

Conclusion: It seems that using nanotechnology could shorten wound healing process to reduce treatment costs and increase compliance of patients.

Introduction

Wounds may occur different occasions in anyone's life and wound healing is a biological process which involves four main phases including: hemostasis, inflammation, proliferation and maturation.[1,2] Nanotechnology as a novel technology focuses on wound healing as well as many other medical complains. Ag, Au, Zn, Cu and NO nalso antibiotic containing nanoparticles are some of those which were used in wound healing.[3] Most of mentioned nanoparticle show antibacterial activity and help to shortened wound healing process. Researchers demonstrated that nanofibers showed effectiveness in skin regeneration based on their structures which are similar to the extracellular matrix.[4] Numerous innovative nanoscale products have emerged for wound healing that are currently under clinical investigation.[5] Nash and Hugh demonstrated that topical ampicillin could help to reduce the incidence of infections after cancer operation of the large intestine also topical ampicillin showed a significant reduction in the frequency of infections after operation for cancer of the colon and rectum and side effects were not reported as well.[6] Based on our knowledge there is no publication in which curcumin and ampicillin nanoparticles together apply via semi solid formulation for burn wound healing, in the present research we tried to evaluate the benefit of this rout of

***Corresponding author:** Solmaz Ghaffari, Email: ghaffari.s@iaups.ac.ir administration. Formulation of suitable dosage form which could be used for in-vivo studies was the main purpose of us. After achieving the optimum formulations, in-vitro, ex-vivo and in-vivo studies were carried out.

Materials and Methods

Preparation of SLNs

Curcumin and ampicillin solid lipid nanoparticles (SLNs) were prepared using high pressure homogenization method which was described by Varshosaz *et al* (2010). with justifications as needed.[7] In brief active substances were dissolved/dispersed in water and tween 80 was added, in other side hot oily phase was prepared which contains cholesterol and ethanol/acetone (in volume ratio of 3/1), then oily phase was added to the watery phase under homogenization (13500 rpm). SLNs were prepared during homogenization and cooling of the mixture to the room temperature. Prepared SLNs were lyophilized using 5% mannitol as cryoprotectant, Varshosaz *et al.* (2012) Particle size, zeta potential, morphology, drug loading efficacy and antibacterial activities as well as drug release profile were investigated after freeze drying too.[8]

Preparation of semisolid formulations

Ointments and gels were selected to be prepared for administering in animals.

Ointment preparation

Petroleum (4.7 g) and Eucerin (4.3 g) were melted and cacao butter and olive oil, 0.2 and 0.6 g respectively, were added, 0.6 g glycerin was added to the mixture and under mixing and cooling condition to the room temperature, 255 and 192 mg lyophilized curcumin and ampicillin SLNs were added which were equal to 70 and 18 mg curcumin and ampicillin respectively. A soft ointment with an acceptable texture was made to apply.

Emulgel Preparation

0.8 g carbopol (971) added to distilled water (q.s 10 ml), then 2 and 3g olive oil and glycerin was added under mixer, after obtaining a soft gel texture, 255 and 192 mg of freeze dried curcumin and ampicillin SLNs was added and mixed to be homogenized.

Both formulations were evaluated for their viscosity using Brookfield DV III + Rheometer (USA).

Antimicrobial evaluation

Muller Hinton's agar plates were used the *in vitro* antimicrobial testing as recommended by clinical and Laboratory Standards Institute. Bacterial strains were sub cultured from frozen stocks. One of three loopful of 24 h old cultures from each test strains were used to prepare 0.5 McFarland standard suspensions. Each bacteria strain (*Escherichia coli, Staphylococcus aureus,* and *Pseudomonas aeruginosa*) were inoculated into Mueller-Hinton agar (MHA) plates to form a bacterial lawn. Then swabs soaked in different formulations and were stretched on the central inoculated MHA agar. The inoculated plates were incubated at 37°C and examined after 18-24 h. The zones of inhibition so obtained were measured and the results were compared. This study was performed in triplicate for each formulation.

Animal studies

Animal Housing and Maintenance for safety studies

Female rabbits were individually housed in separate quarters in solid bottom cages. Individual animals were identified by color coding, the animal number and group number also appeared on the outside of each cage to preclude mix-up. The animal room environment was controlled (targeted ranges: temperature 22°C to 25°C, relative humidity 30-20%) and monitored daily. The photo-cycle was 12 hours light and 12 hours dark .Upon arrival all animals were submitted to a general physical examination and all were found healthy and were admitted. Diet and water were offered ad libitum throughout the acclimatization and study periods. The cage cleaning schedule, air filtration and recirculation, health checks and facility maintenance were carried out in accordance with the IAUPS Standard Operating Procedures, and such activities were recorded in the animal room records.

Animal Selection/Randomization

The test population of animals was selected from newly arrived and the method of randomization was based upon the random selection of numbers generated from a set of numbers without replacement.

Skin Irritation and Corrosion Test

An acute skin irritation and corrosion study of the test article, Curcumin and ampicillin solid lipid nanoparticles (SLNs) was carried out before starting the burn model for topical application. The study was conducted according to OECD 404 protocol, Acute Dermal Irritation and Corrosion Test. The test substance was applied in a single dose to the skin of the first rabbit and untreated skin areas of the test animal serve as the control. The degree of irritation/corrosion was read and scored at specified intervals and was further described in order to provide a complete evaluation of the effects. The duration of the study was sufficient to evaluate the reversibility of the effects observed.

All rabbits received the test article by dermal application according to the test guideline Animals were observed individually at least once during the first 4 hours after dosing, periodically during the first 24, 48, 72 hours (with special attention given during the first 4 hours), and daily thereafter, for a total of 14 days, except where they need to be removed from the study and humanely killed for animal welfare reasons or are found dead. All observations were systematically recorded with individual records being maintained for each animal. Body weights were recorded before initiation of the treatment, and daily until the end of the study.

Animal's manipulation for creating skin burn model

Adult male Wistar rats weighing 200–230 g were obtained from Animal house of Experimental Medicine Research Center of Tehran University of Medical Sciences. These animals were housed with ad libitum access to pellet food and water, under standard room temperature (22±2°C) on the 12hr light/dark cycles. The bedding materials for rats were replaced with new ones every day.

Experimental protocol for generation of burn skin model and burn healing

The animals were anaesthetized with an intraperitoneal injection of Ketamine (80 mg/kg) and xylazine HCL (10 mg/kg). The skin of dorsum was shaved and cleaned with 70% ethanol. An experimental skin burn model was induced on rats by the Edraki method.[9] Second-degree burn wounds on the dorsum of the animals were exposed to ironic cylindrical devices with a surface of 2.5 cm2 for 10 seconds. The devices were heated in boiling water (98 ± 1 °C) at least 20 minutes before application to induce burn injury. Rats were randomly divided into either control or experimental groups. Control group did not receive any treatment. Experimental groups were subdivided into six groups as follows: Group 1 received topical ointment Group 2 received topical gel, Group 3 received blank of ointment formulation which contains all ingredients except desired nanoparticles, Group 4 received blank of gel formulation which contains all ingredients except desired nanoparticles, Group 5 and 6 received solution of curcumin and ampicillin and normal saline respectively. Each Rat treated with equal volume of topical formulation, once daily with regards to the assigned group and continued until 12 h before sample collection.

In order to collect samples for histopathology examination, the animals were euthanized at 7 and 14 days after inducing burn injury. These samples were preserved in 10% formalin for light microscopic study. Photography was also followed until the 21th day on the other wound of rats for wound surface measurements.

Histological assessments

Tissue samples of burn wounds for histopathological analysis were immediately fixed in 10% formalin, and then the sections were embedded in paraffin. The section blocks of 5 μm were prepared and stained with hematoxylin and eosin (H&E) for histopathological examination by light microscopy. All skin tissues were examined in a blinded manner by a pathologist. Inflammation, collagen deposition, angiogenesis, granulation tissue formation and epithelialization were graded as 0-3 to each section.[10] The burn wounds surface area, were photographed at the 0th, 5th, 11th, 14th, 18th and 21th days using a digital camera; then, the healing rate was evaluated by comparison of wound area at each control days with the wound area in the first day.[11]

Results and Discussion

Particle size and morphology evaluation of nanoparticles

SEM photographs demonstrated that most of the particles are spherical even after freeze drying and non-significant size enlargement was seen after freeze drying. Figure 1a and 1b show SEM photographs of the desired nanoparticles.

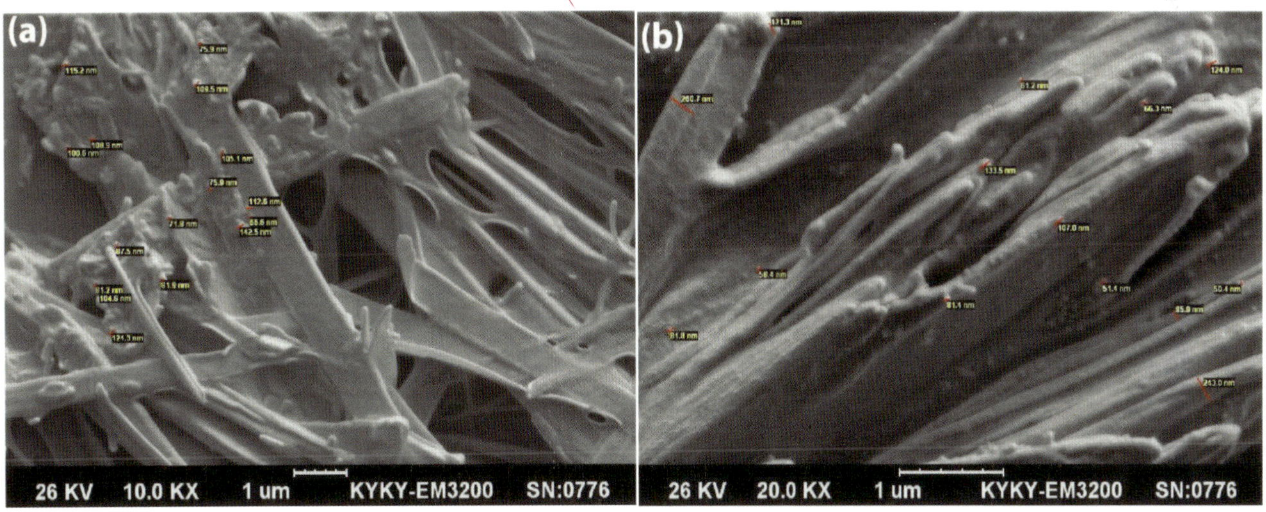

Figure 1. a: Curcumin Solid Lipid Nanoparticles photographs after freeze-drying(left). b: Ampicillin Solid Lipid Nanoparticles photographs after freeze-drying(right)

Antimicrobial efficacy of formulations

As antimicrobial efficacy enhancement using nanotechnology for both curcumin and ampicillin as well as synergic effect of using both nanoparticles containing curcumin and ampicillin were reported previously by Alihoseyni 2014, Jourghanian 2016 and Alihosseini 2016, this benefit of nanotechnology was evaluated in semisolid dosage forms in this project.[12-14] Also previously Varaprasad et al (2011) studied on benefit of using curcumin with Ag hydrogel to enhance antibacterial efficacy. Their study results showed that

curcumin could enhance anti bacterial efficacy of Ag nanoparticles.[15]
The "well diffusion test" was carried out using P.aueroginosa (ATCC 27853), S.aureus (ATTC 25923) and Ecoli (ATCC 25922), results show that antimicrobial effects of active ingredients which were loaded on SLNs remain in the formulation.

Viscosity control

Viscosities of desired formulations were 1187 and 139.5 cps for ointment and gel formulation respectively.

Animal studies

After applying formulations on the burned skin as described in methodology part, wound healing process studied for 14 days. Rate of healing based on wound appearance and diameter was evaluated in comparison with negative and positive controls as well as placeboes. Results show that by applying nano curcumin and nano ampicillin, rate of healing increases significantly. Figures 2(a, b, c, d) show photos of wound healing after using formulations in comparison with placeboes and normal saline. It is obvious that healing rate increases by applying nanoparticles. The pathology studies confirm the above results. Previously efficacy of curcumin on burn wound healing in comparison with silver sulfadiazine was studied by Mehrabani et al. (2017).[16] They demonstrated that curcumin as an available and inexpensive herbal was shown be a suitable substitute in healing of burn wounds. Curcumin was encapsulated into a silane-hydrogel nanoparticle vehicle (curc-np) to overcome native curcumin's poor solubility and investigate its potential as a topical therapy for wound infection by Krausz et al.[17] Curc-np demonstrated efficacy in vitro against methicillin-resistant Staphylococcus aureus and inhibited growth of this bacteria strain and enhanced wound healing in an in vivo burn wound model. These data suggest that curc-np may possess clinical utility as a novel topical antimicrobial and wound healing agent for infected burn wounds.[17] Ahmadi et al demonstrated that using nanotechnology could enhance the rate of burn wound healing. The studied on Ag and tetracycline nanoparticles. Their findings support use of the AgNPs in combination with antibacterial medicine for the treatment of infectious skin wounds.[18] present study is correlated with the Krausz and Ahmadi's researches results.

Pathology studies

Pathology studies confirm that nanotechnology enhances wound healing process. Figure 3(a, b, c, d, e and f) show the results.
As wound healing is a natural but time consuming process, in control groups healing observed but slower than when nanoparticles were applied.

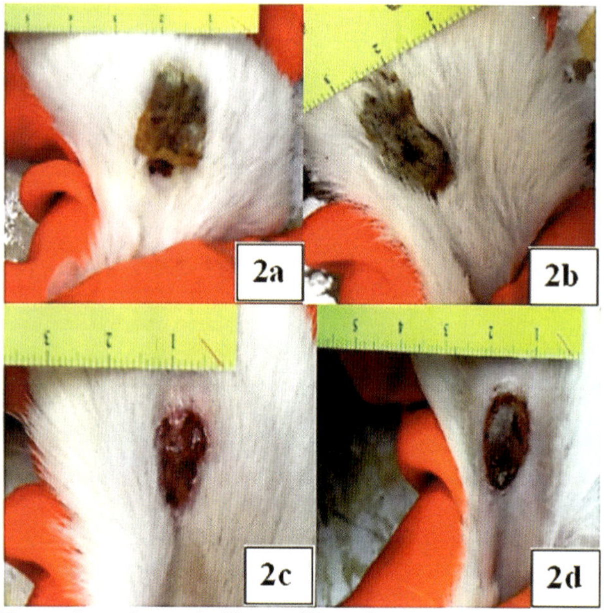

Figure 2. a: Group 1 skin condition after 14 days, **b**: Group 2 skin condition after 14 days. **c**: Skin condition of Group 3 after 14 days, **d**: Group 4 skin condition after 14 days

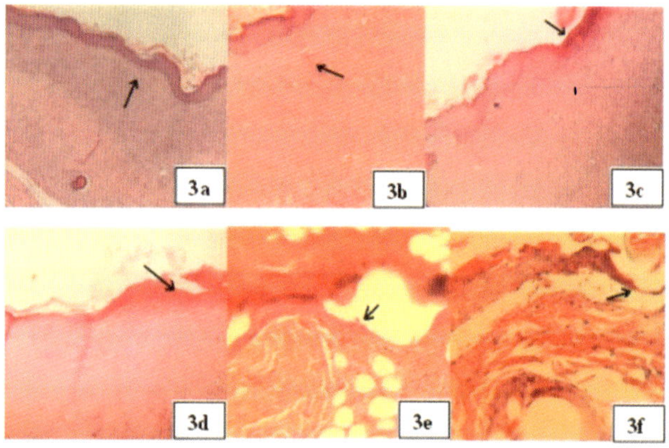

Figure 3. a: belongs to Group 1 after 14 days applying ointment formulation and shows showed tissue healing with complete and mature re-epithelialization, fibroblast proliferation, and collagen fiber. (mag:200×). **b**: belongs to Group 2 after 14 days applying gel formulation and shows complete and mature epithelization. There was severe fibroplasias (arrow) with high level of collagen fiber. (mag:400×). **c**: belongs to Group 3 after 14 days applying placebo of ointment formulation and shows incomplete epithelization(arrow) with severe fibrosis and moderate inflammatory cells infiltration. (mag:200×).**d**: belongs to Group 4 after 14 days applying placebo of gel formulation and shows partial epithelization(arrow).there was moderate fibrosis in wound area. (mag:200×). **e**: is belonging to Group 5 In which Curcumin and ampicillin solution was applied, after 14 days complete, but thin epithelization (mag:400×) was observed. **f**: is belonging to Group 6 in which Normal saline was applied and photograph was taken after 14 days. Revealed partial epithelization.(mag:400×) is obvious

Skin Irritation and Corrosion Test

All animals were examined for signs of erythema and edema, and the responses scored at 60 minutes, and then at 24, 48 and 72 hours after patch removal. For the initial test in one animal, the test site was also examined immediately after the patch had been removed. Dermal reactions were graded and recorded according to the grades in Table 1 as below. If there was damage to skin which could not be identified as irritation or corrosion at 72 hours, observations were continued until day 14 to determine the reversibility of the effects. In addition to the observation of irritation, all local toxic effects, such as defeating of the skin, and any systemic adverse effects (e.g., effects on clinical signs of toxicity and body weight), were fully described and recorded.

Observations of the first examined rabbit were described in Table 1. The proposed SLNs exposed areas didn't show any sign of toxicity after first 4 hrs from dermal application. In long term continuous dermal exposure, very slight erythema and dryness were observed but these mild signs of toxicity were recovered to normal appearance after the removal of the patch in case areas. The mean total score was 4 in treated rabbits therefore the product showed very slight irritant effect without any corrosive response in long term (>24hrs) exposure. After the recovery period all animals had normal appearance and hair growth in treated areas.

Table 1. Mean (SD) skin reactions of 3 rabbits 1 after 3min,1hrs,4 hrs,24 hrs,48 hrs and 72 hrs dermal exposure to proposed Solid Lipid Nanoparticles

Erythema and Eschar Formation	3min	1hr	4hr	24hr	48hr	72hr	Edema	3min	1hr	4hr	24hr	48hr	72hr
No erythema	0	0	0	0	0	0	No edema	0	0	0	0	0	0
Very slight erythema (barely perceptible)	0	0	0	1	1	1	Very slight edema	0	0	0	0	0	0
Well defined erythema	0	0	0	0	0	0	Slight edema	0	0	0	0	0	0
Moderate to severe erythema	0	0	0	0	0	0	Moderate oedema	0	0	0	0	0	0
Severe erythema	0	0	0	0	0	0	Severe edema	0	0	0	0	0	0
Skin dryness	0	0	0	0	1	0	Weight of Animals :3865±108						
Total score:4	0	0	0	1	2	1							

Bodyweight

Individual weights of animals were determined shortly before the test substance was administered and for more two weeks thereafter. Weight changes were calculated and recorded. At the end of the test surviving animals were weighed. No significant weight change was detected in this test.

Based on the foregoing results, the SLNs samples didn't show any sign irritant effects even after long term (>72 hrs) in treated animals when compared with control areas in Albino Rabbit.

Conclusion

In this project, synergic antibacterial effect of ampicillin and curcumin SLNs which was demonstrated previously, was applied to treat burn wound. Two semisolid preparations were designed to use on burned skin. The combination of curcumin and ampicillin nanoparticles was evaluated as wound dressing materials in animal wound models. Application of the dressings showed significant improvement in wound healing. These two nanoparticles have synergistic antibacterial effect together. It seems that using nanotechnology could help to increase rate of wound healing.

Acknowledgments

Research reported in this publication was supported by Elite Researcher Grant Committee under award number [943784] from the National Institutes for Medical Research Development (NIMAD), Tehran, Iran. Authors would like to appreciate Laboratory of veterinary pathology with managing of Dr Hasti Azarabad for pathology studies. Authors also would like to appreciate kind assistance of Mrs. Hedieh Ghaffari for English polishing of the manuscript.

Ethical Issues

The experimental performed during this study were approved by Animal Ethics Committee of Tehran University of Medical Sciences as well as Animal Care Guidelines Published by the Department of Pharmacology, School of Medicine, Tehran University of Medical Sciences.

Conflict of Interest

There is no conflict of interest to declare.

References

1. Rajkumar RJ, Muthukumar Nadar MSA, Selvakumar PM. Nanotechnology in Wound Healing- A Review. *Glob J Nanomed* 2017;3(1):1-4. doi: 10.19080/GJN.2017.03.555605
2. Garraud O, Hozzein WN, Badr G. Wound healing: Time to look for intelligent, 'natural' immunological approaches? *BMC Immunol* 2017;18(Suppl 1):23. doi: 10.1186/s12865-017-0207-y
3. Cortivo R, Vindigni V, Iacobellis L, Abatangelo G, Pinton P, Zavan B. Nanoscale particle therapies for wounds and ulcers. *Nanomedicine (Lond)* 2010;5(4):641-56. doi: 10.2217/nnm.10.32
4. Alberti T, Coelho DS, Voytena A, Pitz H, de Pra M, Mazzarino L, et al. Nanotechnology: A promising tool towards wound healing. *Curr Pharm Des* 2017;23(24):3515-28. doi: 10.2174/1381612823666170503152550

5. Hamdan S, Pastar I, Drakulich S, Dikici E, Tomic-Canic M, Deo S, et al. Nanotechnology-driven therapeutic interventions in wound healing: Potential uses and applications. *ACS Cent Sci* 2017;3(3):163-75. doi: 10.1021/acscentsci.6b00371
6. Nash AG, Hugh TB. Topical ampicillin and wound infection in colon surgery. *Br Med J* 1967;1(5538):471-2.
7. Varshosaz J, Ghaffari S, Khoshayand MR, Atyabi F, Azarmi S, Kobarfard F. Development and optimization of solid lipid nanoparticles of amikacin by central composite design. *J Liposome Res* 2010;20(2):97-104. doi: 10.3109/08982100903103904
8. Varshosaz J, Ghaffari S, Khoshayand MR, Atyabi F, Dehkordi AJ, Kobarfard F. Optimization of freeze-drying condition of amikacin solid lipid nanoparticles using d-optimal experimental design. *Pharm Dev Technol* 2012;17(2):187-94. doi: 10.3109/10837450.2010.529149
9. Edraki M, Akbarzadeh A, Hosseinzadeh M, Tanideh N, Salehi A, Koohi-Hosseinabadi O. Healing effect of sea buckthorn, olive oil, and their mixture on full-thickness burn wounds. *Adv Skin Wound Care* 2014;27(7):317-23. doi: 10.1097/01.ASW.0000451061.85540.f9
10. Abramov Y, Golden B, Sullivan M, Botros SM, Miller JJ, Alshahrour A, et al. Histologic characterization of vaginal vs. Abdominal surgical wound healing in a rabbit model. *Wound Repair Regen* 2007;15(1):80-6. doi: 10.1111/j.1524-475X.2006.00188.x
11. Verma J, Kanoujia J, Parashar P, Tripathi CB, Saraf SA. Wound healing applications of sericin/chitosan-capped silver nanoparticles incorporated hydrogel. *Drug Deliv Transl Res* 2017;7(1):77-88. doi: 10.1007/s13346-016-0322-y
12. Alihoseyni F, Ghaffari S, Dabirsiaghi AR, Haghighat S. Preparation and evaluation of ampicillin solid lipid nanoparticles. *World J Pharm Sci* 2014;2(9):914-20.
13. Jourghanian P, Ghaffari S, Ardjmand M, Haghighat S, Mohammadnejad M. Sustained release curcumin loaded solid lipid nanoparticles. *Adv Pharm Bull* 2016;6(1):17-21. doi: 10.15171/apb.2016.004
14. Alihosseini F, Azarmi S, Ghaffari S, Haghighat S, Rezayat Sorkhabadi SM. Synergic antibacterial effect of curcumin with ampicillin; free drug solutions in comparison with SLN dispersions. *Adv Pharm Bull* 2016;6(3):461-5. doi: 10.15171/apb.2016.060
15. Varaprasad K , Murali Mohan Y, Vimala K, Mohana Raju K. Synthesis and characterization of hydrogel-silver nanoparticle-curcumin composites for wound dressing and antibacterial application. *J Appl Polym Sci* 2011;121(2):784-96. doi.10.1002/app.33508
16. Mehrabani D, Farjam M, Geramizadeh B, Tanideh N, Amini M, Panjehshahin MR. The healing effect of curcumin on burn wounds in rat. *World J Plast Surg* 2015;4(1):29-35.
17. Krausz AE, Adler BL, Cabral V, Navati M, Doerner J, Charafeddine RA, et al. Curcumin-encapsulated nanoparticles as innovative antimicrobial and wound healing agent. *Nanomedicine* 2015;11(1):195-206. doi: 10.1016/j.nano.2014.09.004
18. Ahmadi M, Adibhesami M. The effect of silver nanoparticles on wounds contaminated with pseudomonas aeruginosa in mice: An experimental study. *Iran J Pharm Res* 2017;16(2):661-9.

Effects of Pharmacologic Dose of Resveratrol Supplementation on Oxidative/Antioxidative Status Biomarkers in Nonalcoholic Fatty Liver Disease Patients

Somayyeh Asghari[1], Maryam Rafraf[2*], Laleh Farzin[1], Mohammad Asghari-Jafarabadi[3,4], Seyed-Mostafa Ghavami[5], Mohammad-Hossein Somi[6]

[1] *Students' Research Committee, Faculty of Nutrition and Food Science, Tabriz University of Medical Sciences, Tabriz, Iran.*
[2] *Nutrition Research Center, Department of Community Nutrition, Faculty of Nutrition and Food Science, Tabriz University of Medical Sciences, Tabriz, Iran.*
[3] *Road Traffic Injury Research Center, Tabriz University of Medical Sciences, Tabriz, Iran.*
[4] *Department of Statistics and Epidemiology, Faculty of Health, Tabriz University of Medical Sciences, Tabriz, Iran.*
[5] *Department of Radiology, Paramedical school, Tabriz University of Medical Sciences, Tabriz, Iran.*
[6] *Liver and Gastrointestinal Diseases Research Centre, Tabriz University of Medical Sciences, Tabriz, Iran.*

Keywords:
- Clinical trial
- Nonalcoholic fatty liver disease
- Oxidative stress
- Resveratrol supplementation

Abstract

Purpose: Despite a proposed role for oxidative stress in the pathogenesis of nonalcoholic fatty liver disease (NAFLD), antioxidant approaches have not been sufficiently investigated in human NAFLD management. Resveratrol has been reported to possess a wide range of biological functions, including antioxidant activities. This study aimed to evaluate the effects of resveratrol supplementation on oxidative/anti-oxidative status in patients with NAFLD.

Methods: This randomized, double-blind, placebo-controlled clinical trial was conducted on 60 patients with NAFLD (males and females) aged 20 to 60 years, and body mass index (BMI) of 25-35 kg/m^2. Subjects were randomly assigned to receive a daily dose of 600 mg resveratrol (2×300 mg pure trans-resveratrol capsules; n=30) or placebo capsules (n=30) for 12 wk. Fasting blood samples, anthropometric measurements, and dietary intakes were collected for all patients at baseline and at the end of the trial. Oxidative stress was evaluated by measurement of serum malondialdehyde (MDA), oxidized low-density lipoprotein (ox-LDL), total antioxidant capacity (TAC), and erythrocyte superoxide dismutase (SOD) as well as glutathione peroxidase (GSH-Px) activities. Changes in the outcomes were analyzed using analysis of covariance (ANCOVA).

Results: Resveratrol supplementation did not significantly affect neither serum MDA, ox-LDL, and TAC levels, nor erythrocyte SOD and GSH-Px activities, compared to placebo group (All $P>0.05$). Moreover, changes in serum levels of liver enzymes (ALT, AST, GGT, and ALP) were not significant in neither of the study groups (All P>0.05).

Conclusion: Resveratrol supplementation did not modify oxidative/anti-oxidative status in patients with NAFLD.

Introduction

Non-alcoholic fatty liver disease (NAFLD) is the most common chronic liver disease worldwide, with a prevalence rate of 6-35% in the general population, depending on the assessment methods and the study population.[1] Higher prevalences were found among those afflicted with metabolic disorders such as obesity, type 2 diabetes, and metabolic syndrome.[1,2] NAFLD represents a spectrum of liver diseases from simple hepatic steatosis to nonalcoholic steatohepatitis (NASH), and fibrosis, which may progress to cirrhosis and even hepatocellular carcinoma.[3] Insulin resistance and oxidative stress are among the major important risk factors for this disease, and current therapeutic approaches to NAFLD include strategies that could modify these risk factors.[4] Insulin resistance leads to increased lipolysis and hepatic uptake of free fatty acids (FFA) and enhances hepatic triglyceride synthesis and accumulation.[5] The excessive offer of lipids to the mitochondria would promote production of reactive oxygen species (ROS), which contribute to lipid peroxidation and eventual oxidative stress.[6,7] The most remarkable consequence of oxidative stress is the oxidation of lipids, proteins, DNA, and

***Corresponding author:** Maryam Rafraf, Email: rafrafm@tbzmed.ac.ir enzymes, leading to cellular damage and acceleration of cell death induced by apoptosis and necrosis.[8] Oxidative stress is considered of primary importance in the disease progression from simple steatosis to steatohepatitis and liver damage.[9]

Lipid peroxidation and ROS can also lead to depletion of nonenzymatic antioxidants as well as antioxidant enzymes such as superoxide dismutase (SOD) and glutathione peroxidase (GSH-Px). These antioxidant defenses are particularly important because they represent the direct elimination of free radicals, providing maximum protection against oxidative damages.[10] Multiple clinical studies have demonstrated the elevated levels of circulating products of oxidative stress and lipid peroxidation,[11] as well as decreased antioxidant levels in patients with NAFLD.[12]

The use of compounds with antioxidant activity has been postulated to have favorable effects in prevention and treatment of complications caused by oxidative stress.[13] Despite a proposed role of oxidative stress in the pathogenesis of NAFLD, antioxidant approaches have not been sufficiently investigated in NAFLD therapy. Resveratrol (3, 4', 5- trihydroxystilbene), a natural non-flavonoid phenolic compound found mainly in grapes, berries and red wine, has been known to have a wide array of biological functions.[14] Most animal studies have shown that resveratrol acts as a potent antioxidant agent against oxidative stress.[15-18] Furthermore, resveratrol has been reported to increase the activities of certain antioxidant enzymes,[15,19] decrease lipid peroxidation products,[17,20,21] and elevate the levels of nonenzymatic antioxidant compounds.[22]

Despite the numerous studies in rodents, to date, there have been limited clinical trials with contradictory results on the effects of resveratrol supplementation on NAFLD characteristics.[23] Given the potential antioxidant properties of resveratrol, and the limited human research about its possible effects in NAFLD, we designed this study to investigate whether resveratrol supplementation could improve oxidative/anti-oxidative status in patients with NAFLD.

Materials and Methods

Study subjects

Patients aged 20 to 60 years with body mass index (BMI) ranging 25-35 kg/m^2, were recruited from Golgasht clinic (Tabriz, Iran) between January and June 2016.

In this study, liver ultrasonography was used to diagnose NAFLD. All the trans-abdominal ultrasound measurements of liver steatosis were performed by one radiologist, at baseline and at the end of the study.

Pregnant, lactating and postmenopausal women, as well as professional athletes were excluded from the study. Other exclusion criteria also included smoking, consumption of any alcoholic beverages, suffering from inherited liver disorders, known liver, cardiovascular, kidney and gastrointestinal diseases, diabetes, thyroid dysfunction, or malignancies, using medications such as hepatotoxic drugs, corticosteroids, hormonal drugs, psychotropic and antidepressants, oral anti-diabetic and lipid-lowering drugs, taking any kinds of supplements three months prior to the study and/or during the study period.

Sample size of the study was determined based on the primary information obtained for oxidized-low density lipoprotein (ox-LDL) from Tome-Carneiro study.[24] By considering 95% confidence, 80% power and two-tailed statistical test, the sample size was computed to be 25 per group. In order to cover possible dropouts, the sample size was increased to 30 in each group.

Study Design and Measurements

This study was designed as a randomized, double-blind placebo-controlled clinical trial. Sixty patients (41 males and 19 females) were randomly assigned to receive a daily dose of 600 mg resveratrol (2×300 mg capsules per day of pure trans-resveratrol; n=30) or identical placebos (2×300 mg capsules per day of starch; n=30) for 12 weeks. An independent person not involved in the study process prepared both resveratrol and placebo bottles, and labeled them as A or B. The patients and researchers were all blinded to the treatment assignment until the statistical analyses were completed. Randomization was carried out using block randomization procedure of size 2 and 4, stratified by age (20-40, 40-60 years old), sex (male, female), and BMI (25-30, 30-35 kg/m^2). Random allocation software was used for generating a random sequence, by the study statistician.

At baleline, all patients were educated about the basic principles of a healthy diet and weight control by a nutritionist, based on Food Guide Pyramid and the recommendations of the NIH Obesity Education Initiative Expert Panel. Patients' compliance was monitored by counting the number of returned capsules every two weeks. The patients were excluded from the study if the remaining capsule counts were more than 10% of the expected ones, at the end of the study. At each visit, the patients received a supply of their medications for the next two weeks.

Anthropometric parameters were measured for all patients at baseline and at the end of the study. Height was measured without shoes with a precision of 0.1 cm. Weight was measured in light clothing by a Seca scale to the nearest 0.1 kg. BMI was calculated as weight (kg) divided by squared height (m^2).

To assess daily dietary intakes of the patients, they were asked to complete a consecutive three-day food record questionnaire, including two weekdays and one weekend, at baseline and week 12. Average daily dietary intakes were determined by using the modified Nutritionist 4 software (First Databank, Hearst Corp, San Bruno, CA, USA). Physical activity level was also assessed by using the international physical activity questionnaire (IPAQ),[25] at baseline and week 12.

Blood samples (10cc) were obtained after a 12-h overnight fast, at baseline and at the end of the study. The serum samples were separated from whole blood (9cc) by centrifugation at 3500 rpm for 10 min. The remaining whole blood samples (1cc) were collected and stabilized in EDTA tubes. Both serum and whole blood samples were immediately stored at -70°C until performing the analyses. Biochemical measurements were conducted at Drug Applied Research Center (Tabriz University of Medical Sciences, Tabriz, Iran). Alanine aminotransferase (ALT), aspartate aminotransferase (AST), gamma-glutamyl transferase (GGT), and alkaline phosphatase (ALP) were measured by enzymatic colorimetric assay (Pars Azmoon Inc. kit, Iran) and autoanalyzer set (Alcyon 300, USA). Serum concentration of malondialdehyde (MDA) was determined by thiobarbituric acid reactive substances (TBARS) method described by Bilici et al.[26] Total antioxidant capacity (TAC) was measured using spectrophotometry method, with Randox kit (Randox Laboratories, Ltd., UK). Erythrocyte SOD and GSH-Px activities were measured spectrophotometrically using a Ransod and Ransel kit, respectively (Randox Laboratories, Ltd., UK). Results were expressed as units of SOD and GSH-Px activity per milligram of hemoglobin (Hb). Hb was measured in the hemolysates by the commercial cyanmethemoglobin method (Pars Azmoon Inc. kit, Iran). Serum levels of ox-LDL were measured by enzyme-linked immunosorbent assay (ELISA; Human ox-LDL ELISA kit, Crystal Day Bio-Tec, China).

Statistical Analysis

All statistical analyses were performed by using SPSS software version 17 (SPSS Inc., IL, Chicago, USA). All analyses were done using intention to treat (ITT) principle according to the CONSORT statement.
Kolmogorov–Smirnov test was used to determine normality of the distribution of variables. Data were presented as frequency (percent) for categorical variables, mean (standard deviation (SD)) for numeric normal variables and geometric mean (95% confidence interval) for numeric non-normal variables. Analyses of non-normal variables were performed after log transformation. Comparisons of baseline characteristics were performed using independent samples t-test and chi-squared test, where appropriate. Paired samples t-test was applied for within group comparisons. The effect of the intervention was determined by analysis of covariance (ANCOVA) adjusting for baseline values and confounders. In all analyses, P<0.05 was considered to be statistically significant.

Results and Discussion

Sixty patients were enrolled in the study, and 51 (35 male and 16 female) completed the 12-week intervention: 25 in the resveratrol group and 26 in the placebo group. The reasons for the loss to follow up are described in the study flowdiagram (Figure 1). Participants' compliance was high in both study groups. Capsule counts indicated that more than 90% of the participants took more than 90% of their capsules. No adverse effects or symptoms were reported throughout the study.

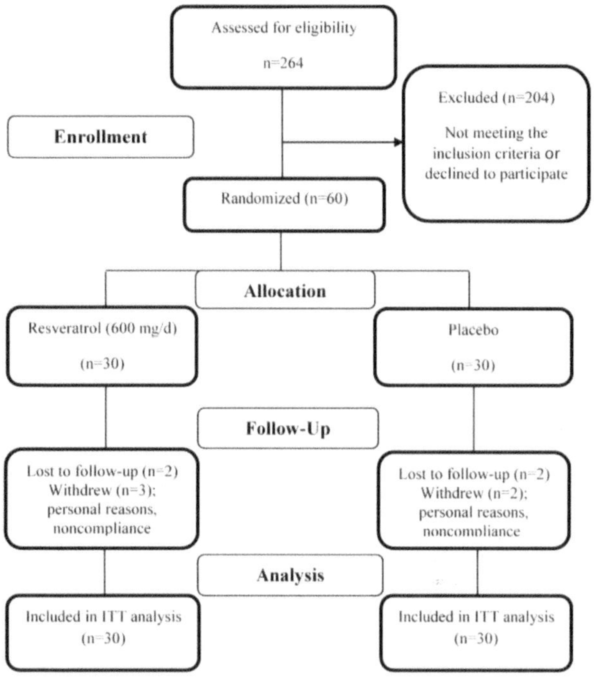

Figure 1. Study flow diagram

Baseline characteristics of the study patients are presented in Table 1. There were no significant differences in age, sex, BMI, liver steatosis grade, or physical activity levels among the study groups at baseline. No significant changes were found in patients' physical activity level and liver steatosis grade throughout the study neither within, nor between the two groups (P>0.05).
The total daily intakes of energy, macronutrients and known antioxidants are shown in Table 2. There were no significant differences between the two study groups in terms of mean daily intake of energy and macronutrients at baseline. Calorie and macronutrient intakes did not change significantly in neither of the groups, throughout the study (P>0.05). Changes in mean daily dietary antioxidants intakes of study subjects were not significant throughout the study neither within, nor between the two groups (P>0.05).
BMI reduced significantly in the resveratrol group compared to the placebo group (MD= -0.31, 95% CI: -0.64 to -0.02), P<0.05) (data not shown). This finding was in accord with a recent study which indicated a significant decrease in BMI of metabolic syndrome patients following administration of 500 mg resveratrol for three months.[27] Some previous animal studies have also shown the antiobesity potential of resveratrol, which might be attributed to its effect on adipogenesis inhibition and lipolysis induction.[28,29] Given the effect of resveratrol on improving mitochondrial biogenesis and function,[30-32] it is probable that resveratrol increases the whole-body energy expenditure; this has been demonstrated in some rodent studies.[31,33] However, several studies have not confirmed the beneficial effects

of resveratrol on body weight[34,35] or energy expenditure.[36,37] Thus, the exact effects of resveratrol on anthropometric indices are still controversial.

Table 1. Baseline characteristics of the study patients

Variables	Control (n=30)	Resveratrol (n=30)	*P*-value
Age (y)*	38.50 (30, 48)	40.00 (22, 58)	
Sex, n (%)			
Male	19 (63.3%)	21 (70.0%)	
Female	11 (36.7%)	9 (30.0%)	
BMI (kg/m²)**	30.41 (3.39)	30.78 (3.10)	
PAL, n (%)			0.43§
light	15 (50.0%)	11 (36.7%)	
moderate	15 (50.0%)	16 (53.3%)	
vigorous	0 (0.0%)	3 (10.0%)	
Grade of liver steatosis, n (%)			0.61§
grade 1	11 (42.3%)	10 (40.0 %)	
grade 2	15 (57.7%)	13 (52.0%)	
grade 3	0 (0.0%)	2 (8.0%)	

BMI: body mass index; PAL: physical activity level
* Data are expressed as median (min, max)
**Data are expressed as mean (standard deviation)
§ Fisher's exact test

Biochemical characteristics of patients at baseline and after the 12 weeks intervention are presented in Figure 2 and Figure 3. There were no significant differences in biochemical values between the two study groups at baseline. Liver enzyme levels (ALT, AST, GGT and ALP) did not change significantly in resveratrol and placebo groups (All $P>0.05$). Results of ANCOVA also showed no significant differences in liver enzymes levels between the two groups after adjusting for the baseline values and mean change of BMI, daily energy intake and physical activity level, at the end of the study (All $P>0.05$; Figure 2).

Previous animal studies have shown that resveratrol protects the liver against steatosis[14,16] and reduces intracellular lipids in the liver.[38] However, similar to our results, Heebøll et al.[39] reported no improvement in intrahepatic lipid content and serum levels of liver enzymes by a daily dose of 1500 mg resveratrol. Administering 3000 mg resveratrol for eight weeks, not only failed to show any significant improvements in NAFLD features, but also increased liver enzymes levels.[40] On the other hand, Faghihzadeh et al.[41] found significant improvements in liver steatosis and ALT levels by 500 mg resveratrol supplementation for three months, in NAFLD patients. A similar study with 600 mg of resveratrol also reported significant improvements in liver enzymes levels without any changes in liver steatosis degree.[42] These inconsistent results may be related to the stage of the disease, method of measuring liver fat content, different dosage of resveratrol administered, or baseline metabolic characteristics of the patients. In the present study, baseline serum values of liver enzymes were in normal range in the study subjects; this might have contributed to the non-significant changes in these variables.

Following 12 weeks intervention, serum MDA, ox-LDL and TAC did not change significantly in resveratrol and placebo groups. No significant changes were observed in the activities of SOD or GSH-Px enzymes in neither of the groups ($P>0.05$). Results of ANCOVA adjusted for baseline values and mean changes of BMI, daily energy intake and physical activity level, showed no significant differences for serum MDA, ox-LDL and TAC as well as SOD and GSH-Px activities between resveratrol and placebo groups, at the end of the intervention (All $P>0.05$; Figure 3).

Extensive evidence has shown that oxidative stress may be one of the key mediators of hepatic injury in NAFLD and play a fundamental role in the progression of simple steatosis towards NASH.[9]

Elevated systemic levels of oxidative stress biomarkers and lipid peroxidation, as well as decreased antioxidant levels, have been found in patients with NAFLD.[11,12]

MDA, a common marker of lipid peroxidation, is generally produced by ROS interaction with polyunsaturated fatty acids, and used to evaluate the oxidative stress status.[8] Ox-LDL is another common serum biomarker of oxidative stress and lipid peroxidation, which we measured. High ox-LDL level may play a major role in atherosclerosis and cardiovascular disease.[43]

In the present study, supplementation with 600 mg of resveratrol for 12 weeks, had no beneficial effects on serum MDA levels. Serum ox-LDL levels did not change significantly, either. To our knowledge, no intervention study has been carried out previously among NAFLD patients, to investigate the levels of these oxidative markers after resveratrol supplementation. In a study on normal-weight healthy subjects performed by Ghanim et al.,[44] a Polygonum cuspidatum extract containing 40 mg resveratrol, induced a significant reduction in ROS generation in mononuclear cells. Schmatz et al.,[8] demonstrated that resveratrol treatment prevented the elevation in TBARS levels in kidney and liver of diabetic rats. In another study on fructose-fed rats, resveratrol induced a significant reduction in TBARS levels, indicating a possible role of resveratrol in free radical inactivation.[45]

Table 2. Daily dietary intakes of energy, macronutrients and known antioxidants of the study patients at baseline and after the 12-wk intervention

Variables		Control (n=30)	Resveratrol (n=30)	P-value
Energy (Kcal/d)	Before	2082.6 (246.2)	2154.4 (307.8)	0.36†
	After	2068.6 (218.8)	2143.7 (355.1)	0.76‡
	P-value§	0.17	0.82	
Carbohydrate (g/d)	Before	321.4 (47.8)	336.1 (58.2)	0.33†
	After	318.0 (34.7)	328.0 (55.4)	0.87‡
	P-value§	0.32	0.28	
Protein (g/d)	Before	83.2 (5.7)	84.8 (12.0)	0.52†
	After	85.3 (9.8)	87.7 (16.7)	0.48‡
	P-value§	0.11	0.12	
Total fat (g/d)	Before	52.8 (3.9)	53.6 (6.3)	0.59†
	After	53.4 (4.9)	54.6 (10.9)	0.85‡
	P-value§	0.10	0.62	
Vitamin E (mg/day)	Before	10.53 (4.32)	11.11 (5.68)	0.66†
	After	8.96 (6.56)	10.05 (5.95)	0.50‡
	P-value§	0.28	0.48	
Vitamin C (mg/day)	Before	86.42 (38.69)	85.53 (38.55)	0.93†
	After	90.33 (42.76)	90.87 (40.90)	0.96‡
	P-value§	0.71	0.61	
β-Carotene (μg/day)	Before	566.17 (231.45)	582.16 (264.13)	0.80†
	After	623.14 (244.20)	630.27 (264.33)	0.91‡
	P-value§	0.36	0.48	
Zinc (mg/day)	Before	8.09 (3.03)	7.68 (3.31)	0.61†
	After	8.28 (3.13)	7.92 (3.09)	0.66‡
	P-value§	0.81	0.77	
Selenium (μg/day)	Before	67.33 (28.50)	65.42 (31.09)	0.81†
	After	67.87 (27.07)	65.24 (28.56)	0.72‡
	P-value§	0.94	0.98	

Data are expressed as mean (standard deviation)
† Independent t-test
‡ Analysis of covariance (ANCOVA) adjusted for baseline values
§ Paired t-test

There is increasing evidence that antioxidant-rich dietary patterns, induce significant reductions in LDL oxidation.[46] A recent trial performed in hypercholesterolemic patients demonstrated that resveratrol at a dose of 8 mg/d significantly reduced serum ox-LDL during 6 months.[24] The evidence suggests that resveratrol exerts its antioxidant activities by scavenging ROS and reactive nitrogen species (RNS) and secondary organic radicals formed as a result of the reaction of biomolecules with ROS and RNS.[47]

The increased lipid peroxidation might be explained by increased oxidative stress as a result of the antioxidant depletion.[48] LDL and other biomolecules are protected from oxidative damage by the action of blood antioxidant capacity.[49] TAC is an indicator of the overall protection of antioxidants against oxidative stress in body fluids and cell components.[50] Plasma antioxidant status includes enzymatic and nonenzymatic antioxidant activities.[49] Enzymatic antioxidants like SOD and GSH-Px are the first line of defense against ROS and play a vital role in scavenging free radicals. SOD catalyzes the conversion of superoxide anion radical to hydrogen peroxide (H_2O_2). H_2O_2 is then degraded to H_2O by the action of GSH-Px, which is one of the body's most potent defenses; it protects cells from damage caused by lipid peroxide radicals and H_2O_2.[48] A decrease in the action of these antioxidant enzymes may lead to an excessive levels of free radicals and H_2O_2 and consequently increased hydroxyl radicals generation, which results in further initiation and promotion of lipid peroxidation.[8]

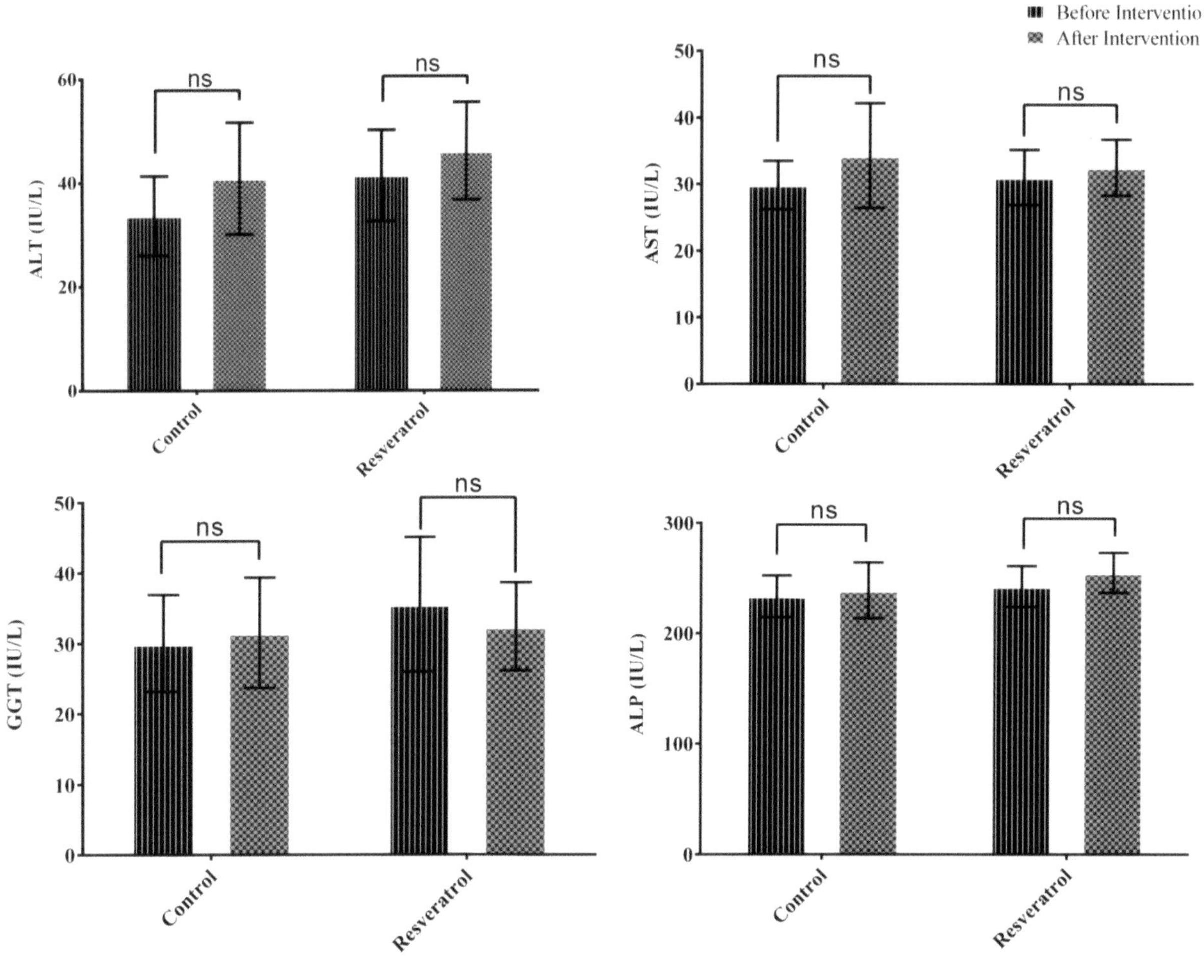

Figure 2. Mean (±95% Confidence interval) of liver enzymes levels in resveratrol and placebo groups after 12 weeks intervention (n=30 per group).
ALT: alanine aminotransferase, AST: aspartate aminotransferase, GGT: gamma-glutamyl transferase, ALP: alkaline phosphatase
Analysis of covariance (ANCOVA) adjusted for baseline values and mean change of BMI, daily energy intake and physical activity level showed no significant differences between resveratrol and placebo groups.

Resveratrol supplementation in our study did not affect erythrocyte SOD and GSH-Px activities. TAC did not change significantly, either. Similar to our findings, Chachay et al.,[40] found no changes in SOD and GSH-Px activities and TAC serum levels after eight-week administration of 3000 mg/d resveratrol in patients with NAFLD. However, in a randomized, double-blind, cross-over trial on healthy adult smokers, 500 mg resveratrol/d for 30 days increased TAC values.[51]

Some rodent studies have demonstrated the effects of resveratrol on regulation of oxidative stress. Zhu et al.,[20] showed decreased ROS levels and increased glutathione (GSH), GSH-Px and SOD levels after resveratrol treatment in KKAy mice, suggesting that resveratrol has a favorable anti-oxidative effect. Schmatz et al.,[8] also demonstrated that resveratrol treatment (10 and 20 mg/kg) prevented the reduction in SOD activity in liver and kidney of streptozotocin-induced diabetic rats. In addition, it has been reported that resveratrol could upregulate mRNA expression of antioxidant enzymes.[52,53]

The main finding of our study was that resveratrol supplementation is not associated with detectable physiological anti-oxidative effects in subjects with NAFLD. In this study, there were no significant differences in daily dietary intakes of macronutrients and known antioxidants between the two groups, by the end of the study. Therefore, dietary factors are not likely to have confounded our results. It is probable that non-significant changes in oxidative stress markers are partly attributed to the clinical and metabolic characteristics of our studied subjects. The severity of existing metabolic abnormalities before treatment seem to be of importance for measurable metabolic benefits of resveratrol supplementation.[54,55] It is possible that the subjects in the present study were relatively 'metabolically healthy' in terms of oxidative/antioxidative status, and were therefore unlikely to experience any improvements after resveratrol supplementation.

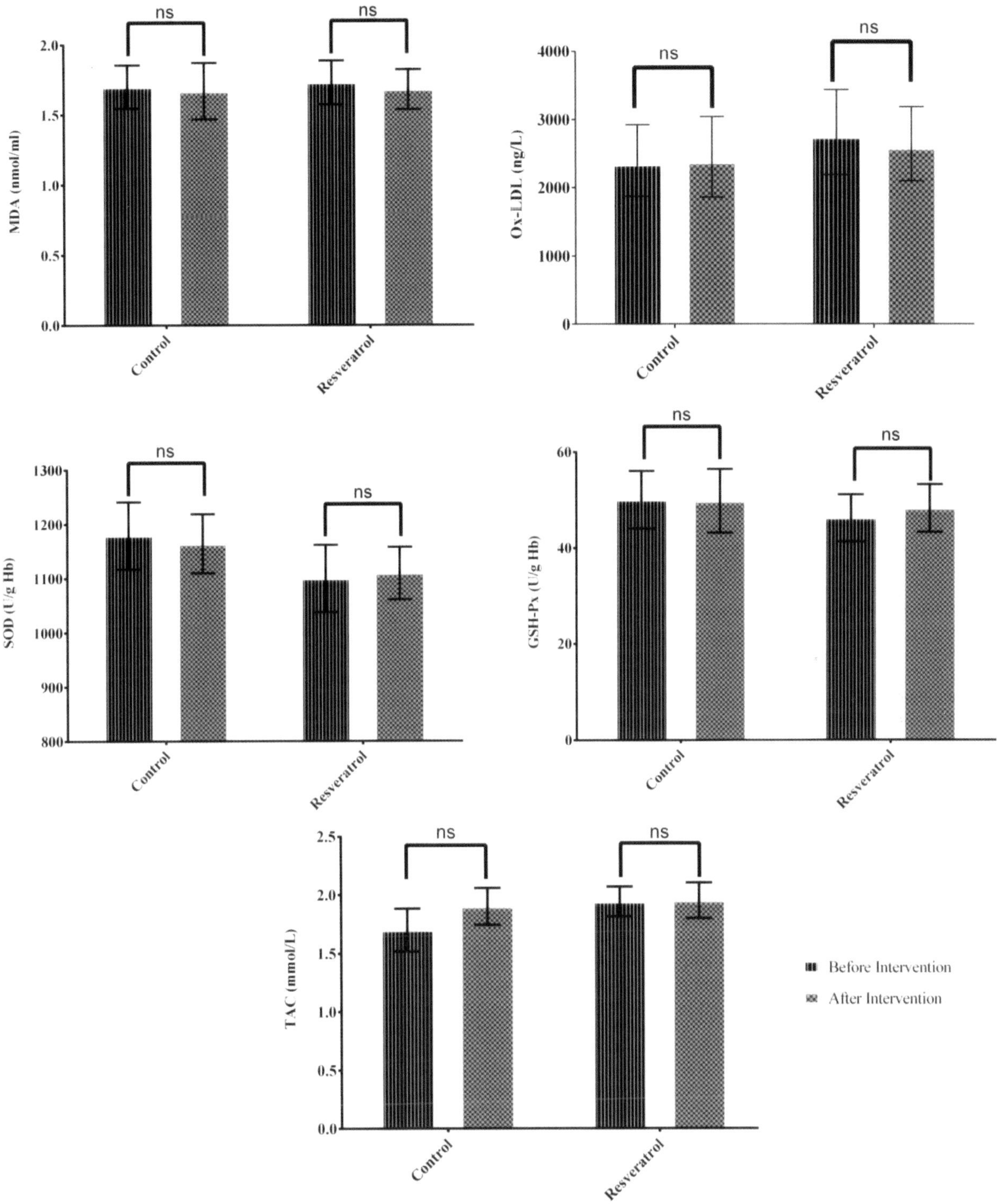

Figure 3. Mean (±95% Confidence interval) of oxidative stress markers in resveratrol and placebo groups after 12 weeks intervention (n=30 per group). Geometric mean (95% confidence interval) was expressed for ox-LDL.

MDA: Malondialdehyde, SOD: Superoxide Dismutase, GSH-Px: Glutathione Peroxidase, TAC: Total Antioxidant Capacity, Ox-LDL: Oxidized Low-density Lipoprotein.

Analysis of covariance (ANCOVA) adjusted for baseline values and mean change of BMI, daily energy intake and physical activity level showed no significant differences between resveratrol and placebo groups.

Another important aspect to be discussed is the dose of resveratrol administered, which may contribute to its antioxidant properties. In the study by Brasnyó et al.,[56] daily dose of 10 mg of resveratrol for four weeks, significantly decreased urinary ortho-tyrosine excretion as a measure of oxidative stress in type 2 diabetic patients. Hassan-Khabbar et al.[57] reported that resveratrol with a dose of 0.2 mg/kg in rats, increased glutathione reductase, SOD, and catalase activities; however, at a high dose (20 mg/kg), became pro-oxidant with a reduced GSH levels and antioxidant enzyme activities. Such pro-oxidant action of resveratrol has been proposed to be involved in anticancer mechanisms of polyphenols.[19] It has been also proposed that resveratrol may act as a pro-oxidant during low oxidative conditions; whereas, it could work as an antioxidant under strong oxidative status.[58] Therefore, its function seems to depend on the dose, different pathological conditions, environmental factors, nutritional status as well as possible interactions with other compounds.[58-60] The differences in bioavailability of various formulations, together with the duration of treatment periods, and metabolic characteristics of the patients included in the studies might also influence the study results. However, the cellular mechanisms linking resveratrol and oxidative stress are not fully understood and remain to be determined.

The current study had several strengths including a high compliance rate and the randomized double-blind, placebo-controlled design which minimized the potential bias and confounding effects of factors other than the study supplement. Use of the liver ultrasound technique as the diagnostic criteria for NAFLD was one of the limitations of our study. However, ultrasonography is currently the preferred non-invasive, inexpensive and widely available method for screening fatty liver in clinical and population-based studies, and is regarded as the first-line diagnostic tool. It should also be noted that the findings of this study are not generalizable to other studies concerning different doses and durations of resveratrol supplementation.

Conclusion

This trial showed that supplementation with 600 mg of resveratrol could not modify oxidative/anti-oxidative status in patients with NAFLD. Further human research is needed to explore potential antioxidant properties of resveratrol in NAFLD, and to elucidate the optimum therapeutic dose.

Acknowledgments

We thank the Research Vice-Chancellor and Nutrition Research Center of Tabriz University of Medical Sciences, Tabriz, Iran, for the financial support. We also appreciate the patients who kindly participated in this study. This article was written based on data set of PhD thesis registered in Tabriz University of Medical Sciences, Iran.

Ethical Issues

The study protocol was approved by the Ethics committee of Tabriz University of Medical Sciences (TBZMED.REC.1394.823) and conducted according to the principles of the Declaration of Helsinki. Informed consent was obtained from participants prior to the study.

Conflict of Interest

The authors report no declarations of interest.

References

1. Vernon G, Baranova A, Younossi ZM. Systematic review: The epidemiology and natural history of non-alcoholic fatty liver disease and non-alcoholic steatohepatitis in adults. *Aliment Pharmacol Ther* 2011;34(3):274-85. doi: 10.1111/j.1365-2036.2011.04724.x
2. Ahmed M. Non-alcoholic fatty liver disease in 2015. *World J Hepatol* 2015;7(11):1450-9. doi: 10.4254/wjh.v7.i11.1450
3. Chalasani N, Younossi Z, Lavine JE, Diehl AM, Brunt EM, Cusi K, et al. The diagnosis and management of non-alcoholic fatty liver disease: Practice guideline by the american association for the study of liver diseases, american college of gastroenterology, and the american gastroenterological association. *Hepatology* 2012;55(6):2005-23. doi: 10.1002/hep.25762
4. Younossi ZM. Review article: Current management of non-alcoholic fatty liver disease and non-alcoholic steatohepatitis. *Aliment Pharmacol Ther* 2008;28(1):2-12. doi: 10.1111/j.1365-2036.2008.03710.x
5. Kawano Y, Cohen DE. Mechanisms of hepatic triglyceride accumulation in non-alcoholic fatty liver disease. *J Gastroenterol* 2013;48(4):434-41. doi: 10.1007/s00535-013-0758-5
6. Bechmann LP, Hannivoort RA, Gerken G, Hotamisligil GS, Trauner M, Canbay A. The interaction of hepatic lipid and glucose metabolism in liver diseases. *J Hepatol* 2012;56(4):952-64. doi: 10.1016/j.jhep.2011.08.025
7. Narasimhan S, Gokulakrishnan K, Sampathkumar R, Farooq S, Ravikumar R, Mohan V, et al. Oxidative stress is independently associated with non-alcoholic fatty liver disease (nafld) in subjects with and without type 2 diabetes. *Clin Biochem* 2010;43(10-11):815-21. doi: 10.1016/j.clinbiochem.2010.04.003
8. Schmatz R, Perreira LB, Stefanello N, Mazzanti C, Spanevello R, Gutierres J, et al. Effects of resveratrol on biomarkers of oxidative stress and on the activity of delta aminolevulinic acid dehydratase in liver and kidney of streptozotocin-induced diabetic rats. *Biochimie* 2012;94(2):374-83. doi: 10.1016/j.biochi.2011.08.005
9. Takaki A, Kawai D, Yamamoto K. Multiple hits, including oxidative stress, as pathogenesis and treatment target in non-alcoholic steatohepatitis

(NASH). *Int J Mol Sci* 2013;14(10):20704-28. doi: 10.3390/ijms141020704

10. Al-Busafi SA, Bhat M, Wong P, Ghali P, Deschenes M. Antioxidant therapy in nonalcoholic steatohepatitis. *Hepat Res Treat* 2012;2012:947575. doi: 10.1155/2012/947575
11. Polimeni L, Del Ben M, Baratta F, Perri L, Albanese F, Pastori D, et al. Oxidative stress: New insights on the association of non-alcoholic fatty liver disease and atherosclerosis. *World J Hepatol* 2015;7(10):1325-36. doi: 10.4254/wjh.v7.i10.1325
12. Yesilova Z, Yaman H, Oktenli C, Ozcan A, Uygun A, Cakir E, et al. Systemic markers of lipid peroxidation and antioxidants in patients with nonalcoholic fatty liver disease. *Am J Gastroenterol* 2005;100(4):850-5. doi: 10.1111/j.1572-0241.2005.41500.x
13. Li S, Tan HY, Wang N, Zhang ZJ, Lao L, Wong CW, et al. The role of oxidative stress and antioxidants in liver diseases. *Int J Mol Sci* 2015;16(11):26087-124. doi: 10.3390/ijms161125942
14. Aguirre L, Portillo MP, Hijona E, Bujanda L. Effects of resveratrol and other polyphenols in hepatic steatosis. *World J Gastroenterol* 2014;20(23):7366-80. doi: 10.3748/wjg.v20.i23.7366
15. Pandey KB, Rizvi SI. Anti-oxidative action of resveratrol: Implications for human health. *Arab J Chem* 2011;4(3):293-8. doi: 10.1016/j.arabjc.2010.06.049
16. Gómez-Zorita S, Fernández-Quintela A, Macarulla MT, Aguirre L, Hijona E, Bujanda L, et al. Resveratrol attenuates steatosis in obese zucker rats by decreasing fatty acid availability and reducing oxidative stress. *Br J Nutr* 2012;107(2):202-10. doi: 10.1017/S0007114511002753
17. Franco JG, Lisboa PC, Lima NS, Amaral TA, Peixoto-Silva N, Resende AC, et al. Resveratrol attenuates oxidative stress and prevents steatosis and hypertension in obese rats programmed by early weaning. *J Nutr Biochem* 2013;24(6):960-6. doi: 10.1016/j.jnutbio.2012.06.019
18. Wenzel E, Soldo T, Erbersdobler H, Somoza V. Bioactivity and metabolism of trans-resveratrol orally administered to wistar rats. *Mol Nutr Food Res* 2005;49(5):482-94. doi: 10.1002/mnfr.200500003
19. de la Lastra CA, Villegas I. Resveratrol as an antioxidant and pro-oxidant agent: Mechanisms and clinical implications. *Biochem Soc Trans* 2007;35(Pt 5):1156-60. doi: 10.1042/BST0351156
20. Zhu W, Chen S, Li Z, Zhao X, Li W, Sun Y, et al. Effects and mechanisms of resveratrol on the amelioration of oxidative stress and hepatic steatosis in kkay mice. *Nutr Metab (Lond)* 2014;11:35. doi: 10.1186/1743-7075-11-35
21. Kavas GO, Ayral PA, Elhan AH. The effects of resveratrol on oxidant/antioxidant systems and their cofactors in rats. *Adv Clin Exp Med* 2013;22(2):151-5.
22. Oyenihi OR, Oyenihi AB, Adeyanju AA, Oguntibeju OO. Antidiabetic effects of resveratrol: The way forward in its clinical utility. *J Diabetes Res* 2016;2016:9737483. doi: 10.1155/2016/9737483
23. Zhang C, Yuan W, Fang J, Wang W, He P, Lei J, et al. Efficacy of resveratrol supplementation against non-alcoholic fatty liver disease: A meta-analysis of placebo-controlled clinical trials. *PLoS One* 2016;11(8):e0161792. doi: 10.1371/journal.pone.0161792
24. Tomé-Carneiro J, Gonzálvez M, Larrosa M, García-Almagro FJ, Avilés-Plaza F, Parra S, et al. Consumption of a grape extract supplement containing resveratrol decreases oxidized LDL and apoB in patients undergoing primary prevention of cardiovascular disease: A triple-blind, 6-month follow-up, placebo-controlled, randomized trial. *Mol Nutr Food Res* 2012;56(5):810-21. doi: 10.1002/mnfr.201100673
25. Moghaddam MHB, Bakhtari Aghdam F, Asghari Jafarabadi M, Allahverdipour H, Dabagh Nikookheslat S, Safarpour S. The Iranian Version of International Physical Activity Questionnaire (IPAQ) in Iran: Content and Construct Validity, Factor Structure, Internal Consistency and Stability. *World Appl Sci* 2012;18(8):1073-80. doi: 10.5829/idosi.wasj.2012.18.08.754
26. Bilici M, Efe H, Köroğlu MA, Uydu HA, Bekaroğlu M, Değer O. Antioxidative enzyme activities and lipid peroxidation in major depression: Alterations by antidepressant treatments. *J Affect Disord* 2001;64(1):43-51. doi: 10.1016/s0165-0327(00)00199-3
27. Méndez-del Villar M, González-Ortiz M, Martínez-Abundis E, Pérez-Rubio KG and Lizárraga-Valdez R. Effect of resveratrol administration on metabolic syndrome, insulin sensitivity, and insulin secretion. *Metab Syndr Relat Disord* 2014;12(10):497-501. doi: 10.1089/met.2014.0082
28. Szkudelski T, Szkudelska K. Anti-diabetic effects of resveratrol. *Ann N Y Acad Sci* 2011;1215:34-9. doi: 10.1111/j.1749-6632.2010.05844.x
29. Fischer-Posovszky P, Kukulus V, Tews D, Unterkircher T, Debatin KM, Fulda S, et al. Resveratrol regulates human adipocyte number and function in a sirt1-dependent manner. *Am J Clin Nutr* 2010;92(1):5-15. doi: 10.3945/ajcn.2009.28435
30. Baur JA, Pearson KJ, Price NL, Jamieson HA, Lerin C, Kalra A, et al. Resveratrol improves health and survival of mice on a high-calorie diet. *Nature* 2006;444(7117):337-42. doi: 10.1038/nature05354
31. Lagouge M, Argmann C, Gerhart-Hines Z, Meziane H, Lerin C, Daussin F, et al. Resveratrol improves mitochondrial function and protects against metabolic disease by activating SIRT1 and PGC-1α. *Cell* 2006;127(6):1109-22. doi: 10.1016/j.cell.2006.11.013
32. Price NL, Gomes AP, Ling AJ, Duarte FV, Martin-Montalvo A, North BJ, et al. SIRT1 is required for

AMPK activation and the beneficial effects of resveratrol on mitochondrial function. *Cell Metab* 2012;15(5):675-90. doi: 10.1016/j.cmet.2012.04.003
33. Dal-Pan A, Blanc S, Aujard F. Resveratrol activates energy metabolism by influencing body temperature, locomotor activity and resting metabolic rate in a non-human primate. *Comp Biochem Physiol A Mol Integr Physiol* 2009;153(2):S147. doi: 10.1016/j.cbpa.2009.04.282
34. Tauriainen E, Luostarinen M, Martonen E, Finckenberg P, Kovalainen M, Huotari A, et al. Distinct effects of calorie restriction and resveratrol on diet-induced obesity and fatty liver formation. *J Nutr Metab* 2011;2011:525094. doi: 10.1155/2011/525094
35. Wang S, Moustaid-Moussa N, Chen L, Mo H, Shastri A, Su R, et al. Novel insights of dietary polyphenols and obesity. *J Nutr Biochem* 2014;25(1):1-18. doi: 10.1016/j.jnutbio.2013.09.001
36. Yoshino J, Conte C, Fontana L, Mittendorfer B, Imai S, Schechtman KB, et al. Resveratrol supplementation does not improve metabolic function in nonobese women with normal glucose tolerance. *Cell Metab* 2012;16(5):658-64. doi: 10.1016/j.cmet.2012.09.015
37. Poulsen MM, Vestergaard PF, Clasen BF, Radko Y, Christensen LP, Stødkilde-Jørgensen H, et al. High-dose resveratrol supplementation in obese men: an investigator-initiated, randomized, placebo-controlled clinical trial of substrate metabolism, insulin sensitivity, and body composition. *Diabetes* 2013;62(4):1186-95. doi: 10.2337/db12-0975
38. Shiozaki M, Hayakawa N, Shibata M, Koike M, Uchiyama Y, Gotow T. Closer association of mitochondria with lipid droplets in hepatocytes and activation of kupffer cells in resveratrol-treated senescence-accelerated mice. *Histochem Cell Biol* 2011;136(4):475-89. doi: 10.1007/s00418-011-0847-6
39. Heebøll S, Kreuzfeldt M, Hamilton-Dutoit S, Kjær Poulsen M, Stødkilde-Jørgensen H, Møller HJ, et al. Placebo-controlled, randomised clinical trial: High-dose resveratrol treatment for non-alcoholic fatty liver disease. *Scand J Gastroenterol* 2016;51(4):456-64. doi: 10.3109/00365521.2015.1107620
40. Chachay VS, Macdonald GA, Martin JH, Whitehead JP, O'Moore-Sullivan TM, Lee P, et al. Resveratrol does not benefit patients with nonalcoholic fatty liver disease. *Clin Gastroenterol Hepatol* 2014;12(12):2092-103.e6. doi: 10.1016/j.cgh.2014.02.024
41. Faghihzadeh F, Adibi P, Rafiei R, Hekmatdoost A. Resveratrol supplementation improves inflammatory biomarkers in patients with nonalcoholic fatty liver disease. *Nutr Res* 2014;34(10):837-43. doi: 10.1016/j.nutres.2014.09.005
42. Chen S, Zhao X, Ran L, Wan J, Wang X, Qin Y, et al. Resveratrol improves insulin resistance, glucose and lipid metabolism in patients with non-alcoholic fatty liver disease: A randomized controlled trial. *Dig Liver Dis* 2015;47(3):226-32. doi: 10.1016/j.dld.2014.11.015
43. Maiolino G, Rossitto G, Caielli P, Bisogni V, Rossi GP, Calò LA. The role of oxidized low-density lipoproteins in atherosclerosis: The myths and the facts. *Mediators Inflamm* 2013;2013:714653. doi: 10.1155/2013/714653
44. Ghanim H, Sia CL, Abuaysheh S, Korzeniewski K, Patnaik P, Marumganti A, et al. An antiinflammatory and reactive oxygen species suppressive effects of an extract of polygonum cuspidatum containing resveratrol. *J Clin Endocrinol Metab* 2010;95(9):E1-8. doi: 10.1210/jc.2010-0482
45. Bagul PK, Middela H, Matapally S, Padiya R, Bastia T, Madhusudana K, et al. Attenuation of insulin resistance, metabolic syndrome and hepatic oxidative stress by resveratrol in fructose-fed rats. *Pharmacol Res* 2012;66(3):260-8. doi: 10.1016/j.phrs.2012.05.003
46. De Lorenzo A, Noce A, Bigioni M, Calabrese V, Della Rocca D, Daniele N, et al. The effects of italian mediterranean organic diet (IMOD) on health status. *Curr Pharm Des* 2010;16(7):814-24. doi: 10.2174/138161210790883561
47. Gerszon J, Rodacka A, Puchała M. Antioxidant properties of resveratrol and its protective effects in neurodegenerative diseases. *Adv Cell Biol* 2014;4(2):97-117. doi: 10.2478/acb-2014-0006
48. Birben E, Sahiner UM, Sackesen C, Erzurum S, Kalayci O. Oxidative stress and antioxidant defense. *World Allergy Organ J* 2012;5(1):9-19. doi: 10.1097/WOX.0b013e3182439613
49. Di Renzo L, Marsella LT, Carraro A, Valente R, Gualtieri P, Gratteri S, et al. Changes in LDL oxidative status and oxidative and inflammatory gene expression after red wine intake in healthy people: A randomized trial. *Mediators Inflamm* 2015;2015:317348. doi: 10.1155/2015/317348
50. Koca K, Yurttas Y, Cayci T, Bilgic S, Kaldirim U, Durusu M, et al. The role of preconditioning and n-acetylcysteine on oxidative stress resulting from tourniquet-induced ischemia-reperfusion in arthroscopic knee surgery. *J Trauma* 2011;70(3):717-23. doi: 10.1097/TA.0b013e3181f30fb0
51. Bo S, Ciccone G, Castiglione A, Gambino R, De Michieli F, Villois P, et al. Anti-inflammatory and antioxidant effects of resveratrol in healthy smokers a randomized, double-blind, placebo-controlled, cross-over trial. *Curr Med Chem* 2013;20(10):1323-31. doi: 10.2174/0929867311320100009
52. Cao Z, Li Y. Potent induction of cellular antioxidants and phase 2 enzymes by resveratrol in cardiomyocytes: Protection against oxidative and electrophilic injury. *Eur J Pharmacol* 2004;489(1-2):39-48. doi: 10.1016/j.ejphar.2004.02.031
53. Leonard SS, Xia C, Jiang BH, Stinefelt B, Klandorf H, Harris GK, et al. Resveratrol scavenges reactive oxygen species and effects radical-induced cellular

responses. *Biochem Biophys Res Commun* 2003;309(4):1017-26. doi: 10.1016/j.bbrc.2003.08.105

54. de Ligt M, Timmers S, Schrauwen P. Resveratrol and obesity: Can resveratrol relieve metabolic disturbances? *Biochim Biophys Acta* 2015;1852(6):1137-44. doi: 10.1016/j.bbadis.2014.11.012
55. Timmers S, de Ligt M, Phielix E, van de Weijer T, Hansen J, Moonen-Kornips E, et al. Resveratrol as add-on therapy in subjects with well-controlled type 2 diabetes: A randomized controlled trial. *Diabetes Care* 2016;39(12):2211-7. doi: 10.2337/dc16-0499
56. Brasnyó P, Molnár GA, Mohás M, Markó L, Laczy B, Cseh J, et al. Resveratrol improves insulin sensitivity, reduces oxidative stress and activates the akt pathway in type 2 diabetic patients. *Br J Nutr* 2011;106(3):383-9. doi: 10.1017/S0007114511000316
57. Hassan-Khabbar S, Cottart CH, Wendum D, Vibert F, Clot JP, Savouret JF, et al. Postischemic treatment by trans-resveratrol in rat liver ischemia-reperfusion: A possible strategy in liver surgery. *Liver Transpl* 2008;14(4):451-9. doi: 10.1002/lt.21405
58. Gadacha W, Ben-Attia M, Bonnefont-Rousselot D, Aouani E, Ghanem-Boughanmi N, Touitou Y. Resveratrol opposite effects on rat tissue lipoperoxidation: Pro-oxidant during day-time and antioxidant at night. *Redox Rep* 2009;14(4):154-8. doi: 10.1179/135100009X466131
59. Marques FZ, Morris BJ. Commentary on resveratrol and hormesis: Resveratrol--a hormetic marvel in waiting? *Hum Exp Toxicol* 2010;29(12):1026-8. doi: 10.1177/0960327110383640
60. Calabrese EJ, Mattson MP, Calabrese V. Resveratrol commonly displays hormesis: Occurrence and biomedical significance. *Hum Exp Toxicol* 2010;29(12):980-1015. doi: 10.1177/0960327110383625

Enhanced Intestinal Permeation of Doxorubicin Using Chitosan Nanoparticles

Marziyeh Zare[1], Soliman Mohammadi Samani[1], Zahra Sobhani[2]*

[1] *Faculty of Pharmacy, Shiraz University of Medical Sciences, Shiraz, Iran.*
[2] *Department of Quality Control, Faculty of Pharmacy, Shiraz University of Medical Sciences, Shiraz, Iran.*

Keywords:
- Doxorubicin
- Chitosan nanoparticles
- Oral delivery
- Intestinal permeation
- Everted rat gut method

Abstract

Purpose: Due to limited oral bioavailability of doxorubicin (Dox) many efforts during the last decades focused on the development of novel delivery systems to overcome these limitations. In the present study, Dox encapsulated chitosan nanoparticles were prepared to evaluate the intestinal permeation of Dox via oral administration.

Methods: Nanoparticles were fabricated based on ionic gelation method using tripolyphosphate. Some physicochemical properties, such as nanoparticle size and morphology, loading efficiency and in *vitro* drug release in 3 different pH values (5.0, 6.8 & 7.4) were evaluated. Intestinal permeations of free Dox and Dox loaded in nanoparticles were assessed using rat intestinal sac model.

Results: The nanoparticles were spherical shape with average size of 150 $\pm$ 10 nm. The entrapment and loading efficiency of Dox were up to 40% and 23%, respectively. According to the release profiles, up to 30% of loaded drug was released within 6hrs and the remaining amount of Dox was released more gradually, but this pattern was related to pH of the medium. The amount of drug released at acidic condition (pH 5.0) was greater than other pHs. The intestinal permeation of Dox increased nearly up to 90% by loading in chitosan nanoparticles.

Conclusion: Using chitosan nanoparticles presents a potential safe drug delivery system for oral administration of Dox. *In vivo* studies and the determined pharmacokinetic and pharmacodynamic of Dox loaded chitosan nanoparticles after oral administration are planned for future studies.

Introduction

Oral administration of drugs is one of the most common approaches. It has many advantages in comparison with intravenous rout, such as better safety, ease of administration, lower cost, convenience and patient compliance.[1-3] The common regimen for chemotherapy consists of the administration of anticancer drugs through i.v. injection or infusion. The poor physicochemical and biopharmaceutical properties of various anticancer drugs and biological barriers in the GI tract restrict the oral administration of these drugs.[4] Utilizing pharmaceutical approaches, such as nanocarriers can improve the oral absorption of such drugs.[3]

Polymeric nanoparticles, particularly chitosan nanoparticles have special features that can improve the oral absorption of drugs. Chitosan is the polycationic derivative of chitin with mucopolysaccharide structure similar to cellulose.[5-9] Chitosan nanoparticles have many advantages over natural polymers. The preparation methods of chitosan nanoparticles are simple and mild, and the resulting particles have good stability, and low toxicity (LD50>16g/kg). This nanoparticles can be used for different purposes. Hence, they are being considered as a drug delivery carrier, especially in recent years. Chitosan has a linear structure with a number of free amine groups, and can easily form ionic cross-linkage with multivalent anions.[10] The mucoadhesive properties of chitosan increase the contact time of a drug with the absorption site, leading to increased absorption. This property is based on the interaction between the positive charge of the chitosan and the negative charge of the mucin in the intestine.[11] Furthermore, many studies have shown that chitosan can affect the tight junctions and induce their temporary opening, which increases the permeation of drugs through the intestinal epithelium.[3,10-13] The effect of chitosan and its derivatives on the oral absorption of some anticancer drugs has been studied.[10,12]

Dox is an anticancer drug with excellent properties, which is being used to treat several malignancies, such as lymphoma, osteosarcoma and other sarcomas, carcinomas, and melanoma.[14-17] Dox is an anthracycline glycoside antibiotic that inhibits the DNA synthesis and cell proliferation. Dox is one of the essential drugs in cytotoxic and adjuvant medicine of 20th WHO essential

***Corresponding author:** Zahra Sobhani, Email: sobhani@sums.ac.ir medicine list (EML) for adult and 6th for children. It is administered through IV infusion. However, there is the possibility of unwanted side effects due to high initial concentration or its toxicity followed by fast decay if its administered below the minimum therapeutic level.[13,18] A relatively longer systemic exposure time with less fluctuation, can lead to lower toxicity and improved efficacy, which can be provided by oral delivery of this drug.[13,18]

During this project chitosan nanoparticles were prepared by ionic gelation method and the effect of some parameters, such as polymer concentration, poly anionic agent concentration, mixing speed, etc. on particle size were analyzed. Dox was loaded in the selected nanoparticles, and the intestinal permeability studies were carried out by intestinal sac model.

Materials and Methods

Low-molecular weight chitosan and pentasodium tripolyphosphate (TPP) were purchased from a domestic supplier of Sigma-Aldrich (USA) in Iran. Doxorubicin hydrocloride was obtained as a 2mg/ml solution in 0.9% (w/v) sodium chloride from EBEWE Pharma (Austria). All other chemicals, solvents and reagents used were of chemical or analytical grade as needed, which were used without further purification. All aqueous solutions were prepared with deionized water.

Preparation of Dox loaded chitosan nanoparticles

Chitosan nanoparticles loaded Dox (Dox-Cs-NPs) were prepared using an ionic gelation method. Nanoparticles were formed spontanously, by dropwise adding of TPP aqueous solution to the chitosan aqueous solution (in 1% v/v acetic acid) under stirring at room temperature. Probe sonicator or magnet stirrer were used to mix chitosan and TPP solutions. The effect of chitosan and TPP solutions concentration, and different mixing methods on the particle size and size distribution were analyzed. Selected formulations with the particle size less than 300 nm [3] and narrow size distribution were used for loading experiments. Dox was added into chitosan solution at different drug: polymer ratio (w:w) prior to adding TPP solution. The suspension was centrifuged at 15000 rpm for 30 min, and sedimented nanoparticles were washed with deionized water and lyophilized before storage.

Characterization of NPs

Particle size and particle shape analysis

Nanoparticle sizes were determined using a laser diffraction particle size analyzer (Microtrac, Nano-flex 180°, USA) at room temperature.

The shape and surface characteristics of the nanoparticles were observed by scanning electron microscopy (SEM) (TESCAN vega3,Czech).

Drug loading and encapsulation efficiency

The encapsulation efficiency of Dox-Cs-NPs was determined by indirect method. Dox-Cs-NPs were separated from the suspension by ultracentrifugation (Hettich, Model Mikro220R, Germany) at 15000 rpm and 4°C for 30 min. The amount of free Dox in the supernatant was analyzed by HPLC.[19-22] The encapsulation efficiency (EE) was calculated by equation 1:

$$EE\% = ((T-F)/T)*100 \qquad \text{(eq. 1)}$$

And drug loading amounts (LA) were determined using equation 2:

$$LA\% = ((T-F)/W)*100 \qquad \text{(eq. 2)}$$

Where F is the free amount of drug in the supernatant, T is the total amount of drug added into the chitosan solution, and W is the weight of Dox-Cs-NPs. All formulations were carried out in triplicate.

The chromatographic system for Dox analysis consist of a Hichrom C18 column (250 × 4 mm, UK) and a Cecil instrument (Adept series and CE 4200 UV/Vis Detector, England). The mobile phase consisted of acetonitrile: distilled water (30:70 v/v) and the pH of the mobile phase adjusted to 3 using phosphoric acid. The flow rate was set to 1 mL/min and Dox was quantified at 233 nm. The HPLC method validation showed the linearity of method ($r^2 = 0.9993$) in the range of 1–50 µg/ mL. CV% was less than 9% and the accuracy was more than 88% within this range of concentrations (1–50 µg/ mL). The specificity was tested in the presence of the nanoparticles components.

In vitro drug release study

Profile of Dox release from the nanoparticles was analyzed in three different pH values of 5.0, 6.8 and 7.4 in phosphate buffer solution. Dox-Cs-NPs were suspended in 0.5 mL buffer solution in the microtubes. The tubes were put into shaker incubator (BIOER Mixing Block MB-102, China) and temperature was set to 37°C. At scheduled time points, the nanoparticles were separated by centrifugation at 10000 rpm for 10 min, and the released drug in the supernatant was measured by HPLC method as described earlier. Following supernatant decantation, the same volume of fresh pre-warmed buffer solution was replaced. All measurements were performed in triplicate. The release percentage at each time was calculated and cumulative released curves are depicted.

Analysis of release data

To describe the drug release mechanism, release data were analyzed using the Ritger and Peppas equation:

$$M_t / M_\infty = Kt^n \qquad \text{(eq. 3)}$$

Where M_t represents the amount of drug released in time t, M_∞ is the total amount of drug that should be released at infinite time, K is constant and "n" is the release exponent indicating the type of drug release mechanism.[23]

To assay the release kinetic, data were evaluated by zero order, first order, and Higuchi model. For zero order release kinetic, the cumulative percent of released drug versus time was assessed. In the cases of first order kinetic and Higuchi model, the logarithm of the amounts of the remaining drug to be released versus time, and the cumulative percent of released drug versus square root of time were evaluated, respectively. The relevant correlation coefficients were used to determine the best model.

Intestinal permeation studies by intestinal sac model

Preparation of everted intestinal sac

Permeation of free Dox and Dox loaded chitosan nanoparticles across the intestinal wall was studied. Everted and normal intestinal sacs were prepared according to the standard procedure.[24-26]

Male Sprague Dawley rats (250-300g) were used for the intestinal permeation experiments. Animals were sacrificed and a longitudinal segment as long as 30 cm of the upper section of intestine was removed and rinsed with cold oxygenated physiological Ringer solution and cut into segments of 2 cm length. Each sac tied to a cotton thread and filled with 2 mL Ringer solution. For everting the intestine segment a glass rod was carefully used and the serosal side of the intestine was filled with 0.5 mL Ringer solution (acceptor part). Sacs were placed in a jacket glass tubes containing 40 mL physiologic Ringer solution that were continually bubbled with 95% O_2 and 5% CO_2 kept at 37°C (donor chamber).

Intestinal permeation

After equilibration at 37°C for 5 min, the exact volume of Dox solution or nanosuspension of Dox-Cs-NPs were added to the donor chamber. At scheduled time points after adding the drug to the donor chamber five intestinal sacs were removed. The liquid inside the sacs were centrifuged and analyzed with HPLC method. In the case of adding Dox-Cs-NPs to the donor chamber, the liquid inside the sacs at first was treated with acetic acid 1% and then ultrasonicated for 45 min to dissolve chitosan and to extract the entrapped drug within the nanoparticles. Finally, the solution was centrifuged and analyzed with HPLC.

Results and Discussion

Preparation of Dox-Cs-NPs

Preparation of chitosan nanoparticles was performed by using various concentrations of chitosan (0.2-0.5mg/mL) and TPP solutions (0.2-0.5mg/mL).[27] Chitosan nanoparticles were prepared through ionic gelation technique. This method is based on electrostatic interaction between the positive charge of amine groups of chitosan and negative charge groups of polyanion, such as tripolyphosphate. This technique is simple and performed in the aqueous medium. By adding TPP to the chitosan solution, nanoparticles were spontaneously formed during stirring at room temperature. For mixing the nanosuspension the effects of magnetic stirring and ultrasonic wave on the particle size and size distribution were analyzed. The results of particle size are shown in Table 1. Dispersion of the NPs with probe sonicator was much better than magnetic stirrer, and the homogenisity of the particle size improved when probe sonicator was used.

Table 1. Particle size of nanoparticles obtained by two methods of mixing. Data were reported as mean (n=3)

Formulation No	Chitosan Conc (W/V%)	TPP Conc (W/V%)	Nanoparticle Mean Size (nm)- Number size	Nanoparticle Mean Size (nm)- Volume size	Mixing Methods
F_1	0.2	0.2	52.4	418	Magnet Stirrer
F_2	0.3	0.2	49.3	572	
F_3	0.5	0.2	228.2	285.3	
F_4	0.2	0.3	2449	2521	
F_5	0.3	0.3	2582	2691	
F_6	0.5	0.3	39.7	503	
F_7	0.2	0.5	1765	1822	
F_8	0.3	0.5	6000	6000	
F_9	0.5	0.5	3470	3520	
F_{10}	0.5	0.1	440	738	Probe Sonicator
F_{11}	0.5	0.25	418	781	
F_{12}	**0.5**	**0.3**	**152.675**	**341.75**	
F_{13}	0.5	0.5	Unread	-	

The poly dispersity of obtained NPs with two methods is shown in Figure 1. The selected formulation had the minimum size (volume diameter 152.6 nm) and was prepared by adding 2 mL of TPP (0.3%w/v) to 3 mL of chitosan solution (0.5%w/v) and sonicated for 120 sec by 75% amplitude. This formulation was selected for Dox loading. Dox was added into chitosan solution at different drug: polymer ratio (w:w) prior to the addition of TPP solution.

Drug loading and encapsulation efficiency is shown in Figure 2. Dox were successfully entrapped into chitosan nanoparticles with the encapsulation efficiency up to 23% and loading amount of 40%.

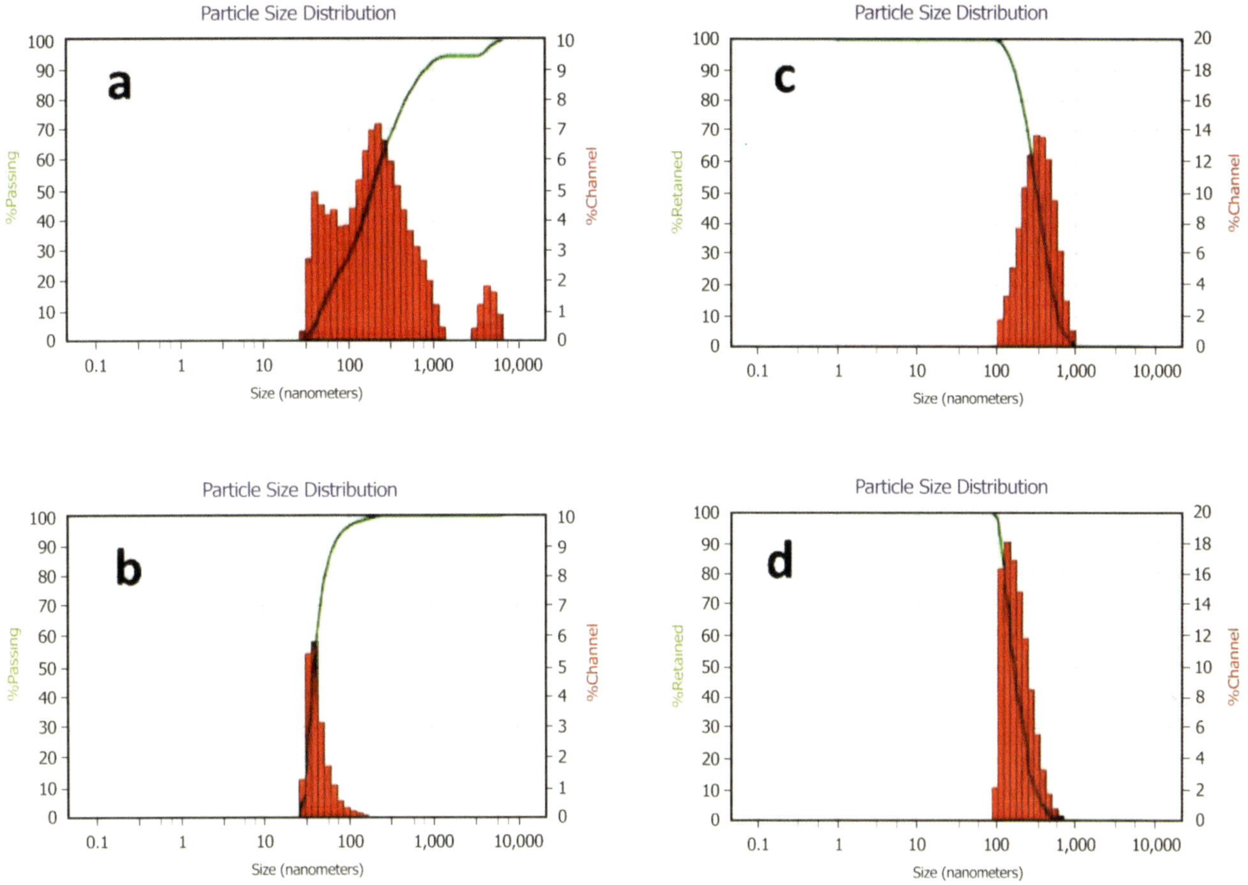

Figure 1. Volume (top) and number (bottom) size and size distribution of nanoparticle obtained by magnetic stirrer (a,b) and probe sonicator (c,d)

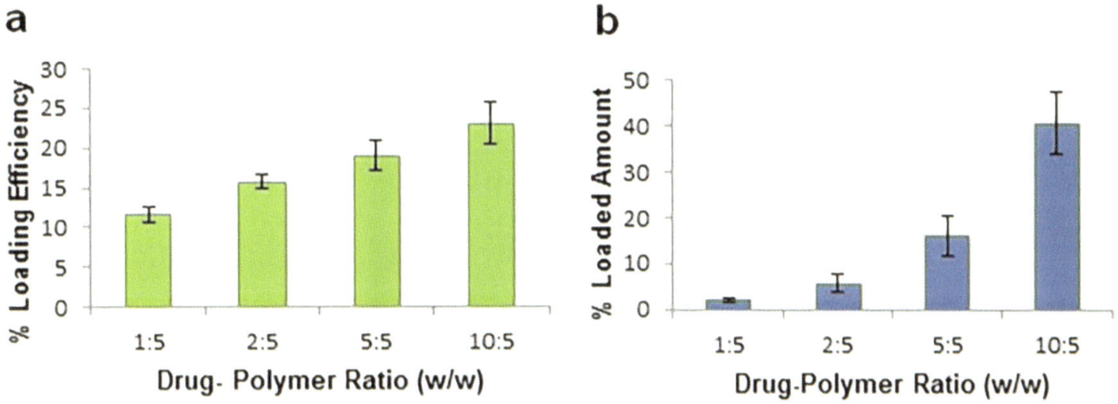

Figure 2. Loading efficiency (a) and loaded amount (b) of Dox in chitosan nanoparticles. Data were reported as mean ± SD (n=3)

Characterization of Preparation of Dox

Morphology studies

The morphology of Dox-CS-NPs was assessed by SEM and the results are shown in Figure 3. As it can be seen, the particles are spherical with smooth surface. No aggregation was detected and the particle size in the micrographs confirms the results of laser diffraction particle size analysis.

In vitro drug release

The release profile of Dox from Dox-Cs-NPs at three different pH values is shown in Figure 4. A quick release was seen from Dox-Cs-NPs in the first 6 hrs (approximately 30% of the drug was released at pH 5.0) and a relatively slow and sustained release was observed in the following days. By decreasing the pH from 7.4 to 5.0, the percentage of the released drug increased, but by changing the pH of the release medium to 6.8 the amount of drug released was reduced. The amount of drug released at acidic condition (pH 5.0) was greater than other pHs. This phenomenon is suitable for drug release at tumor region.[28] Another positive aspect of these nanoparticles is the release profile at pH 6.8. At this pH, the lowest amount of drug was released. Since in the *in vivo* condition the range of intestine pH is similar to this point, the Dox-Cs-NPs will have slight release before absorption. These differences in the release behavior at three pH media could be explained as the influence of protonation of amine groups of Dox, chitosan and changing the solubility of drug and polymer in these conditions.[28]

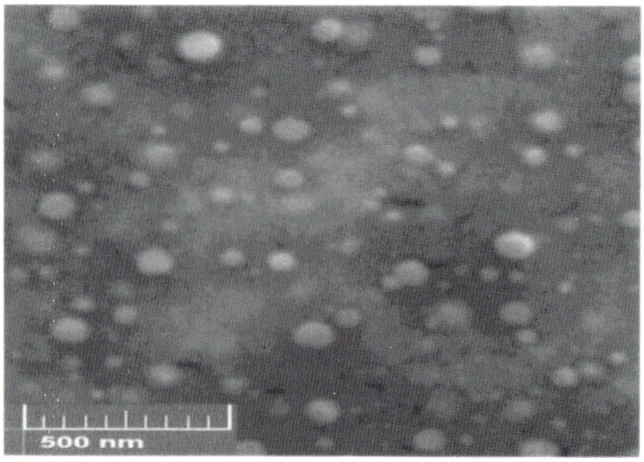

Figure 3. Scanning electron microscopic image of Dox-Cs-NPs

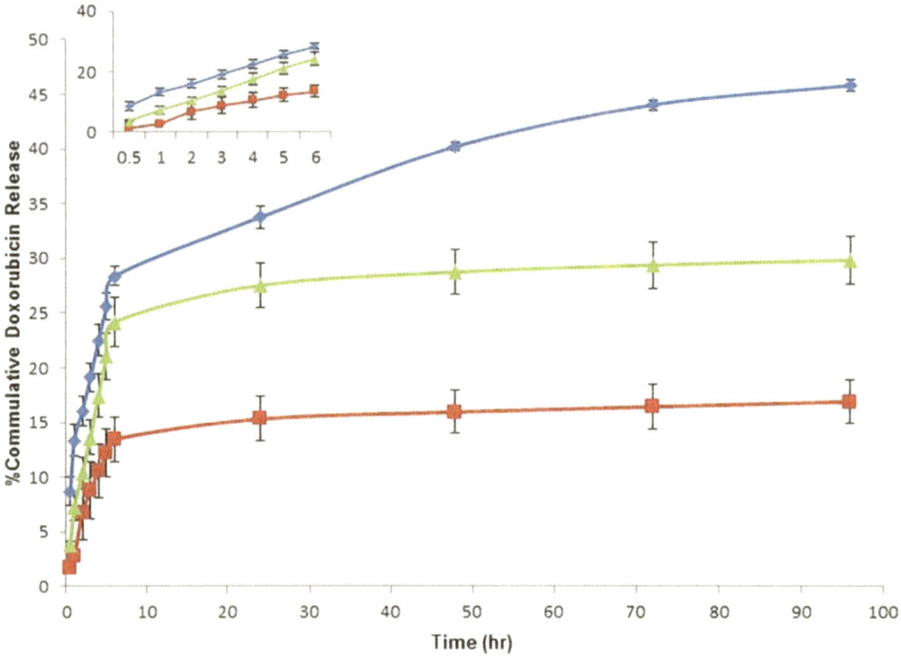

Figure 4. In vitro release profile of Dox from Dox-Cs-NPs in three different pH values. Blue line is related to pH 5, green to pH 7.4 and red to pH 6.8

According to the Figure 4 the release of Dox from chitosan nanoparicles occurred in 2 different manners. At first, a fast release profile was observable showing that some part of Dox was absorbed on the surface of the nanoparticles and this part was released at the beginning up to the first 6 hrs showing a burst release, and the second part of the drug could be released up to 96 hrs from the beginning. In this regards release kinetics were assessed in two different time intervals. Release kinetic was evaluated for 0-6 hrs and 6-96 hrs, separately. Release kinetic was calculated by data fitting to zero order, first order, Higuchi model, and Ritger and Peppas equation. The relevant correlation coefficients were used to determine the best model (Table 2). According to the results, the drug release followed the Higuchi model. The mechanism of drug release is highly related to the pH. It seems that Fickian diffusion at pH 5.0 and anomalous mechanism (Fickian diffusion and polymer relaxation) at pH 7.4 and 6.8 are the major drug release mechanisms. In addition, erosion of the chitosan nanoparticles at pH 6.8 is also involved.

Intestinal permeation

To evaluate the role of chitosan nanoparticles in the intestinal permeation of Dox, everted rat gut sac technique was employed. This is a simple and accurate model.[24,26,27] Permeation of Dox from simple solution and Dox-Cs-NPs across the everted and not- everted gut is shown in Figure 5. The transport of Dox encapsulated in the nanoparticles was significantly higher than the free Dox (approximately12.7 folds). When Dox solution was placed at the mucosal surface of intestine, the very low amount of drug (7%) transported across the intestinal wall (Figure 5a). In spite of the proper log P of Dox (log P=1.3) for diffusion across the intestinal wall, presence of P-glycoprotein pumps (P-gp pumps) as an efflux pumps in the luminal part of the enterocytes could show this discrepancy. In contrast, Dox can diffuse from the serosal site to mucosal site of intestine. Assessment of the Dox loaded Cs-NPs permeation via everted gut and bypassing the P-gp pump showed that permeation of the drug will be increased profoundly up to 89% (Figure 5b). The presence of chitosan nanoparticles increased the intestinal permeation of Dox approximately by 12.7 folds. This observation also showed that when Dox is entrapped into the chitosan nanoparticles, it is not available for P-gp pumps and can be transported across the intestinal wall. In addition, this significant increase in the intestinal permeation could be explained by the effect of chitosan on the opening of tight junctions and facilitation of the paracellular transport of Dox. However, in the not everted gut experiment, simple diffusion of drug was inhibited by entrapping the drug into the nanoparticles. Therefore, no Dox could be transport from serosal to mucosal site.

Table 2. Results of release kinetics according to various equations

R^2 Correlation of Doxorubicin Chitosan Nanoparticles Release Data								
Release Model	Zero Order		First Order		Higuchi		n*	
pH	0-6 (hr)	6-96 (hr)	0-6 (hr)	6-96 (hr)	0-6 (hr)	6-96 (hr)	0-6 (hr)	6-96 (hr)
5	0.9804	0.9476	0.9846	0.9374	0.9882	0.9885	0.4393	0.1793
6.8	0.935	0.7891	0.9641	0.7893	0.9806	0.9051	0.9127	0.07
7.4	0.9957	0.7492	0.9971	0.7563	0.9846	0.88	0.7074	0.0707

n*: Pepas mechanism slope equation line

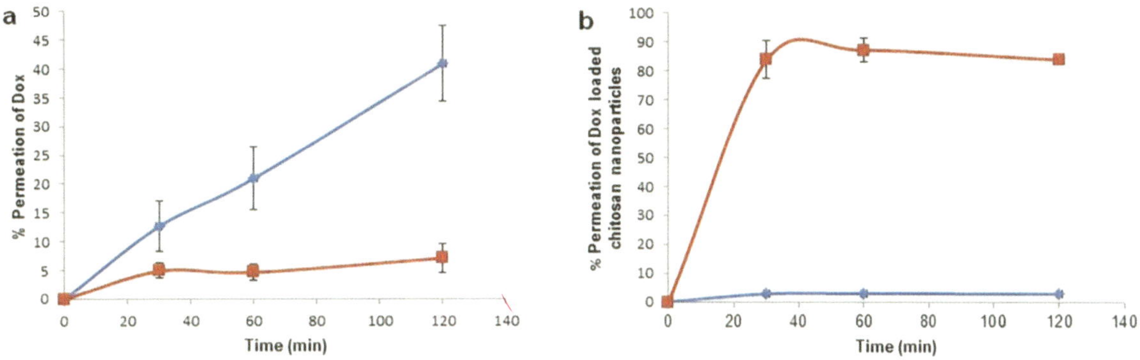

Figure 5. Intestinal permeation of Dox solution (a) and Dox loaded in chitosan nanoparticles (b) across the everted (red line) and not-everted (blue line) rat gut

Conclusion

By using the chitosan nanoparticles, the intestinal permeation of Dox approximately reached to 90%. Considering this effect, chitosan nanoparticles can present a promising platform for the development of oral delivery of poorly absorbable drugs. *In vivo* studies and determination the pharmacokinetic and pharmacodynamic of Dox loaded chitosan nanoparticles after oral administration are planned for future studies.

Acknowledgments

This project was part of Pharm. D thesis of the Marziyeh Zare. The authors would like to thank Shiraz University of Medical Sciences, Vice Chancellor of Research for their financial support (grant No 11114). They also wish to thank Mr. H. Argasi at the Research Consultation Center (RCC) of Shiraz University of Medical Sciences for his invaluable assistance in editing this manuscript.

Ethical Issues

The protocol of the animal study was approved by the local Ethics Committee of Shiraz University of Medical Sciences (approval number 11114).

Conflict of Interest

Authors state that there is no conflict of interest.

References

1. Aulton ME, Taylor K. Aulton's pharmaceutics: The design and manufacture of medicines. Churchill Livingstone/Elsevier; 2013.
2. Schoener CA, Peppas NA. Oral delivery of chemotherapeutic agents: Background and potential of drug delivery systems for colon delivery. *J Drug Deliv Sci Technol* 2012;22(6):459-68. doi: 10.1016/S1773-2247(12)50081-X
3. Thanki K, Gangwal RP, Sangamwar AT, Jain S. Oral delivery of anticancer drugs: Challenges and opportunities. *J Control Release* 2013;170(1):15-40. doi: 10.1016/j.jconrel.2013.04.020
4. Montaseri H, Mohammadi-Samani S, Zarea B, Sobhani Z, Ahmadi F. Enhanced oral bioavailability of paclitaxel by concomitant use of absorption enhancers and P-glycoprotein inhibitors in rats. *J Chemother* 2013;25(6):355-61. doi: 10.1179/1973947813Y.0000000088

5. Chen MC, Mi FL, Liao ZX, Hsiao CW, Sonaje K, Chung MF, et al. Recent advances in chitosan-based nanoparticles for oral delivery of macromolecules. *Adv Drug Deliv Rev* 2013;65(6):865-79. doi: 10.1016/j.addr.2012.10.010
6. Ensign LM, Cone R, Hanes J. Oral drug delivery with polymeric nanoparticles: The gastrointestinal mucus barriers. *Adv Drug Deliv Rev* 2012;64(6):557-70. doi: 10.1016/j.addr.2011.12.009
7. Kurita K. Chitin and chitosan: Functional biopolymers from marine crustaceans. *Mar Biotechnol (NY)* 2006;8(3):203-26. doi: 10.1007/s10126-005-0097-5
8. Mourya V, Inamdar NN. Chitosan-modifications and applications: Opportunities galore. *React Funct Polym* 2008;68(6):1013-51. doi: 10.1016/j.reactfunctpolym.2008.03.002
9. Dodane V, Vilivalam VD. Pharmaceutical applications of chitosan. *Pharm Sci Technolo Today* 1998;1(6):246-53. doi: 10.1016/S1461-5347(98)00059-5
10. Derakhshandeh K, Fathi S. Role of chitosan nanoparticles in the oral absorption of gemcitabine. *Int J Pharm* 2012;437(1-2):172-7.doi: 10.1016/j.ijpharm.2012.08.008
11. Sailaja AK, Amareshwar P, Chakravarty P. Chitosan nanoparticles as a drug delivery system. *Res J Pharm Biol Chem Sci* 2010;1(3):474-84.
12. Feng C, Sun G, Wang Z, Cheng X, Park H, Cha D, et al. Transport mechanism of doxorubicin loaded chitosan based nanogels across intestinal epithelium. *Eur J Pharm Biopharm* 2014;87(1):197-207. doi: 10.1016/j.ejpb.2013.11.007
13. Kalaria DR, Sharma G, Beniwal V, Ravi Kumar MN. Design of biodegradable nanoparticles for oral delivery of doxorubicin: In vivo pharmacokinetics and toxicity studies in rats. *Pharm Res* 2009;26(3):492-501. doi: 10.1007/s11095-008-9763-4
14. Jain AK, Swarnakar NK, Das M, Godugu C, Singh RP, Rao PR, et al. Augmented anticancer efficacy of doxorubicin-loaded polymeric nanoparticles after oral administration in a breast cancer induced animal model. *Mol Pharm* 2011;8(4):1140-51. doi: 10.1021/mp200011f
15. Lacy CF, Armstrong LL, Lance LL, Goldman MP. Drug information handbook: A comprehensive resource for all clinicians and healthcare professionals. Lexi-Comp; 2012.
16. Di Marco A, Gaetani M, Scarpinato B. Adriamycin (NSC-123,127): A new antibiotic with antitumor activity. *Cancer Chemother Rep* 1969;53(1):33-7.
17. Alldredge BK, Corelli RL, Ernst ME, Koda-Kimble MA, Guglielmo BJ, Jacobson PA, et al. Koda-kimble and young's applied therapeutics: The clinical use of drugs. Lippincott Williams & Wilkins; 2012.
18. Kim JE, Yoon IS, Cho HJ, Kim DH, Choi YH, Kim DD. Emulsion-based colloidal nanosystems for oral delivery of doxorubicin: Improved intestinal paracellular absorption and alleviated cardiotoxicity. *Int J Pharm* 2014;464(1-2):117-26. doi: 10.1016/j.ijpharm.2014.01.016
19. Han J, Zhang J, Zhao H, Li Y, Chen Z. Simultaneous determination of doxorubicin and its dipeptide prodrug in mice plasma by hplc with fluorescence detection. *J Pharm Anal* 2016;6(3):199-202. doi: 10.1016/j.jpha.2015.12.005
20. Reddy LH, Meda N, Murthy RR. Rapid and sensitive hplc method for the estimation of doxorubicin in dog blood--the silver nitrate artifact. *Acta Pharm* 2005;55(1):81-91.
21. Ricciarello R, Pichini S, Pacifici R, Altieri I, Pellegrini M, Fattorossi A, et al. Simultaneous determination of epirubicin, doxorubicin and their principal metabolites in human plasma by high-performance liquid chromatography and electrochemical detection. *J Chromatogr B Biomed Sci Appl* 1998;707(1-2):219-25. doi: 10.1016/S0378-4347(97)00610-5
22. Farvadi F, Tamaddon AM, Abolmaali SS, Sobhani Z, Yousefi GH. Micellar stabilized single-walled carbon nanotubes for a ph-sensitive delivery of doxorubicin. *Res Pharm Sci* 2014;9(1):1-10.
23. Samani SM, Montaseri H, Kazemi A. The effect of polymer blends on release profiles of diclofenac sodium from matrices. *Eur J Pharm Biopharm* 2003;55(3):351-5. doi: 10.1016/S0939-6411(03)00030-4
24. Ritschel WA, Kearns GL. Handbook of basic pharmacokinetics- including clinical applications. American Pharmaceutical Association; 1999.
25. Borchardt RT, Smith PL, Wilson G. Models for assessing drug absorption and metabolism. Springer; 1996.
26. Gamboa JM, Leong KW. In vitro and in vivo models for the study of oral delivery of nanoparticles. *Adv Drug Deliv Rev* 2013;65(6):800-10. doi: 10.1016/j.addr.2013.01.003
27. Sobhani Z, Mohammadi Samani S, Montaseri H, Khezri E. Nanoparticles of chitosan loaded ciprofloxacin: Fabrication and antimicrobial activity. *Adv Pharm Bull* 2017;7(3):427-32. doi: 10.15171/apb.2017.051
28. Unsoy G, Khodadust R, Yalcin S, Mutlu P, Gunduz U. Synthesis of doxorubicin loaded magnetic chitosan nanoparticles for ph responsive targeted drug delivery. *Eur J Pharm Sci* 2014;62:243-50. doi: 10.1016/j.ejps.2014.05.021

Permissions

All chapters in this book were first published in APB, by Tabriz University of Medical Sciences; hereby published with permission under the Creative Commons Attribution License or equivalent. Every chapter published in this book has been scrutinized by our experts. Their significance has been extensively debated. The topics covered herein carry significant findings which will fuel the growth of the discipline. They may even be implemented as practical applications or may be referred to as a beginning point for another development.

The contributors of this book come from diverse backgrounds, making this book a truly international effort. This book will bring forth new frontiers with its revolutionizing research information and detailed analysis of the nascent developments around the world.

We would like to thank all the contributing authors for lending their expertise to make the book truly unique. They have played a crucial role in the development of this book. Without their invaluable contributions this book wouldn't have been possible. They have made vital efforts to compile up to date information on the varied aspects of this subject to make this book a valuable addition to the collection of many professionals and students.

This book was conceptualized with the vision of imparting up-to-date information and advanced data in this field. To ensure the same, a matchless editorial board was set up. Every individual on the board went through rigorous rounds of assessment to prove their worth. After which they invested a large part of their time researching and compiling the most relevant data for our readers.

The editorial board has been involved in producing this book since its inception. They have spent rigorous hours researching and exploring the diverse topics which have resulted in the successful publishing of this book. They have passed on their knowledge of decades through this book. To expedite this challenging task, the publisher supported the team at every step. A small team of assistant editors was also appointed to further simplify the editing procedure and attain best results for the readers.

Apart from the editorial board, the designing team has also invested a significant amount of their time in understanding the subject and creating the most relevant covers. They scrutinized every image to scout for the most suitable representation of the subject and create an appropriate cover for the book.

The publishing team has been an ardent support to the editorial, designing and production team. Their endless efforts to recruit the best for this project, has resulted in the accomplishment of this book. They are a veteran in the field of academics and their pool of knowledge is as vast as their experience in printing. Their expertise and guidance has proved useful at every step. Their uncompromising quality standards have made this book an exceptional effort. Their encouragement from time to time has been an inspiration for everyone.

The publisher and the editorial board hope that this book will prove to be a valuable piece of knowledge for researchers, students, practitioners and scholars across the globe.

List of Contributors

Anayatollah Salimi, Najme Hedayatipour and Eskandar Moghimipour
Nanotechnology Research Center, Department of Pharmaceutics, Ahvaz Jundishapur University of Medical Sciences, Ahvaz, Iran

Nastaran Faghihi and Mohammad Taghi Mohammadi
Department of Physiology and Biophysics, Faculty of Medicine, Baqiyatallah University of Medical Sciences, Tehran, Iran

Hadi Valizadeh and Hamed Hamishekar
Drug Applied Research Center, Tabriz University of Medical Sciences, Tabriz, Iran

Mehran Mesgari Abbasi
Drug Applied Research Center, Tabriz University of Medical Sciences, Tabriz, Iran
Students Research Committee, Tabriz University of Medical Sciences, Tabriz, Iran

Leila Mohammadnejad
Immunology Research Center, Tabriz University of Medical Sciences, Tabriz, Iran

Parvin Zakeri-Milani
Liver and Gastrointestinal Diseases Research Center and Faculty of Pharmacy, Tabriz University of Medical Sciences, Tabriz, Iran

Simin Janitabar-Darzi and Kamal Yavari
Radiopharmaceutical Research and Development Laboratory, Nuclear Science and Technology Research Institute, Tehran, Iran

Reza Rezaei
Department of biochemistry, Faculty of Science, Zanjan University, Zanjan, Iran

Swati Jagdale and Apoorva Chandekar
Department of Pharmaceutics, MAEER's Maharashtra Institute of Pharmacy, MIT Campus, S. No. 124, Kothrud, Pune 411038, Savitribai Phule Pune University, India

Zahra Mardhiah Adib
Research Center for Pharmaceutical Nanotechnology and Students' Research Committee, Tabriz University of Medical Sciences, Tabriz, Iran

Saeed Ghanbarzadeh
Zanjan Pharmaceutical Nanotechnology Research Center, Department of Pharmaceutics, Faculty of Pharmacy, Zanjan University of Medical Sciences, Zanjan, Iran

Maryam Kouhsoltani
Department of Oral and Maxillofacial Pathology, Faculty of Dentistry, Tabriz University of Medical Sciences, Tabriz, Iran

Ahmad Yari Khosroshahi
Biotechnology Research Center and Faculty of Pharmacy, Tabriz University of Medical Sciences, Tabriz, Iran

Hamed Hamishehkar
Drug Applied Research Center, Tabriz University of Medical Sciences, Tabriz, Iran

Afsaneh Vazin, Iman Karimzadeh*, Atiyeh Zand, Nazafarin Hatami-Mazinani, Dena Firouzabadi
Department of Clinical Pharmacy, Faculty of Pharmacy, Shiraz University of Medical Sciences, Shiraz, Iran.

Ebrahim Salehifar
Pharmaceutical Research Center, Faculty of Pharmacy, Mazandaran University of Medical Sciences, Sari, Iran

Shima Ebrahim
Student Research Committee, Faculty of Pharmacy, Mazandaran University of Medical Sciences, Sari, Iran

Mohammad-Reza Shiran
Immunogenetics Research Center, Faculty of Medicine, Mazandaran University of Medical Sciences, Sari, Iran

Fatemeh Faramarzi and Razieh Avan
Student Research Committee, Department of Clinical Pharmacy, Mazandaran University of Medical Sciences, Sari, Iran

Hossein Askari Rad
Faculty of Pharmacy, Mazandaran University of Medical Sciences, Sari, Iran

Asadollah Mohseni Kiasari
Faculty of Medicine, Mazandaran University of Medical Sciences, Sari, Iran

Pouneh Ebrahimi
Department of Chemistry, Faculty of Basic Sciences, Golestan University, Gorgan, Iran

Farhad Mohammadi
Department of Pharmaceutics, School of Pharmacy, Shiraz University of Medical Sciences, Shiraz, Iran

Soliman Mohammadi Samani and Fatemeh Ahmadi
Department of Pharmaceutics, School of Pharmacy, Shiraz University of Medical Sciences, Shiraz, Iran
Research Center for Nanotechnology in Drug Delivery, School of Pharmacy, Shiraz University of Medical Sciences, Shiraz, Iran

Nader Tanideh
Department of Pharmacology, Stem Cell and Transgenic Research Center, Shiraz University of Medical Sciences, Shiraz, Iran

Saieede Soltani
Drug Applied Research Center, Tabriz University of Medical Sciences, Tabriz, Iran

Mitra Jelvehgari and Hadi Valizadeh
Drug Applied Research Center, Tabriz University of Medical Sciences, Tabriz, Iran
Faculty of Pharmacy, Tabriz University of Medical Sciences, Tabriz, Iran

Sanam Ziapour
Biotechnology Research center, Tabriz University of Medical Sciences, Tabriz, Iran
Student Research Committee, Tabriz University of Medical Sciences, Tabriz, Iran

Mahdieh Rahmani
Student Research Committee, Tabriz University of Medical Sciences, Tabriz, Iran

Seyed Hassan Montazam
Department of Microbiology, Bonab Branch, Islamic Azad University, Bonab, Iran

Parisa Jourghanian
Department of Chemical Engineering, Shahrood Branch, Islamic Azad University, Shahrood, Iran

Solmaz Ghaffari
Department of Medical Nanotechnology, Faculty of Advanced Sciences and Technology, Pharmaceutical Sciences Branch, Islamic Azad University, (IAUPS), Tehran, Iran
Young Researchers and Elite Club, Pharmaceutical Sciences Branch, Islamic Azad University, (IAUPS), Tehran, Iran

Mehdi Ardjmand
Department of Chemical Engineering, South Tehran Branch, Islamic Azad University, Tehran, Iran.

Setareh Haghighat
Department of Microbiology, Faculty of Advanced Sciences and Technology, Pharmaceutical Sciences Branch, Islamic Azad University (IAUPS), Tehran, Iran

Mahdieh Mohammadnejad
Quality Control Department, Tofigh Daru Research and Engineering Co. Tehran, Iran

Mandana Rastegar, Haji-Amin Marjani, Yaghoub Yazdani, Majid Shahbazi, Masoud Golalipour and Touraj Farazmandfar
Medical Cellular and Molecular Research Center, Golestan University of Medical Sciences, Gorgan, Iran

Arash Khodaei1 Soheila Bolandnazar and Hadi Valizadeh
Drug Applied Research Center and Faculty of Pharmacy, Tabriz University of Medical Sciences, Tabriz, Iran

Leila Hasani
Department of Biological Sciences, Institute for Advanced Studies in Basic Sciences, Zanjan, Iran

Parvin Zakeri-Milani
Liver and Gastrointestinal Diseases Research Center and Faculty of Pharmacy, Tabriz University of Medical Sciences, Tabriz, Iran

Mehdi Hassanpour Aghdam
Research Center for Pharmaceutical Nanotechnology, and Students' Research Committee, Tabriz University of Medical Sciences, Tabriz, Iran

Saeed Ghanbarzadeh
Zanjan Pharmaceutical Nanotechnology Research Center, and Department of Pharmaceutics, Faculty of Pharmacy, Zanjan University of Medical Sciences, Zanjan, Iran
Drug Applied Research Center, Tabriz University of Medical Sciences, Tabriz, Iran

Hamed Hamishehkar
Drug Applied Research Center, Tabriz University of Medical Sciences, Tabriz, Iran

Yousef Javadzadeh
Biotechnology Research Center and Department of Pharmaceutics, Faculty of Pharmacy, Tabriz University of Medical Sciences, Tabriz, Iran

Alireza Farnam, Arezoo MehrAra*, Hossein Dadashzadeh, Golamreza Chalabianlou and Salman Safikhanlou
Research Center of Psychiatry and Behavioral Sciences, Razi Hospital, Tabriz University of Medical Sciences, Tabriz, Iran

Vinit K. Srivastava, Abhishek Mishra, Sunil Sharma and Raj Kumar
Apollo Hospitals Bilaspur, Chhattisgarh, India

Sanjay Agrawal
Himalayan Institute of Medical Sciences, Dehradun, India.

Sanjay Kumar
Sanjay Gandhi Postgraduate Institute of Medical Sciences, Lucknow, India

Karla Veloso Gonçalves Ribeiro
Núcleo de Microscopia e Microanálise, Universidade Federal de Viçosa, 36570-900, Viçosa, Minas Gerais, Brasil
Departamento de Biologia Geral, Universidade Federal de Viçosa, 36570-900, Viçosa, Minas Gerais, Brasil

Cleberson Ribeiro, Roberto Sousa Dias, Sérgio Oliveira de Paula and Leandro Licursi de Oliveira
Departamento de Biologia Geral, Universidade Federal de Viçosa, 36570-900, Viçosa, Minas Gerais, Brasil

Silvia Almeida Cardoso
Departamento de Medicina e Enfermagem, Universidade Federal de Viçosa, 36570-900, Viçosa, Minas Gerais, Brasil

Jose Cola Zanuncio
Departamento de Entomologia, Universidade Federal de Viçosa, 36570-900, Viçosa, Minas Gerais, Brasil

Fereshteh Dehbashi
Toxicology Research Center, Ahvaz Jundishapur University of Medical Sciences, Ahvaz, Iran

Hojatolla Nikravesh, Mohammad Javad Khodayar, Masoud Mahdavinia and Leila Zeidooni
Toxicology Research Center, Ahvaz Jundishapur University of Medical Sciences, Ahvaz, Iran
Department of Toxicology, School of Pharmacy, Ahvaz Jundishapur University of Medical Sciences, Ahvaz, Iran

Esrafil Mansouri
Cellular and Molecular Research Center, Department of Anatomical Sciences, School of Medicine, Ahvaz Jundishapur University of Medical Sciences, Ahvaz, Iran

Fatemeh Sheikhbahaei
Department of Anatomy, Afzalipour School of Medicine, Kerman University of Medical Sciences, Kerman, Iran

Mozafar Khazaei
Fertility and Infertility Research Center, Kermanshah University of Medical Sciences, Kermanshah, Iran

Seyed Noureddin Nematollahi-Mahani
Physiology Research Center, Institute of Neuropharmacology, Kerman University of Medical Sciences, Kerman, Iran

Smriti Ojha
Vishveshwarya Group of Institutions, Department of Pharmacy, G.B. Nagar, Uttar Pradesh 203207

Babita Kumar
Sanskar Educational Group, Department of Pharmacy, Ghaziabad, Uttar Pradesh 201302

Goltaj Bayrami, Alireza Alihemmati and Mustafa Mohammadi1
Drug Applied Research Center, Tabriz University of Medical Sciences, Tabriz, Iran

Rana Keyhanmanesh
Drug Applied Research Center, Tabriz University of Medical Sciences, Tabriz, Iran
Department of Physiology, Faculty of Medicine, Tabriz University of Medical Sciences, Tabriz, Iran

Reza Badalzadeh
Drug Applied Research Center, Tabriz University of Medical Sciences, Tabriz, Iran
Department of Physiology, Faculty of Medicine, Tabriz University of Medical Sciences, Tabriz, Iran
Molecular Medicine Research Center, Tabriz University of Medical Sciences, Tabriz, Iran

Pouran Karimi
Neurosciences Research Center, Tabriz University of Medical Sciences, Tabriz, Iran

Aniseh Javadi
Cardiovascular Research Center, Tabriz University of Medical Sciences, Tabriz, Iran
Student Research Committee, Tabriz University of Medical Sciences, Tabriz, Iran

Milad Zadi-Heydarabad
Student Research Committee, Tabriz University of Medical Sciences, Tabriz, Iran

Sara Shojaei Zarghani
Student Research Committee, Urmia University of Medical Sciences, Urmia, Iran

Samin Abbaszadeh and Hamid Soraya
Cellular and Molecular Research Center, Department of Pharmacology, Faculty of Pharmacy, Urmia University of Medical Sciences, Urmia, Iran

Mohammad Alizadeh
Department of Nutrition, Food and Beverages Safety Research Center, Faculty of Medicine, Urmia University of Medical Sciences, Urmia, Iran

Maryam Rameshrad and Alireza Garjani
Department of Pharmacology and Toxicology, Faculty of Pharmacy, Tabriz University of Medical Sciences, Tabriz, Iran

Faezeh Alihosseini and Ahoo Afshar Nasab
Pharmaceutical Sciences Research Center, Pharmaceutical Sciences Branch, Islamic Azad University (IAUPS), Tehran, Iran

Solmaz Ghaffari
Pharmaceutical Sciences Research Center, Pharmaceutical Sciences Branch, Islamic Azad University (IAUPS), Tehran, Iran
Young Researchers and Elite Club, Pharmaceutical Sciences Branch, Islamic Azad University (IAUPS), Tehran, Iran

Seyed Mahdi Rezayat Sorkhabadi
Pharmaceutical Sciences Research Center, Pharmaceutical Sciences Branch, Islamic Azad University (IAUPS), Tehran, Iran
Department of Medical Nanotechnology, School of Advanced Sciences and Technology in Medicine, Tehran University of Medical Sciences (TUMS), Tehran, Iran
Department of Pharmacology and Toxicology, Pharmaceutical Sciences Branch, Islamic Azad University, (IAUPS), Tehran, Iran

Sepideh Arbabi Bidgoli
Pharmaceutical Sciences Research Center, Pharmaceutical Sciences Branch, Islamic Azad University (IAUPS), Tehran, Iran
Department of Toxicology, Pharmaceutical Sciences Branch, Islamic Azad University (IAUPS), Tehran, Iran

Nooshin Kianvash
Young Researchers and Elite Club, Pharmaceutical Sciences Branch, Islamic Azad University (IAUPS), Tehran, Iran

Seyyedeh Elaheh Mousavi
Department of Pharmacology, School of Medicine, Tehran University of Medical Sciences, Tehran, Iran

Setareh Haghighat
Department of Microbiology, Faculty of Advanced Sciences and Technology, Pharmaceutical Sciences Branch, Islamic Azad University (IAUPS), Tehran, Iran

Somayyeh Asghari and Laleh Farzin
Students' Research Committee, Faculty of Nutrition and Food Science, Tabriz University of Medical Sciences, Tabriz, Iran

Maryam Rafraf
Nutrition Research Center, Department of Community Nutrition, Faculty of Nutrition and Food Science, Tabriz University of Medical Sciences, Tabriz, Iran

Mohammad Asghari-Jafarabadi
Road Traffic Injury Research Center, Tabriz University of Medical Sciences, Tabriz, Iran
Department of Statistics and Epidemiology, Faculty of Health, Tabriz University of Medical Sciences, Tabriz, Iran

Seyed-Mostafa Ghavami
Department of Radiology, Paramedical school, Tabriz University of Medical Sciences, Tabriz, Iran

Mohammad-Hossein Somi
Liver and Gastrointestinal Diseases Research Centre, Tabriz University of Medical Sciences, Tabriz, Iran

Marziyeh Zare and Soliman Mohammadi Samani
Faculty of Pharmacy, Shiraz University of Medical Sciences, Shiraz, Iran

Zahra Sobhani
Department of Quality Control, Faculty of Pharmacy, Shiraz University of Medical Sciences, Shiraz, Iran

Index

A
Abnormal Hypersynchronous, 9
Acetaminophen, 136, 140, 142-144
Acinetobacter, 51, 53-54, 56-57
Acinetobacter Baumannii, 51, 56-57
Angiogenesis, 58, 63, 91-93, 95-97, 145-146, 151-153, 185

B
Bile Canalicula, 17
Brachytherapy Agent, 28
Breast Carcinoma, 26, 32
Buccal, 75-76, 78-79, 81, 85-86

C
Carbonyl Stretching, 1, 3
Cartilage Regeneration, 66-67, 73
Cellulose Acetate, 34-36, 42, 86
Cetirizine, 17-24
Chitosan, 34-43, 66, 74, 86, 91, 161, 188, 200-206
Colistin, 51-57
Colistinus Subspecies, 51
Collagen, 66-73, 145, 152, 185-186
Curcumin, 87-91, 161, 183-188

D
Denaturation, 1-2, 4-7, 93
Deracination, 25
Dexmedetomidine, 118-119, 121-124
Diffusion Coefficient, 1, 4, 6-7
Digoxin, 17-23

E
Empirical Therapy, 51, 54
Endothelial Cell, 93, 146, 153
Endothermic Transition, 5
Epilepticus, 9-10, 14-16
Escherichia Coli, 53, 125-126, 128-134, 184

G
Gemfibrozil, 136, 143-144
Glucuronidation, 61, 136

H
Haemodynamics, 118, 123
Hepatocellular Carcinoma, 92, 96-97, 162
Hippocampal Neuronal Death, 10
Hyaluronic Acid, 66, 73, 82
Hybrid Scaffold, 66
Hydroxypropyl Methylcellulose, 73, 76

I
Implantable Disk, 66, 71-72
Intestinal Permeability, 17, 19, 21-23, 201
Intra-peritoneal Injection, 164
Ischemic Postconditioning, 163-164, 167, 169, 171-173
Itraconazole, 105-112

L
Lipid Fluidization, 1-2, 4, 7

M
Metformin, 92-97, 174-182
Methylprednisolone, 34-35, 37-38, 42-43
Metoclopramide, 75-77, 80, 82-83
Micellization, 71
Mucoadhesive, 75-76, 78-81, 85-86, 200
Mucosa, 76, 78-79, 81-82, 85

N
Naproxen, 1-4, 6-8, 49, 98-103
Nephrotoxicity, 52-55, 57, 143-144
Nitrosative Damage, 9, 13, 15

O
Oleic Acid, 1
Osteoarthritis, 66-68, 73
Oxidative Damage, 9, 15, 141-142, 193

P
P-glycoprotein, 17, 22-24, 205
Pentylenetetrazol, 9-10, 15
Permeability, 1-3, 6-7, 17-24, 50, 73, 83, 87, 90, 105, 136, 141-142, 154, 162, 170, 172, 201
Pharmacodynamic, 58, 60-61, 63-64, 200, 205
Pharmacokinetic, 23, 51, 53, 55, 58-64, 87, 98, 100, 154, 156, 159-160, 200, 205
Pharmacokinetic Dosing Method, 51, 53
Pitavastatin, 9-16
Poloxamer, 46, 67, 71-73
Poly Amidoamine, 25
Polydispersity, 89, 154-155
Polymorphism, 58, 62-65
Polyoxypropylene Core, 71
Prednisolone, 35, 66-68, 71-72, 74

Propranolol, 58-64
Propylene Glycol, 1-4, 6-7, 76

R
Radioisotope, 28
Radionuclidic Purity, 25-26, 28
Rapamycin, 50, 92-99, 104
Reperfusion Injury, 15, 144, 163-164, 168, 171-173
Rheumatoid Arthritis, 68, 145
Rhodamine B, 45-47

S
Sertraline, 113-117
Sirolimus, 97-104, 111
Solid Lipid Nanoparticle, 45
Stratum Corneum, 1-4, 7-8, 45, 47, 49, 76
Sumatriptan, 75-77, 80, 82-83, 85
Superoxide Dismutase, 9-10, 12, 16, 189-190, 195

T
Thermotropic Behavior, 1-2, 4-5
Transdermal Drug Delivery, 1-2, 7, 49, 111
Transmucosal, 75-76, 79